A Physician's Guide to Clinical Forensic Medicine

FORENSIC SCIENCE AND MEDICINE

***Steven B. Karch,** MD,* Series Editor

Toxicology and Clinical Pharmacology of Herbal Products,
edited by ***Melanie Johns Cupp,*** *2000*

Criminal Poisoning: *Investigational Guide for Law Enforcement, Toxicologists, Forensic Scientists, and Attorneys,*
by ***John H. Trestrail, III,*** *2000*

A Physician's Guide to Clinical Forensic Medicine,
edited by ***Margaret M. Stark,*** *2000*

Brain Imaging in Substance Abuse: *Research, Clinical, and Forensic Applications,*
edited by ***Marc J. Kaufman,*** *2000*

A PHYSICIAN'S GUIDE to CLINICAL FORENSIC MEDICINE

Edited by

Margaret M. Stark, LLM, MB, BS, DGM, DMJ, DAB

The Forensic Medicine Unit, St George's Hospital Medical School, London, UK

Humana Press **Totowa, New Jersey**

999 Riverview Drive, Suite 208
Totowa, New Jersey 07512

This publication is printed on acid-free paper. ∞
ANSI Z39.48-1984 (American Standards Institute) Permanence of Paper for Printed Library Materials.

Cover design by Patricia F. Cleary.

For additional copies, pricing for bulk purchases, and/or information about other Humana titles, contact Humana at the above address or at any of the following numbers: Tel: 973-256-1699; Fax: 973-256-8341; E-mail: humana@humanapr.com, or visit our Website at www.humanapress.com

Printed in the United States of America. 10 9 8 7 6 5 4 3 2 1

Library of Congress Cataloging in Publication Data

Preface

Clinical Forensic Medicine, a term now commonly used to refer to that branch of medicine involving an interaction among the law, the judiciary, and the police, and usually concerning living persons, is emerging as a speciality in its own right. There have been enormous developments in the subject in the last decade, with an increasing amount of published research that needs to be brought together in a handbook such as *A Physician's Guide to Clinical Forensic Medicine*. The role of the healthcare professional in this field must be independent, professional, courteous, and nonjudgmental, as well as well-trained and informed. This is essential for the care of victims and suspects, for the criminal justice system, and for society as a whole.

As we enter the 21st century it is important that healthcare professionals are "forensically aware." Inadequate or incorrect diagnosis of a wound, for example, may have an effect on the clinical management of an individual, as well as a significant influence on any subsequent criminal investigation and court proceedings. A death in police custody resulting from failure to identify a vulnerable individual is an avoidable tragedy. Although training in clinical forensic medicine at the undergraduate level is variable, once qualified, every doctor will have contact with legal matters to a varying degree.

A Physician's Guide to Clinical Forensic Medicine concentrates on the clinical aspects of forensic medicine, as opposed to the pathological, by endeavoring to look at issues from fundamental principles, including recent research developments where appropriate. It is written primarily for physicians and nurses working in the field of clinical forensic medicine—forensic medical examiners, police surgeons, accident and emergency room physicians, pediatricians, gynecologists, and forensic and psychiatric nurses—but such other health care professionals as social workers and the police will also find the contents of use.

The history and development of clinical forensic medicine worldwide is outlined, with highlighting being accorded the variable standards of care for detainees and victims. Because there are currently no international standards of training or practice, we have discussed fundamental principles of consent, confidentiality, note-keeping, court reports, and attendance at court.

The primary clinical forensic assessment of complainants and those suspected of sexual assault should only be conducted by those doctors and nurses who have acquired specialist knowledge, skills, and attitudes during both theoretical and practical training. All doctors should be able accurately to describe and record injuries, although the correct interpretation requires considerable skill and expertise, especially in the field of non-accidental injury in children, where a multidisciplinary approach is required.

Avoidance of a death in police custody is a priority, as is the assessment of fitness-to-be-detained, which must include information on a detainee's general medical problems as well as the identification of high risk individuals, i.e., mental health and substance misuse problems. Deaths in custody include rapid unexplained death occurring during restraint and/or during excited delirium. The recent introduction of chemical crowd control agents means that health professionals also need to be aware of the effects of the common agents, as well as the appropriate treatments.

Custodial interrogation is an essential part of criminal investigations. However, in recent years there have been a number of well-publicized miscarriages of justice in which the conviction depended on admissions made during interviews that were subsequently shown to be untrue. Recently, a working medical definition of fitness-to-be-interviewed has been developed, and it is now essential that detainees be assessed to determine whether they are risks to provide unreliable information.

The increase in substance abuse means that detainees in police custody are often now seen exhibiting the complications of drug intoxication and withdrawal, medical conditions that need to be managed appropriately in the custodial environment. Furthermore, in the section on traffic medicine, not only are medical aspects of fitness-to-drive covered, but also provided is detailed information on the effects of alcohol and drugs on driving, as well as an assessment of impairment to drive.

In the appendices of *A Physician's Guide to Clinical Forensic Medicine*, the relevant ethical documents relating to police, nurses, and doctors are brought together, along with alcohol assessment questionnaires, the mini mental-state examination, and the role of appropriate adults; the management of head-injured detainees, including advice for the police; the Glasgow Coma Scale and an example of a head injury warning card; guidance notes on US and UK statutory provisions governing access to health records; a drink/drugs impairment assessment form, along with a table outlining the peak effect, half life, duration of action, and times for detection of common drugs.

Margaret M. Stark

Acknowledgments

I am grateful to Steven B. Karch, MD (Series Editor) and Paul Petralia (Humana) for their support and advice in the preparation of this book. I am indebted to my husband Martin for his help and support. Chapter 2 was reviewed by Carol Henderson, J.D., Professor of Law, and Kathy Cerminara, J.D., LLM, Assistant Professor of Law from Nova Southeastern University, Fort Lauderdale, FL to add information relevant to a US audience. Their insight is very much appreciated.

To Martin and Feline Friends

Contents

List of Figures

Chapter 9

Chapter 10

List of Tables

Chapter 1

Chapter 6

Chapter 7

Chapter 8

Chapter 9

Chapter 10

Contributors

DR. KARI BLAHO • Department of Emergency Medicine and Clinical Toxicology, UT Medical Group, Memphis TN
PROFESSOR JACK CRANE • The Queen's University of Belfast and Northern Ireland Office, State Pathologist's Department, Institute of Forensic Medicine, Belfast, UK
DR. STEVEN KARCH • Oakland, CA
MRS. MARY NEWTON • The Forensic Science Service, London, UK
DR. GUY NORFOLK • Stockwood Health Centre, Bristol, UK
DR. ROY N. PALMER • London, UK
DR. JASON PAYNE-JAMES • London, UK
DR. DEBORAH ROGERS • The Forensic Medicine Unit, St. George's Hospital Medical School, London, UK
DR. RICHARD SHEPHERD • The Forensic Medicine Unit, St. George's Hospital Medical School, London, UK
DR. MARGARET M. STARK • The Forensic Medicine Unit, St. George's Hospital Medical School, London, UK
DR. AMANDA THOMAS • Department of Community Paediatrics, St. James's University Hospital, Leeds, UK
DR. IAN F WALL • Wellingborough, UK

Chapter 1

The History and Development of Clinical Forensic Medicine Worldwide

Jason Payne-James

1. Introduction

Clinical forensic medicine is a term that has become widely used only in the last two decades or so, although the phrase has been in use at least since 1949 when the Association of Police Surgeons—a UK-based body—was first established. It is now commonly used to refer to the branch of medicine that involves an interaction among the law, the judiciary, and the police generally in respect to living persons. Thus clinical forensic medicine must be distinguished from the other major branch of forensic medicine: forensic pathology. A forensic pathologist does not (in general) deal with living individuals, whereas a forensic physician's role may be much broader.

The practitioners of clinical forensic medicine have been given many different names over the years, but the term *forensic physician* has become accepted. Other names that have been used include police surgeon, forensic medical officer, and forensic medical examiner, but names such as these refer more to the appointed role than to the work done. Table 1 illustrates the variety of roles a forensic physician may be asked to play. Some practitioners of clinical forensic medicine may only perform some of these functions, whereas others may play a more extensive role, depending on geographic location (in terms

From: *Forensic Science: A Physician's Guide to Clinical Forensic Medicine*
Edited by: M. M. Stark © Humana Press, Inc., Totowa, NJ

Table 1
Typical Roles of a Forensic Physician[a]

Normal roles
- Determine fitness to be detained in custody
- Determine fitness to be released
- Determine fitness to be charged: competence to comprehend charge
- Determine fitness to transfer
- Determine fitness to be interviewed by the police or detaining body
- Meet the requirement of an independent person to ensure rights for the vulnerable or mentally disordered
- Assess alcohol and drug intoxication and withdrawal
- Perform comprehensive examination to assess a person's ability to drive a motor vehicle
- Undertake intimate body searches for drugs
- Make precise documentation and interpretation of injuries
- Take forensic samples
- Assess and treat personnel injured while on duty, including needle stick injuries
- Pronounce life extinct at a scene of death and undertake preliminary advisory role
- Perform mental state examinations
- Examine adult complainants of serious sexual assault and the alleged perpetrators
- Examine alleged child victims of neglect or physical or sexual abuse
- Examine victims and assailants in alleged police assaults

Additional roles
- Give expert opinion in courts and tribunals
- Conduct death in custody investigation
- Act in a pressure group and as an independent investigator for ethical and moral issues
  - Victims of torture
  - War crimes
  - Female genital mutilation

For all these examinations a forensic physician must accurately document findings and when needed produce written reports for appropriate civil or criminal courts or other agencies. The forensic physician will also be ready to present the information orally to a court, other tribunal, or forum.

[a]This table illustrates the role of police surgeons/forensic medical examiners in the United Kingdom; roles vary according to geographic location. Adapted from ref. *30*.

of country and state), local statute, and judicial systems. Forensic physicians must have a good knowledge of *medical jurisprudence*: the application of medical science to the law within their own jurisdiction. The extent and range of the role of a clinical forensic medicine practitioner is variable; many may limit themselves to specific aspects of clinical forensic medicine, for example, sexual assault or child abuse. At present the role and scope of the specialty of clinical forensic medicine is ill-defined in global terms, unlike other medical specialties such as gastroenterology or cardiology. In many cases doctors practicing clinical forensic medicine or medical jurisprudence may only take on these functions as subspecialties within their own general workload.

2. Historical References

The origins of clinical forensic medicine go back many centuries, although it is true to say that "forensic medicine [cannot be thought of] as an entity. . . until a stage of civilization is reached in which we have . . . a recognizable legal system . . . and an integrated body of medical knowledge and opinion" *(1)*.

The specific terms *forensic medicine* and *medical jurisprudence* in the English language date back to the early 19th century. In 1840 Thomas Stuart Traill *(2)*, referring to the connection between medicine and legislation, pointed out that "it is known in Germany, the country in which it took its rise, by the name of State Medicine, in Italy and France it is termed Legal Medicine; and with us [in the United Kingdom] it is usually denominated Medical Jurisprudence or Forensic Medicine." However, there are many previous references to the use of medical experts to assist the legal process in many other jurisdictions; these physicians would be involved in criminal or civil cases as well as public health (referred to frequently and somewhat confusingly in the 19th century as "Medical Police"). There is much dispute as to when medical expertise in the determination of legal issues was first utilized. In 1975 Chinese archaeologists discovered a number of bamboo pieces dating from about 220 B.C. (Qin dynasty) with rules and regulations for examining injuries inscribed on them. Other historical examples of the link between medicine and the law can be found around the world.

Amundsen and Ferngren *(3)* assessed the evidence for the role of physicians as expert witnesses in ancient Greece; they concluded that forensic medicine was used by Athenian courts and other public bodies and that the testimony of physicians in matters of a medical nature was given particular credence. They also point out that this use of physicians as expert witnesses was "loose and ill-defined" *(4)*, as it was in the Roman courts. In the Roman Republic the "Lex Duodecim Tabularum" (laws drafted on 12 tablets and accepted as a single statute in 449 B.C.) had minor references to medicolegal matters, including length of gestation (to determine legitimacy), disposal of the dead, punishments dependent on the degree of injury caused by an assailant, and poisoning *(5)*. Papyri related to Roman Egypt dating from the latter part of the 1st to the latter part of the 4th century A.D. contain information about forensic medical examinations or investigations *(6)*.

Although the interaction between medicine and the law in these periods is undoubted, the specific role of forensic medicine, as interpreted by historical documents, is open to dispute; the degree and extent of forensic medical input acknowledged appears to depend on the historian undertaking the assessment.

It is now generally agreed that a specific role for the medical expert as a provider of impartial opinion for the judicial system was identified clearly by the Justinian Laws between 529 and 564 A.D. Traill *(2)* states that "Medical Jurisprudence as a science cannot date farther back than the 16th century." He identifies George, Bishop of Bamberg, who proclaimed a penal code in 1507, as the originator of the first codes in which medical evidence was a necessity in certain cases. However, the "Constitutio Criminalis Carolina," the code of law published and proclaimed in 1553 in Germany by Emperor Charles V, is considered to have originated Legal Medicine as a specialty: expert medical testimony became a requirement rather than an option in cases of murder, wounding, poisoning, hanging, drowning, infanticide, and abortion *(1)*. Medicolegal autopsies were well documented in parts of Italy and Germany five centuries before the use of such procedures by English coroners. The use of such expertise was not limited to deaths or to mainland Europe. Cassar *(7)*, for example, describes the earliest recorded Maltese medicolegal report (1542): medical evidence established that the male partner was incapable of sexual intercourse and this resulted in a marriage annulment.

2.1. Late 18th Century Onward

Beginning in the latter part of the 18th century, a number of books and treatises were published in English concerning forensic medicine and medical jurisprudence. What is remarkable is that the issues addressed by many of the authors would not be out of place in a contemporary setting. It seems odd that many of these principles are restated today as though they are new.

In 1783 William Hunter *(8)* published essays on the murder of bastard children; this may be the first true "forensic medicine" publication from England. The first larger work was published in 1788 by Samuel Farr—*Elements of Medical Jurisprudence*—itself translated from the 1767 publication *Elemental Medicinae Forensis* by Fazelius of Geneva. Davis *(9)* refers to these and to *Remarks on Medical Jurisprudence* by William Dease of Dublin, as well as the *Treatise on Forensic Medicine or Medical Jurisprudence* by

O. W. Bartley of Bristol. Davis considers the latter two works of poor quality, stating that the "first original and satisfactory work" was George Male's *Epitome of Juridical or Forensic Medicine*, published in 1816 (second edition, 1821). Male was a physician at Birmingham General Hospital and is often considered the father of English Medical Jurisprudence.

Texts on forensic medicine began to appear more rapidly and with much broader content. John Gordon Smith *(10)* stated in *The Principles of Forensic Medicine Systematically Arranged and Applied to British Practice* (1821) that "Forensic Medicine—Legal, Judiciary or Juridical Medicine—and Medical Jurisprudence are synonymous terms." Having referred in the Preface to the earlier books, he notes, "It is but justice to mention that the American schools have outstripped us in attention to Forensic Medicine"; he may have been referring to the work of Theodric Romeyn Beck and others. Beck published the first American textbook 2 years later *(5)*. Prior to this, in 1804 J. A. Stringham, who was trained in Edinburgh, was appointed as a lecturer in medical jurisprudence at the College of Physicians and Surgeons of New York and given a Chair in 1813 *(11)*.

John Gordon Smith *(10)* wrote that "Every medical practitioner being liable to a subpoena, should make it his business to know the relations of physiological and pathological principles to the facts on which he is likely to be interrogated, and likewise the principal judiciary bearings of the case. The former of these are to be found in works on Forensic Medicine; the latter in those on Jurisprudence." Alfred Taylor *(12)* in his *A Manual of Medical Jurisprudence* defined medical jurisprudence as ". . . that science, which teaches the application of every branch of medical knowledge to the purpose of the law."

There was a clear demand for such books and Traill's *(2) Outlines of a Course of Lectures on Medical Jurisprudence*, published in 1840 when Traill was Regius Professor of Jurisprudence and Medical Police at Edinburgh, was the second edition of a book initially published in 1834 *(13)*. The first Chair of Forensic Medicine was established in the UK in Edinburgh in 1807 [although Andrew Duncan Senior had lectured there on forensic medicine topics since 1789 *(14)*], with subsequent nonprofessorial academic forensic medicine posts set up at Guy's Hospital and Charing Cross Hospital, London. In 1839 and 1875, respectively, academic chairs of medical jurisprudence were created in Glasgow and Aberdeen *(15)*.

The relevant areas of interest to forensic medicine and medical jurisprudence were gradually becoming better defined. Table 2 summarizes the chapter contents of *Principles of Forensic Medicine* by William Guy *(16)*, Professor of Forensic Medicine at King's College, London in 1844. It will be noted that

Table 2
Chapter Contents of Guy's 1884 Text,
Principles of Forensic Medicine

1.	Medical Evidence
2.	Personal Identity
	Identity
	Age
	Sex
3.	Impotence
	Rape
	Pregnancy
	Delivery
4.	Foeticide, or Criminal Abortion
	Infanticide
	Legitimacy
5.	Life Assurance
	Feigned Diseases
6.	Unsoundness of Mind
7.	Persons Found Dead
	Real & Apparent Death
	Sudden Death
	Survivorship
8.	Death by Drowning
	Death by Hanging
	Death by Strangulation
	Death by Suffocation
9.	Wounds
10.	Death by Fire
	Spontaneous Combustion
	Death by Lightning
	Death from Cold
	Death from Starvation
11.	Toxicology
	Specific Poisons

much of this material is relevant to forensic physicians and forensic pathologists working today.

Thus, by the end of the 19th century, a framework of forensic medicine that persists today had been established in Europe, the United Kingdom, America, and related jurisdictions.

3. Contemporary Clinical Forensic Medicine

Even though medicine and law interact much more frequently in cases of living individuals, forensic pathology has long been established as the academic basis for forensic medicine. It is only in the last two decades that research and academic interest in clinical forensic medicine has become an area of much more focused research. The following working definition has been suggested: "... clinical forensic medicine includes all medical [healthcare] fields which may relate to legal, judicial and police systems" *(17)*.

The recent growth in awareness of abuses of human rights and civil liberties has directed attention to the conditions of detention of prisoners and to the application of justice to both victim and suspect. Examples of injustice and failure to observe basic human rights or rights enshrined in statute in which the input of medical professionals may be considered at least of poor quality and at worst criminally negligent have occurred and continue to occur worldwide. The death of Steve Biko in South Africa, the conviction of Carole Richardson in England, and the deaths of native Australians in prison are widely publicized instances of such problems. Reports from the European Committee for the Prevention of Torture and Inhuman and Degrading Treatment in the early 1990s drew attention to the problem of lack of independence of some police doctors. The conflicting needs and duties of those involved in the judicial system are clear, and it is sometimes believed that recognition of such conflicts is comparatively recent, which would be naïve and wrong.

The differing roles that a forensic physician may play when attending a prisoner have been recognized by identifying three facets of medical care that may conflict: first, the role of medicolegal expert for a law enforcement agency; second, the role of a treating doctor; and third, the examination and treatment of detainees who allege that they have been mistreated by the police during their arrest, during interrogation, or during the various stages of police custody *(18)*. This conflict is well recognized by forensic physicians. G. Grant *(19)*, a police surgeon appointed to the Metropolitan Police in the East End of London just over a century ago, records the following incident: "One night I was called to Shadwell [police] station to see a man charged with being drunk and disorderly, who had a number of wounds on the top of his head ... I dressed them] ... and when I finished he whispered 'Doctor, you might come with me to the cell door' ... I went with him. We were just passing the door of an empty cell, when a police constable with a mop slipped out and struck the man a blow over the head ... Boiling over with indignation I hurried to the Inspector's Office [and] told him what had occurred." Dr. Grant records that the offender was dealt with immediately.

Clearly Dr. Grant perceived that he had moral, ethical, and medical duties to his patient, the prisoner. In England and Wales, the Human Rights Act 1998—whose purpose is to make it unlawful for any public authority to act in a manner incompatible with a right defined by the European Convention of Human Rights—is likely to emphasize (in England and Wales at least) the need for doctors to be very aware of those human rights issues that touch on prisoners and that doctors can influence. It is worth noting that this law was enacted almost 50 years after publication of the European Convention of Human Rights and Fundamental Freedoms.

Dr. Grant was one of the earlier "police surgeons" in England, the first "Superintending Surgeon" having been appointed to the Metropolitan Police Force on April 30, 1830. The Metropolitan Police Surgeons Association was formed in 1888 with 156 members. In 1949 the Association was reconstituted as a national body under the leadership of Ralph Summers, so that improvements in the education and training for clinical forensic medicine could be made. The Association of Police Surgeons remains the leading professional body of forensic physicians worldwide, with over 1000 members.

4. Clinical Forensic Medicine Around the World

How are clinical forensic medical workloads dealt with around the world? Table 3 is a summary of responses to a questionnaire on various aspects of clinical forensic medicine sent in mid-1997 to specialists in different countries *(20)*. It shows the range of standards and procedures in a number of the most important aspects of clinical forensic medicine. The questionnaire responses were all from individuals familiar with the police/forensic medicine and judicial procedures within their own country. Although the sample is small, the responses can be summarized by a number of key points illustrating the current state of clinical forensic medicine around the world at the beginning of the 21st century:

No clear repeatable patterns of clinical forensic medicine practice may be seen on an international basis.
Several countries have informal/ad hoc arrangements to deal with medical and forensic care of detainees and victims.
The emphasis in several countries appears to be on the alleged victim rather than the alleged suspect.
The standard of medical care of detainees in police custody is variable.
There are no international standards of practice or training.
There are apparent gaps in the investigation of police complaints in some countries.
Death in custody statistics are not always in the public domain.

There is, however, increasing awareness that clinical forensic medicine needs to be considered a specialty. In Tunisia, where forensic medicine itself is a specialty only 30 years old, there is a strong emphasis on the clinical aspects of the training program, including teaching in judicial medicine, medical law and ethics, and human rights *(21)*. In countries where forensic medicine has a much longer history such as Greece, forensic pathologists are routinely responsible for medical examinations in certain circumstances, e.g. rape, although nonspecialists may sometimes be used *(22)*. In some countries such as Japan where many chairs of forensic medicine exist, interest in clinical forensic medicine is sometimes limited because of an absence of incentives in terms of training or remuneration *(23)*. The use of general practitioners (primary care physicians) with a special interest in clinical forensic medicine is common; England, Wales, Northern Ireland, Scotland, Australasia, and the Netherlands all being heavily dependent on such professionals. The role may vary in its emphasis on various aspects of clinical forensic medicine, for example, assessments of adult and child sexual assault victims or suspects are only occasionally undertaken by Dutch police surgeons, in contrast to Scotland, where most of these assessments are undertaken by police surgeons, although police surgeon training has been longer established in the Netherlands *(24)*.

Despite the global absence of specific clinical forensic medicine training, a number of recent appointments [a chair in Clinical Forensic Medicine in the Netherlands, honorary senior lecturer posts in Clinical Forensic Medicine in the UK, full-time forensic physicians in Australia *(25)*] reveal the importance of the specialty. The Department of Emergency Medicine at the University of Louisville School of Medicine (Kentucky) established a clinical forensic medicine training program and in 1991 incorporated formal training in clinical forensic medicine into the core curriculum of the academic emergency medicine training program *(26)*.

Specific qualifications related to clinical forensic medicine are few. The Diploma of Medical Jurisprudence (Society of Apothecaries, London, England), and the Diploma of Forensic Medicine (University of Glasgow, Scotland) are basic qualifications, with only the Mastership of Medical Jurisprudence representing a higher qualification in the subject. Monash University in Victoria, Australia, has recently introduced a course leading to a Graduate Diploma in Forensic Medicine, intended to "prepare practitioners for clinical forensic practice, teaching and research activities" *(27)*. The Department of Forensic Medicine has also pioneered a distance-learning Internet-based continuing education program *(28)* that is also serialized in the *Journal of Clinical Forensic Medicine*. Many forensic physicians undertake higher training in law

Table 3

Summary of Responses to Questionnaire Concerning Clinical Forensic Medicine[a]

	1	2	3	4	5	6	7	8	9	10	11	12
	Formal system for assessment in custody?	**Who assesses detainees in custody?**	**Examined if thought under influence?**	**Specific codes for welfare in custody?**	**Who assesses adult sexual assault cases?**	**Are "same sex" doctors available?**	**Who assesses child victims?**	**Assess mentally disordered cases?**	**Who assesses cases of alleged police assault?**	**Is there a body to investigate complaints against police?**	**Who investigates deaths in police custody?**	**Are deaths in custody statistics published?**
Cayman Islands	No		No	No	Medical officer at casualty department / Gynecologist	Yes	Medical officer at casualty department - Pediatrician	Yes	Forensic pathologist / Government Medical Officer / Prisoner's choice of private practitioner	Police appointed body	Police + forensic pathologist (none in recent years)	No incident in recent years
England & Wales	Yes	Forensic physician (police surgeons) paid for by police but professionally independent	Yes	Yes	Forensic physician	Generally yes	Forensic physician + Pediatrician	Yes	Forensic physician	Police Complaints Authority	Police Complaints Authority + the coroner	Yes
France	Yes. Emergency Forensic Units (large towns); GPs / Forensic physicians in others	Independent of police	Yes	Yes	Forensic physician / Gynecologist / GP	Yes - in larger units. Not always possible	Forensic physician / Gynecologist / GP	Yes	Forensic physician	Police / Gendarmerie - appointed by government / Army	Forensic physicians	Not known
Germany	Yes	Employed by police or under contract	Yes	Yes	Institute of Forensic Medicine / Gynecologist	Victims - yes; suspects - no	Institutes of Forensic Medicine + Pediatrician	Yes		No specific body – handled by appropriate Commissioners Dept.	Institute of Forensic Medicine - all must undergo autopsy	No
Indonesia	Yes	Employed by police	No	No	Medical doctor / Forensic pathologist / Gynecologist	No	Medical doctors	Yes	Military police	Government	Military police	No
Japan	Yes	Private practitioners who contract their medical services to local police	Yes	Yes	Gynecologist	Theoretically	Gynecologist / Pediatrician	Yes	Police officer / Private practitioner	Local government	Forensic pathologist	Yes

	1	2	3	4	5	6	7	8	9	10	11	12
	Formal system for assessment in custody?	**Who assesses detainees in custody?**	**Examined if thought under influence?**	**Specific codes for welfare in custody?**	**Who assesses adult sexual assault cases?**	**Are "same sex" doctors available?**	**Who assesses child victims?**	**Assess mentally disordered cases?**	**Who assesses cases of alleged police assault?**	**Is there a body to investigate complaints against police?**	**Who investigates deaths in police custody?**	**Are deaths in custody statistics published?**
Netherlands	Yes	Medical Officer of Public Health	Yes	Yes	Medical Officer of Public Health	Yes	Medical Officer of Public Health	Unaware	Medical Officer of Public Health	Rijksrecherche – organization which polices the police	Medical Officer of Public Health in consultation with Prosecutor	?
People's Republic of China	Yes. Full-time doctor for police custody	Forensic medical worker employed by police / courts	Yes	Yes	Female forensic medical worker	Yes, if victim is female	Forensic medical worker in police station	Yes	Forensic medical worker	Local court	Forensic medical worker	No
Scotland	Yes	Forensic physician (police surgeon) paid for by police but professionally independent	Yes	Yes	Forensic physician	Dependent on availability	Pediatrician + Forensic physician	Yes	Forensic physician	Procurator Fiscal	Procurator Fiscal / Fatal Accident Inquiry	Yes
Singapore	Yes	Predominantly medical officers employed by Ministry of Health	Yes	Yes	O & G specialist for female / Surgeon for male	Yes	Pediatrician / O & G specialists	Yes	Medical Officer	Yes	Police from another division / CID / Forensic pathologist	
Sweden	Yes	Forensic medicine specialist at National Board of Forensic Medicine	No	?	Any doctor / Forensic medicine specialist	Probably	Any doctor / Forensic medicine specialist	No	Any doctor / Forensic medicine specialist	Attorney General and Regional Police Office	Forensic medicine specialist at National Board of Forensic Medicine	?

Full text of questions in columns 1–12:

1. Is there a formal system in your country/state by which the police and judicial system can get immediate medical and/or forensic assessment of individuals in police custody?
2. Who examines/assesses police prisoners to determine whether they are medically fit to be detained in police custody?
3. If a prisoner is suspected of being under the influence of drugs or alcohol in police custody, would they usually be examined to determine whether they remain in custody?
4. Does your country/state have specific codes/laws/statutes making provision for the welfare of individuals in custody?
5. Who assesses forensically victim and suspects in adult sexual assault cases?
6. Is it possible for an individual to have a same sex examining doctor?
7. Who assesses child victims?
8. Is there a means by which those suspected of having mental disorder or learning disability may be assessed?
9. In cases of alleged police assault who examines a) the officers, b) the complainant?
10. Is there a body that investigates complaints against police?
11. Who investigates deaths in police custody?
12. Are deaths in police custody statistics published?

[a] Adapted from ref. *20*.

or medical ethics in addition to their basic medical qualifications, and also psychiatrists, accident and emergency physicians, genitourinary specialists, and pediatricians may often undertake a clinical forensic medical role.

In addition to medical professionals, others may have a direct involvement in matters of a clinical forensic medical nature, in particular when the number of medical professionals with a specific interest is limited. The International Association of Forensic Nurses has increased awareness of the role of specialist nurses in the assessment and care of individuals, particularly those who are victims of sexual or other crimes of violence. Forensic nurses have a high profile in North America, and a large number of sexual assault referral centers have been established, staffed, and run by such health care professionals *(29)*.

5. Conclusions

Having reviewed the links between medicine and law over many centuries, it is possible to identify three key issues that clinical forensic medicine specialists must address in the near future:

1. Clinical forensic medicine needs to be recognized as a distinct subspecialty with its own full-time career posts, with an understanding that it will be appropriate for those undertaking the work part-time to receive appropriate training and postgraduate education.
2. Forensic physicians and other forensic health care professionals must ensure that the term *clinical forensic medicine* is recognized as synonymous with knowledge, fairness, independence, impartiality, and the upholding of basic human rights.
3. Forensic physicians and others practicing clinical forensic medicine must be of an acceptable and measurable standard.

If these three issues continue to be addressed and acted on, forensic physicians and others involved in clinical forensic medicine will be able to ensure that no individual in contact with legal, police, or judicial systems will suffer in medical, legal, or judicial terms because of lack of availability of appropriately skilled practitioners. The ability to work in close collaboration with forensic pathologists and scientists as part of a multidisciplinary team will underpin the role of clinical forensic medicine in the future *(31)*.

References

1. Smith, S. (1951) The history and development of forensic medicine. *BMJ*. 599–607.
2. Traill, T. S. (1840) *Outlines of a Course of Lectures on Medical Jurisprudence*, 2nd ed., Adam & Charles Black, Edinburgh.
3. Amundsen, D. W. and Ferngren, G. B. (1977) The physician as an expert witness in Athenian Law. *Bull Hist Med.* **51,** 202–213.

4. Amundsen, D. W. and Ferngren, G. B. (1979) Forensic role of physicians in Roman law. *Bull Hist Med.* **53,** 39–56.
5. Brittain, R. P. (1967) Origins of legal medicine. Roman law: Lex Duodecim Tabularum. *Medico-Legal J.* **35,** 71–72.
6. Amundsen, D. W. and Ferngren, G. B. (1978) The forensic role of physicians in Ptolemaic and Roman Egypt. *Bull Hist Med.* **52,** 336–353.
7. Cassar, P. (1974) A medicolegal report of the sixteenth century from Malta. *Med Hist.* **18,** 354–359.
8. Hunter, W. (1783) *On the Uncertainty of the Signs of Murder in the Case of Bastard Children*. London.
9. Davis, B. T. (1974) George Edward Male, M. D., the father of English medical jurisprudence. *Proc R Soc Med.* **67,** 117–120.
10. Smith, J. G. (1821) *The Principles of Forensic Medicine Systematically Arranged and Applied to British Practice*. Thomas & George Underwood, London.
11. Forbes, T. R. (1985) *Surgeons at the Bailey: English Forensic Medicine to 1878.* Yale University Press, New Haven.
12. Taylor, A. S. (1844) *A Manual of Medical Jurisprudence.* John Churchill, London.
13. Traill, T. S. (1834) *Outlines of a Course of Lectures on Medical Jurisprudence.* Adam & Charles Black, Edinburgh.
14. Cordner, S. M., Ranson, D. L., and Singh, B. (1992) The practice of forensic medicine in Australasia: a review. *Aust NZ J Med.* **22,** 477–485.
15. Gee, D. J. and Mason, J. K. (1990) *The Courts & the Doctor*. Oxford University Press, Oxford.
16. Guy, W. A. (1844) *Principles of Forensic Medicine*. Henry Renshaw, London.
17. Payne-James, J. J. (1994) Clinical forensic medicine. *J Clin Forensic Med.* **1,** 1.
18. Editorial (1993) Three-faced practice: doctors and police custody. *Lancet.* **341,** 1245–1247.
19. Grant, G. (1920) *The Diary of a Police Surgeon*. C. Arthur Pearson, London.
20. Payne-James, J. J. (1997) *Questionnaire on 'Global Clinical Forensic Medicine,'* 4th Annual Clinical Forensic Medicine Postgraduate Conference, Louisville, KY.
21. Chadly, A. (1998) Forensic medicine training in Tunisia. *J Clin Forensic Med.* **5,** 69–71.
22. Michalodimitrakis, M. and Tsatsakis, A. (1997) The changing status of forensic medicine in Greece. *J Clin Forensic Med.* **4,** 159–162.
23. Tsunenari, S., Yonemitsu, K., Kibayashi, K., and Miyakita, S. (1994) Forensic medicine: education and practice in Japan. *J Clin Forensic Med.* **1,** 3–7.
24. Turnbull, J. A., Hannaford, P. F., and Busuttil, A. (1996) Dutch & Scottish clinical forensic medicine: a comparison. *J Clin Forensic Med.* **3,** 15–19.
25. Howitt, J. B. (1995) Clinical forensic medical services: London and Melbourne contrasted. *J Clin Forensic Med.* **2,** 17–24.
26. Smock, W. S. (1994) Development of a clinical forensic medicine curriculum for emergency physicians in the USA. *J Clin Forensic Med* **1,** 27–30.
27. Wells, D. and Cordner, S. (1998) Postgraduate education in clinical forensic medicine: a Graduate Diploma. *J Clin Forensic Med.* **5,** 187–190.

28. Gall, J. A. (1997) Continuing education in forensic medicine: an exercise in distance learning. *J Clin Forensic Med.* **4,** 117–120.
29. McNair, S. M. and Finigan, A. B. (1996) The role of a forensic clinical nurse specialist in a sexual assault treatment program. *J Clin Forensic Med.* **3,** 29–30.
30. Howitt, J. and Stark, M. M. (1996) *The Role of the Independent Forensic Physician.* Education & Research Committee of the Association of Police Surgeons. Association of Police Surgeons, Harrogate.
31. Payne-James, J. J., Busuttil, A., and Smock, W. (2000) *Forensic Medicine: Clinical and Pathological Aspects.* Greenwich Medical Media, London, UK.

Chapter 2

Fundamental Principles

Roy N. Palmer

1. Introduction

Although medicine is an international discipline, practiced in much the same way throughout the English-speaking world, laws vary considerably from country to country. Much of the law applicable in the United States and in the countries of the Commonwealth derives from the English common law, but medical practitioners may not assume that the laws of their own countries or states will necessarily apply in other countries or states even if medical practices are indistinguishable. In this chapter the author attempts to set out principles of general applicability; however, it is written from the perspective of the law applicable in England and Wales and should be read with that in mind.

In recent years in the United Kingdom and elsewhere, a great many statutes relevant to medical practice have been enacted. Ignorance of the law is no defense, and today's doctors are at risk of prosecution for breaches of the law as no previous generation has been. Yet the teaching at the undergraduate level of forensic (or legal) medicine is now patchy and variable, so today's doctors are seldom well-informed about laws that govern their daily practices. It is hoped that this chapter will go some small way to help redress that position but, in the space available, only a brief outline of some relevant law can be offered. Doctors are advised to continue to subscribe to one of the traditional medical defense organizations (MDU, MPS or MDDUS in the United Kingdom, CMPA in Canada, or one of the Australian defense bodies), to an equiva-

From: *Forensic Science: A Physician's Guide to Clinical Forensic Medicine*
Edited by: M. M. Stark © Humana Press, Inc., Totowa, NJ

lent organization elsewhere, or to take out adequate insurance to ensure that they have access to advice and legal representation for medicolegal problems arising from their professional work—and, of course, indemnity for any adverse awards of costs and damages for professional negligence.

1.1. Ethical Principles

Doctors who practice as forensic medical examiners (FMEs, sometimes referred to as "police surgeons") have a very special responsibility toward detainees, subjects whose liberty is already infringed and who are at serious risk of future curtailment of their liberty. Although enactments in Europe, such as the Human Rights Act 1998, will afford better protection of the rights and liberties of citizens, the FME has a real part to play in acting honorably, by ensuring that the rights of the detainee are upheld in accordance with medical professional codes of ethics. An FME who believes that the rights of the detainee are being ignored or abused may have a duty to report the concern to a person or body in authority.

It is not always appreciated that forensic medical examiners (FMEs) have two roles. First, they are independent medical assessors of victims and/or perpetrators of crimes and, as such, no conventional therapeutic relationship exists. It is most important that this be made clear to the victims or detainees by the FME, so that properly informed consent is secured for the proposed examination. Second, a therapeutic relationship may arise when advice or treatment or other therapeutic intervention is offered, but the nature of the therapeutic relationship will be constrained by the circumstances and by the FME's duty to pass information to police officers who will be responsible for observing the detainee or victim. Great care is necessary over issues of consent and confidentiality in such circumstances.

Some ethical codes are national, drawn up by such bodies as national medical associations and medical boards or councils set up by the state (such as the British Medical Association [BMA] and the General Medical Council [GMC] in the United Kingdom). Other codes of ethics are regional (for example, the European Convention on Human Rights), whereas still others are international, such as the many codes and declarations prepared and published by the World Medical Association (WMA) (*see* Appendix 1).

Most of the ethical principles will be familiar to doctors who practice in countries that derive their laws from the Anglo-American common law system, but the detail of local rules and regulations will vary from nation to nation, state to state.

2. CONSENT

"Even when his or her life depends on receiving medical treatment, an adult of sound mind is entitled to refuse it. This reflects the autonomy of each individual and the right of self-determination. Lest reiteration may diminish the impact of this principle, it is valuable to recognise the force of the language used when the right of self determination was most recently considered in the House Of Lords." (1)

"It is well established English law that it is unlawful, so as to constitute both a tort (a civil wrong) and the crime of battery, to administer medical treatment to an adult who is conscious and of sound mind without his consent. Such a person is completely at liberty to decline to undergo treatment even if the result of his doing so will be that he will die." (2)

"The principle of self-determination requires that respect must be given to the wishes of the patient, so that if an adult patient of sound mind refuses, however unreasonably, to consent to treatment or to care by which his life would or might be prolonged, the doctors responsible for his care must give effect to his wishes, even though they do not consider it to be in his best interests to do so . . . To this extent, the principle of the sanctity of human life must yield to the principle of self-determination . . . and, for present purposes perhaps more important, the doctor's duty to act in the best interests of his patient must likewise be qualified." (3)

"Any treatment given by a doctor to a patient which involves any interference with the physical integrity of the patient is unlawful unless done with the consent of the patient: it constitutes the crime of battery and the tort of trespass to the person." (4)

"A doctor has no right to proceed in the face of objection, even if it is plain to all, including the patient, that adverse consequences and even death will or may ensue." (5)

The author can do no better than to open a discussion of the topic of consent by quoting the powerful and unambiguous language of the law lords in a recent leading case. The underlying reason for this position

"is that English law goes to great lengths to protect a person of full age and capacity from interference with his personal liberty. We have too often seen freedom disappear in other countries not only by coups d'etat

but by gradual erosion; and often it is the first step that counts. So it would be unwise to make even minor concessions." (6)

The foregoing applies to all mentally competent adults; where a patient lacks the capacity to make decisions about whether to consent to treatment (e.g., when he or she is unconscious or suffering from mental disability) the medical practitioners responsible for his or her treatment must act in the patient's best interests and, if appropriate, may carry out major invasive treatments without express consent *(7)*.

2.1. Requisites for Consent

To intervene without consent may give rise to criminal proceedings (for alleged trespass to the person) and may also give rise to tortious liability (a civil claim for damages). To protect against such proceedings the medical practitioner should ensure that the patient is capable of giving consent, has been sufficiently well informed to understand and therefore to give a true consent, and has then expressly and voluntarily consented to the proposed investigation, procedure, or treatment. In the United Kingdom the GMC has produced a booklet *(8)* setting out guidance for doctors about seeking patients' consent with which any doctor who practices in the United Kingdom must comply.

2.1.1. Capacity

If there is serious doubt about the capacity of the patient (to give consent) it should be assessed as a matter of priority. The patient's general practitioner (GP) or other responsible doctor may be sufficiently qualified to make the assessment, but in serious or complex cases involving difficult issues about the future health and well-being, or even the life, of the patient, the issue of capacity to consent should be assessed by an independent psychiatrist (in England, ideally, but not necessarily, one approved under s.12 of the Mental Health Act, 1983) *(9)*. If, following assessment, serious doubts remain about the patient's competence (e.g., the patient is incapable by reason of mental disorder of managing his or her property or affairs), it may be necessary to seek the involvement of the courts.

2.1.2. Understanding; Risks and Warnings

A signature on a form is not, of itself, a valid consent. For a valid, or true, or real consent in law the patient must be sufficiently well informed to understand that to which he or she is asked to give consent. The doctor must be satisfied that the patient

1. Can comprehend and retain the relevant information;
2. Believes the information; and
3. Can weigh in the balance the *pros and cons* in order to arrive at a choice *(10)*.

To defend a doctor against a civil claim alleging lack of consent based on a failure adequately to warn, it is necessary to have more than a signature on a standard consent form. Increasingly in medical negligence actions it is alleged that risks were not explained nor warnings given about possible adverse outcomes. It is therefore essential for the doctor (or any other healthcare professional) to spend adequate time explaining the nature and purpose of the intended investigation, procedure, or treatment in terms that the patient can understand. Risks and adverse outcomes should be discussed. The patient's direct questions must be answered frankly and truthfully (as was made clear in the Sidaway case *[11]*) and thus the discussions should be undertaken by those with adequate knowledge and experience to deal with them; ideally the clinician who is to perform the operation or procedure.

English law differs from the law in other common-law jurisdictions (e.g., Australia, Canada, the United States) regarding the nature of the information that must be imparted in order for the consent to be "informed" and, therefore, valid. Increasingly, world-wide, the courts will decide what the doctor should warn a patient about—applying objective tests, such as what a "prudent patient" would wish to know before agreeing. For example, in the leading Australian case *(12)* the court imposed a duty to warn about risks of very remote (1 in 14,000) but serious complications of elective eye surgery, even though professional opinion in Australia at the time gave evidence that they would not have warned of so remote a risk.

In the United States and Canada, the law about the duty to warn of risks and adverse outcomes has long been much more stringent. Many (but not all) US courts recognize a duty on a doctor to warn a patient of the risks inherent in the treatment proposed. In the leading case *(13)* the District of Columbia appeals court imposed an objective "prudent patient" test and enunciated four principles:

1. Every human being of adult years and sound mind has a right to determine what shall happen to his or her body.
2. Consent is the informed exercise of choice, and that entails an opportunity to evaluate knowledgeably the options available and their attendant risks.
3. The doctor must therefore disclose all "material risks."
4. The doctor must retain a "therapeutic privilege."

A "material risk" was held to be one that a reasonable person, in what the doctor knows or should know to be the patient's position, would likely attach significance to in deciding whether to forego the proposed treatment—this test is known as the "prudent patient test." However, the court held that a doctor has a therapeutic privilege by which he or she is entitled to withhold from the patient information about risk if full disclosure would pose a serious threat of psychological detriment to the patient. In the Canadian leading case *(14)* broad agreement was expressed with the propositions expressed in the American case.

English law continues to allow the doctor discretion in deciding what information is to be imparted to the particular patient being advised. The practitioner is not required to make an assessment based on the information to be given to an abstract "prudent patient;" rather the actual patient being consulted must be assessed to determine what that patient should be told. However, the Sidaway and Bolitho *(15)* cases make clear that doctors must be supported by a body of professional opinion that is not only responsible, but also scientifically and soundly based as determined by the court.

The message for the medical and allied health-care professions is that medical paternalism has no place where consent to treatment is concerned; patients' rights to self determination and personal autonomy based on full disclosure of relevant information is the legal requirement for consent.

2.1.3. Voluntary Agreement

Consent obtained by fraud or duress is not valid. A doctor must be satisfied that the patient is giving a free, voluntary agreement to the proposed investigation, procedure, or treatment.

Consent may then be given expressly or by implication. Express consent is given when the patient agrees in clear terms, verbally or in writing. A verbal consent is legitimate, but because disputes may arise about the nature and extent of the explanation and warnings about risks, often months or years after the event, it is strongly recommended that, except for minor matters, consent be recorded in written form. In the absence of a contemporaneous note of the discussions leading to the giving of consent, any disputed recollections will fall to be decided by a lengthy, expensive legal process. The matter then becomes one of evidence, with the likelihood that the patient's claimed perfect recall will be persuasive to the court in circumstances in which the doctor's truthful concession is that he or she has no clear recollection of what was said to this particular patient, one of hundreds of consultations undertaken.

A contemporaneous note should be made by the doctor of the explanation given to the patient and of warnings about risks and possible adverse outcomes. It is helpful to supplement (but not to substitute) the verbal explanation with a printed information leaflet or booklet about the procedure or treatment. The explanation should be given by the clinician who is to undertake the procedure—it is not acceptable to "send the nurse or junior hospital doctor" to "consent the patient."

For more complex and elective procedures, it is wise to give the patient some time to reflect on the advice and on the choices, offering to meet him or her again, later, before a final decision is made and to respond to any interim questions that the patient might wish to pose. For simple procedures (e.g., taking blood pressure, performing a venepuncture) it may be sufficient for consent to be implied—by the patient proffering an arm for the purpose. However, in circumstances in which the procedure has a forensic rather than a therapeutic content and the doctor is not the patient's usual medical attendant but may be carrying out tasks that affect the liberty of the individual (e.g., as a FME or as an assessor in a civil claim), it is prudent to err on the side of caution. If no assumptions are made by the doctor and express agreement is invariably sought from the patient—and documented contemporaneously—there is less chance of misunderstandings and allegations of duress or of misleading the individual.

2.2. Incompetent Adult Patients

Since the implementation of the 1983 Mental Health Act in England and Wales (and the equivalent in Scotland) no parent, relative, guardian, or court can give consent to the treatment of a mentally incompetent adult patient *(16)*. The House of Lords had to consider a request to sterilize a 36-year-old woman with permanent mental incapacity and a mental age of 5 years who had formed a sexual relationship with a fellow patient. The court held that no one, not even the courts, could give consent on behalf of an incompetent adult. (This is because the 1983 act removed the *parens patriae* jurisdiction of the courts in England and Wales; those jurisdictions in which courts retain *parens patriae* powers will retain the ability to provide consent in such circumstances.) However, the House of Lords made clear that doctors could act in the best interests of their adult, incompetent patients by treating them in accordance with a responsible body of professional opinion (i.e., in accord with the Bolam *[17]* principle).

2.3. Age of Consent

In England, section 8 of the Family Law Reform Act 1969 provides that any person (of sound mind) who has attained 16 years of age may give a valid consent to surgical, medical, or dental treatments. The consent of a parent or guardian is not required. For those under 16 years of age the House of Lords decided *(18)* that valid consent could be given by minors provided that they understood the issues. The case concerned the provision of contraceptive advice to girls under 16 in circumstances in which a parent objected. The House of Lords held that parental rights to determine whether a child under 16 years received treatment terminated if and when the child achieved a sufficient understanding and intelligence to enable him or her to comprehend the issues involved. It is the capacity to understand, regardless of age or of status, that is the determinant factor.

2.4. Intimate Samples; Intimate Searches

Section 62 of the Police and Criminal Evidence Act 1984 (and the equivalent statute in Scotland) provides that intimate samples can only be taken from an individual if authorized by a police superintendent (or higher ranking police officer) and if consent is obtained. For this purpose the age of consent is 17 (not 16) years. For those between 14 and 17 years of age the consents of both the detainee and of the parent or guardian is required and for those under 14 years of age only the consent of the parent or guardian is statutorily required.

Section 55 of the Police and Criminal Evidence Act (and an equivalent provision in Scotland) provides that an intimate search of an individual may be conducted on the authority of a police officer of at least the rank of superintendent only if there are grounds for suspecting that an individual has secreted about him or her either an object that might be used to cause physical injury while he is detained or a class A controlled drug. A doctor called upon to conduct an intimate search will be wise to consider carefully whether a detainee is likely to be able to give a free and voluntary consent in such circumstances; an intimate search should not be conducted unless the doctor is thoroughly satisfied that the individual has given valid consent. An intimate search might, exceptionally, be conducted by a doctor if he or she believes it necessary to remove a concealed object that is of immediate danger to the life or personal safety of those responsible for the detainee's supervision.

2.5. Video and Audio Recordings

The GMC issued guidance in 1997 *(19)* requiring doctors to inform patients before making a video or audio recording and (except in situations in which consent may be understood from a patient's co-operation with a procedure, e.g., radiographic investigation) to obtain their explicit consent. Doctors may make recordings without consent in exceptional circumstances, such as when it is believed that a child has been the victim of abuse.

If a recording has been made in the course of investigation or treatment of a patient but the doctor now wishes to use it for another purpose, the patient's consent must first be obtained. Recordings are not to be published or broadcast in any form without the explicit, written consent of the patient. Consent is required before recordings are published in textbooks or journals or before the public is allowed access to them.

The GMC states that if patients can be identified from recordings a doctor must ensure that the interests and well-being of the patient takes precedence over all other considerations. This is especially so for the mentally ill or disabled, the seriously ill, children, or other vulnerable people. When disability prevents patients from giving informed consent, the GMC advises the doctor to get agreement from a close relative or caregiver; where children lack the understanding to consent, the permission of the parent or guardian is recommended.

2.6. Recording Telephone Calls

Many countries have laws or regulations designed to protect the rights of individuals that govern the electronic recording of telephone conversations. Commonly, a provision will be included stating that persons whose telephone calls are being recorded must be informed of the fact—the details vary from country to country. In the United Kingdom, for example, the Telecommunications Act 1984 requires that the person making a recording shall make "every reasonable effort to inform the parties" of doing so. "Every reasonable effort" is not defined statutorily but the Office of Telecommunications ("Oftel"—a government-appointed regulatory body) has issued guidance. Reasonable effort may be achieved by the use of warning tones, by pre-recorded messages, by warnings spoken by a telephone operator, or by written warnings in publicity material.

A recording may be an invaluable aid for forensic evidence or to help to refute a complaint or claim for compensation, but practitioners who make electronic recordings of telephone calls must ensure that they comply with local laws and codes of practice.

2.7. Emergencies

Before leaving the topic of consent it is necessary to state clearly that in a medical emergency in which a patient is unconscious and thus unable to give or withhold consent, and there is no clear instruction to the contrary in the form of a valid, extant advance directive made by the patient, treatment may—indeed should—be given that is clearly essential to save life or prevent serious harm. However, nonurgent treatment should be deferred until the patient is able to give consent.

3. Confidentiality

". . . And whatsoever I shall see or hear in the course of my profession, as well as outside my profession in my intercourse with men, if it be what should not be published abroad, I will never divulge, holding such things to be holy secrets . . ." (20)

". . . I will respect the secrets which are confided in me, even after the patient has died . . ." (21)

". . . A physician shall preserve absolute confidentiality on all he knows about his patient even after the patient has died . . ." (22)

Information acquired by a medical practitioner from or about a patient in the course of his or her professional work is confidential and must never be disclosed to others without either the consent of the patient or other proper justification.

Confidentiality is primarily a professional conduct matter for the medical practitioner but patients also have a legal right to confidentiality, protected by law. The GMC in the United Kingdom and other medical councils and medical boards world-wide have published guidance to doctors making it clear that a breach of confidentiality is a serious professional offense. The GMC's current guidance *(23)* requires doctors to

"treat information about patients as confidential. If in exceptional circumstances you feel you should pass on information without a patient's consent, or against a patient's wishes, you should follow our guidance on confidentiality and be prepared to justify your decision".

A separate GMC booklet *(24)* sets out more detailed guidance, including the principles of confidentiality and exceptions to the general rule.

Doctors are responsible for the safekeeping of confidential information against improper disclosure when it is stored, transmitted to others, or disposed of. If a doctor plans to disclose information about a patient to others, he or she must first inform the patient of that intention and make clear that the patient has an opportunity to withhold permission for its disclosure. Patients' requests for confidentiality must be respected, except for exceptional circumstances (such as where the health or safety of others would otherwise be at serious risk).

If confidential information is disclosed the doctor should release only as much as is necessary for the purpose and must always be ready and willing to justify the disclosure—e.g., to the relevant medical council or board, or to the courts. Where confidential information is to be shared with healthcare workers or others, the doctor must ensure that they, too, respect confidentiality.

3.1. Death and Confidentiality

The duty of confidentiality extends beyond the death of the patient. The extent to which information may properly be disclosed after the death of a patient will depend on the circumstances. In general it is prudent to seek the permission of all the personal representatives of the estate of the deceased patient (such as the executors or administrators) before any information is disclosed. They, in turn, should be advised of the foreseeable consequences of disclosure. A doctor in any doubt should take advice from the appropriate protection or defense organization.

3.2. Detention and Confidentiality

An FME or police surgeon (or equivalent) should exercise particular care over confidentiality when examining persons who are detained in custody. When taking the medical history and when examining the detainee it is common for a police or other detaining official to be in attendance, as a "chaperone" or simply as a person in attendance, in close proximity to be able to overhear the conversation. Such officials will not owe to the detainee the same duty of confidentiality that is owed by a medical or nurse practitioner, nor be subject to similar professional sanctions for a breach of confidentiality.

The doctor called upon to examine a detainee must take great care to ensure that those being examined understand clearly the role of the FME/police surgeon and the implications for confidentiality. The detainee must understand and agree to the terms of the consultation before any medical information is gathered, preferably giving written consent.

The examining doctor should do everything possible to maintain the confidentiality of the consultation. An accused's right of silence, the presumption of innocence, rights under Human Rights legislation and so forth may produce areas of conflicting principle. The doctor's code of professional conduct may conflict with statutory codes binding upon custody officials (e.g., the duty on a police officer to record events). It may be essential to take the medical history in strict confidence, commensurate with adequate safeguards against violent behavior by the prisoner and to insist on a neutral chaperone for a physical examination. In the space available in this chapter it is possible only to highlight the issues; their resolution will vary according to local rules and circumstances. In the United Kingdom guidance for FMEs is available from their professional bodies *(25)*.

3.3. Exceptions to the General Duty of Confidentiality

Under several circumstances the doctor may legitimately disclose information gained about a patient during his or her professional work. For a full consideration the reader is referred to the GMC guidance or equivalent locally relevant guidance. In summary, the main exceptions are listed in Sections 3.3.1. to 3.3.5.

3.3.1. The Patient's Permission

The confidences are those of the patient, not those of the doctor, so if a patient requests or consents to their disclosure the information may perfectly properly be disclosed, within the terms of the patient's permissions.

Consent to disclose confidential information may be given by the patient in a wide range of circumstances. These include employment and insurance purposes; housing and welfare; testimonials and references; or legal proceedings (whether civil or criminal or family law matters, and so on). However, care must be taken to ensure that disclosure is limited strictly to the terms of the patient's permission and that there is no disclosure to parties with whom the patient may be in contention unless the patient expressly agrees to it. (The classic pitfalls are disclosure to the advisers of the other spouse or other party in contested divorce, child custody, or personal injury cases).

3.3.2. The Patient's Best Interests

In circumstances in which a patient is incapable of giving consent because of incapacity, immaturity, and so forth, and has refused to allow the doctor to speak to other appropriate persons, a doctor may disclose information to other appropriate persons if convinced that it is in the patient's best medical interests. If a doctor believes that a patient is the victim of physical or sexual abuse or of neglect, he or she may disclose relevant information to an appropriate person or statutory agency in an attempt to prevent further harm to the patient.

Another example of this exception is when a doctor believes that seeking permission for the disclosure would be damaging to the patient but that a close relative should know about the patient's condition—e.g., terminal or some psychiatric illnesses.

The doctor must always act in the patient's best medical interests and be prepared to justify his or her decision. Advice may be taken from appropriate colleagues and/or from a protection or defense organization.

3.3.3. The Public Interest, Interest of Others, or Violent or Dangerous Patients

Disclosure in the interests of others may be legitimate when they are at risk because a patient refuses to follow medical advice. Examples include patients who continue to drive when unfit to do so and against medical advice or who place others at risk by failing to disclose a serious communicable disease. Each case demands careful consideration and doctors who are in any doubt regarding how best to proceed should not hesitate to seek appropriate counsel.

Doctors may also be approached by the police for information to assist them in apprehending the alleged perpetrator of a serious crime. A balance must be struck between the doctor's duty to preserve the confidences of a patient and his or her duty as a citizen to assist in the solving of serious crime where he or she has information that may be crucial to a police inquiry. In cases of murder, serious assaults, and rape in which the alleged assailant is still at large, the doctor might be persuaded that there is a duty to assist in the apprehension of the assailant by providing information acquired professionally that will be likely to assist the police in identifying and apprehending the prime suspect(s). Where the accused person is already in custody, however, the doctor would be wise not to disclose confidential information without the agreement of the patient or legal advisers, or an order from the court. Each case must be weighed on its own facts and merits and the doctor may wish to seek advice from an appropriate source, such as a protection or defense organization.

The violent or dangerous patient poses particular dilemmas for the doctor. In the course of a consultation a patient may tell a doctor that he or she intends to perpetrate some serious harm on another person—perhaps a close relative or friend or someone with whom there is a perceived need to "settle an old score." Each case must be carefully assessed on its own facts and merits and careful clinical judgement exercised; however, under some circumstances a doctor may feel obligated to override the duty of confidentiality to the individual and to disclose confidential information to the intended victim, the police, or another person in authority with the power to take appropriate action. Indeed, a failure to act in such circumstances has led to adverse judicial rulings, as in the Californian Tarasoff *(26)* case, in which a specialist psychologist failed to give a warning to the girlfriend of a patient who later murdered her. The court decided that although no general common law duty exists to protect or warn third parties, a special relationship might impose such a duty.

In the United Kingdom a psychiatrist was sued because he had released, without the consent of a violent patient, a report prepared at the request of the patient's solicitors in connection with an application for release from detention.

The psychiatrist advised against release and the solicitors decided not to make use of his report. The psychiatrist was so concerned about his findings that he released a copy of the report to the relevant authorities and, as a consequence, the patient's application for release was refused. The patient's subsequent civil claim for compensation was rejected by the courts *(27)*, which held that the psychiatrist was entitled, under the circumstances, to put his duty to the public above the patient's right to confidentiality.

3.3.4. Medical Teaching, Research, and Audit

In general data should be made anonymous. Every reasonable effort must be made to inform the patients concerned and to obtain their permission to disclose or publish case histories, photographs, and other information. Where consent cannot be obtained, the matter should be referred to a research ethics committee for guidance. The GMC and similar bodies give guidance *(8,23)* and reputable medical journals have strict codes of practice, requiring that appropriate consent be obtained before even anonymous data are published, but the topic is not discussed here.

3.3.5. Judicial and Statutory Exceptions

Statutory provisions may require a doctor to disclose information about patients. In the United Kingdom they include, for example, notifications of births, miscarriages, and deaths, notifications of infectious diseases, notifications of industrial diseases and poisonings, and notifications under the provisions of the Abortion Act 1967.

A doctor may be required to attend court and to answer questions if ordered to do so by the presiding judge, magistrate, or sheriff. When in the witness box the doctor may explain that he or she does not have the consent of the patient to disclose the information (or indeed that the patient has expressly forbidden the doctor to disclose it) but the court may rule that the interests of justice require that the information held by the doctor about the patient be disclosed to the court. The doctor must then answer or risk being charged with contempt of court.

However, disclosure should only be made in judicial proceedings in one of two situations; first, when the presiding judge directs the doctor to answer, or second, when the patient has given free and informed consent. A request by any other person (whether police officer, court official, or lawyer) should be politely but firmly declined. As always, the doctor's protection or defense organization will be pleased to advise in any case of doubt.

Other statutory provisions of forensic relevance exist, but they are peculiar to individual countries or states and are not included here.

4. Notekeeping

All doctors should keep objective, factual records of their consultations with patients and of other professional work. Not only is this desirable *per se*, it is now also a professional requirement. Current GMC guidance *(23)* states that in providing care doctors must keep clear, accurate, and contemporaneous patient records that record the relevant findings, the decisions made, the information given to the patient, and any drugs or other treatment provided.

Good notes assist in the care of the patient, especially when doctors work in teams or partnership and share the care of patients with colleagues. Notes then help to keep colleagues well informed. Good notes are invaluable for forensic purposes, when the doctor faces a complaint, a claim for compensation, or an allegation of serious professional misconduct or poor performance. The medical protection and defense organizations have long explained that an absence of notes may render indefensible that which might otherwise have been defensible. The existence of good notes is often the key factor in preparing and mounting a successful defense to allegations against a doctor or the institution in which he or she works.

Notes should record facts objectively and dispassionately; they must be devoid of pejorative comment, wit, invective, or defamatory comments. Patients and their advisers now have increasing rights of access to their records and rights to request corrections of inaccurate or inappropriate information.

5. Access to Health Records

Access to medical and other health records, which is provided for by statute law, varies considerably from one jurisdiction to another. In English law patients have enjoyed some rights of access to their medical records since the passage of the Administration of Justice Act 1970. Those provisions are now contained in sections 33 and 34 of the Supreme Court Act 1981 and allow for access to medical records in cases of anticipated civil proceedings for personal injury or death. Since then, however, a number of other statutory provisions have made further provision for access to medical records. These include the Data Protection Act 1984, the Access to Medical Reports Act 1988, the Access to Health Records Act 1990, the Data Protection Act 1998, and the Human Rights Act 1998. Space here does not permit consideration of the detailed statutory provisions and readers are respectfully referred to local legal provisions in their country of practice. A more detailed review of the rules applicable in the United Kingdom is set out in Appendix 2.

6. Preparation of Reports

Doctors are frequently asked to prepare reports for medicolegal reasons. It is very important to understand the nature of the request and what is required—a simple report of fact, a report on present condition and prognosis following a medical examination, an expert opinion, or a combination of these. The fact that a doctor possesses expertise does not necessarily make him or her an expert witness every time a report is requested.

A report may be required for a variety of reasons, and its nature and content must be directed to the purpose for which it is sought. Is it a report of the history and findings on examination some time previously because there is now a criminal prosecution or civil claim? Is an expert opinion being requested based on the clinical notes made by others? Is it a request to examine the patient and to prepare a report on present condition and prognosis? Is it a request for an expert opinion on the management of another practitioner for the purposes of a medical negligence claim?

The request should be studied carefully to ascertain what is required and clarification sought where necessary in the case of any ambiguity. The fee to be paid or at least the basis on which it is to be set should also be agreed in advance of the preparation of the report. If necessary, the appropriate consents should be obtained and issues of confidentiality addressed.

Care must be taken in the preparation of any report. A medicolegal report may affect the liberty of an individual in a criminal case or compensation in a personal injury or negligence action. A condemnatory report about a professional colleague may cause great distress and a loss of reputation; it may even be relied upon by the prosecuting authorities to decide whether to bring homicide charges, for murder ("euthanasia") or manslaughter (by gross negligence). Reports must be fair and balanced; the doctor is not an advocate for a cause but should see his or her role as providing assistance to the lawyers and to the court in their attempt to do justice to the parties. It must always be borne in mind that a report may be disclosed in the course of legal proceedings and that the author may be crossexamined about its content.

A negligently prepared report may lead to proceedings against the author, and perhaps even criminal proceedings in exceptional cases. Certainly a civil claim can be sought if a plaintiff's action is settled on disadvantageous terms as a result of a poorly prepared opinion. There is also the attendant risk of adverse judicial comment and press publicity.

The form and content of the report will vary according to circumstances, but it should always be well presented on professional notepaper with relevant dates and details carefully documented in objective terms. Care should be taken to address the questions posed in the letter of instructions from those who commissioned it. If necessary, the report may be submitted in draft before it is finalized but the doctor must always ensure that the final text represents his or her own professional views and must avoid being persuaded by counsel or solicitors to make amendments with which he or she is not content: it is the doctor who will have to answer questions in the witness box and this may be a most harrowing experience if he or she makes claims outside the area of expertise or in any way fails to "come up to proof" (i.e., departs from the original statement).

7. Attendance at Court

Courts are, broadly, of two types—criminal and civil. Additionally, the doctor will encounter the Coroners Courts (or the Procurators Fiscal and Sheriffs in Scotland), which is, exceptionally, inquisitorial and not adversarial in its proceedings. A wide range of other special courts and tribunals exists, from ecclesiastical courts to social security tribunals; these will not be described here.

A doctor may be called to any court to give evidence. The type of court to which he or she is called is likely to depend on the doctor's practice, specialty, and seniority. The doctor may be called to give purely factual evidence of the findings when he or she examined a patient (in which case the doctor is simply a professional witness of fact) or to give an opinion on some matter (in which case the doctor is an expert witness). Sometimes a doctor will be called to give both factual and expert evidence.

Usually the doctor will receive fair warning that attendance in court is required and he or she may be able to negotiate with those calling him or her over suitable dates and times. Many requests to attend court will be made relatively informally, but more commonly a witness summons will be served. A doctor who shows any marked reluctance to attend court may well receive a formal *subpoena ad testificandum*, which compels him or her to attend or to face arrest and proceedings for contempt of court if he or she refuses.

If the doctor adopts a reasonable and responsible attitude he or she will usually receive the sympathetic understanding and co-operation of the lawyers and the court in arranging a time to give evidence that least disrupts his or her practice. However, any exhibition of belligerence by the doctor can induce a rigid inflexibility in lawyers and court officials—who always have the ability to "trump" the doctor by the issuance of a subpoena. So, be warned and be reasonable!

Evidence in court is given on oath or affirmation. A doctor will usually be allowed to refer to any notes made contemporaneously in order to "refresh his memory", although it is courteous to seek the court's agreement.

7.1. Demeanor in Court

In the space available it is not possible to do more than to outline good practice when giving evidence. Court appearances are serious matters; an individual's liberty may be at risk or large awards of damages and costs may turn upon the evidence given. The doctor's dress and demeanor should be appropriate to the occasion and he or she should speak clearly and audibly.

As with an oral examination for medical finals, or the defense of a written thesis, listen carefully to the questions posed. Think carefully about the reply before opening your mouth and allowing words to pour forth. Answer the question asked (not the one you would like it to have been) concisely and carefully and then wait for the next question. There is no need to fill all silences with words; the judge and others will be making notes and it is as well to keep an eye on the judge's pen and adjust the speed of your words accordingly. Pauses between questions allow the judge to finish writing or counsel to think up his or her next question. If anything you have said is unclear or more is wanted from you, be assured that you will be asked more questions.

Be calm and patient and never show a loss of temper or control, however provoking counsel may be. An angry or flustered witness is a gift to any competent and experienced counsel, as is a garrulous or evasive witness.

Try to use simple language devoid of jargon, abbreviations, and acronyms. Stay well within your area of skill and expertise and do not be slow to admit that you do not know the answer. Your frankness will be appreciated, whereas an attempt to bluff or obfuscate or overreach yourself will almost certainly be detrimental to your position.

Doctors usually seek consensus and try to avoid confrontation (at least in a clinical setting). They should remember that lawyers thrive on the adversarial process and are out to win their case, not to engage upon a search for truth. Thus lawyers will wish to extract from witnesses answers that best support the case of the party by whom they are retained. The medical witness, however, is not in court to "take sides" but rather to assist the court, to the best of the expert witness' ability, to do justice in the case. The witness should therefore adhere to his or her evidence where it is right to do so but must be prepared to be flexible and to make concessions if appropriate—for example, because further evidence has emerged since the original statement was prepared, making it appropriate to cede points. The doctor should also recall the terms of the oath or affirmation—to tell the truth, whole truth and nothing but—and give evidence accordingly.

8. *The Duties of Expert Witnesses*

Some medical practitioners have made a career from giving expert opinions, and a few have brought the profession into disrepute by being demonstrably partisan or by giving opinion evidence that is scientifically unsupportable. The courts have now laid down guidance *(28)* for expert witnesses and the UK Expert Witness Institute has prepared a code of practice *(29)* for experts.

The essential requirements for experts are these:

- Expert evidence presented to the court should be and should be seen to be the independent product of the expert, uninfluenced regarding form or content by the exigencies of litigation *(30)*.
- Independent assistance should be provided to the court by way of objective unbiased opinion regarding matters within the expertise of the expert witness *(31)*. An expert witness in the court should never assume the role of advocate.
- Facts or assumptions upon which the opinion was based should be stated together with material facts that could detract from the concluded opinion.
- An expert witness should make clear when a question or issue falls outside his or her expertise.
- If the opinion was not properly researched because it was considered that insufficient data were available, that should be stated with an indication that the opinion is provisional. If the expert cannot assert that the report contains the truth, the whole truth, and nothing but the truth, that qualification should be stated on the report *(32)*.
- If, after an exchange of reports, an expert witness changes an opinion the change of view/opinion should be communicated to the other parties through legal representatives without delay and, when appropriate, to the court.

The Expert Witness Institute *(33)* has also produced an expert's declaration for use by experts that follows the form recommended by Lord Woolf MR in his review of civil justice procedures and that incorporates the legal principles set out above.

In England and Wales, new Civil Procedure Rules for all courts came into force on April 16, 1999 *(34)* and Part 35 sets out rules governing experts. The expert has an overriding duty to the court, overriding any obligation to the person who calls or pays him or her. An expert report in a civil case must end with a statement that the expert understands and has complied with the expert's duty to the court. The expert must answer questions of clarification at the request of the other party and now has a right to ask the court for directions to assist him in carrying out the function as an expert. The new rules make radical changes to the previous use of expert opinion in civil actions.

9. Pitfalls

The potential pitfalls of forensic medical practice are many. Most pitfalls may be avoided by an understanding of the legal principles and forensic processes—a topic of postgraduate rather than undergraduate education now. The normal "doctor–patient" relationship does not apply; the FME/detained person relationship requires that the latter understands the role of the former and that the former takes time to explain it to the latter.

Meticulous attention to detail and a careful documentation of facts is required at all times. You will never know when a major trial will turn on a small detail that you once recorded (or, regrettably, failed to record). Your work will have a real and immediate impact on the liberty of the individual and may well be highly influential in assisting the prosecuting authorities to decide whether to charge the detained person with a criminal offense.

You may well be the only person who can retrieve a medical emergency in the cells—picking up a subdural hematoma, diabetic ketoacidosis, or coronary thrombosis that the detaining authority has misinterpreted as drunkenness, indigestion, or simply "obstructive behavior." Get it right and you will assist in the proper administration of the judicial process, with proper regard for human rights and the liberty of the individual. Get it wrong and you may not only fail to prevent an avoidable death but may lay yourself open to criminal, civil, and disciplinary proceedings.

You clearly owe a duty of care to those who engage your services, for that is well-established law. A question arose recently regarding whether an FME owes a wider duty to the victims of alleged crime and the point was decided in the English Court of Appeal during 1999 *(35)*. An FME examined the victim of an alleged offense of rape and buggery. The trial of the man accused of the offenses was fixed and all prosecution witnesses were warned and fully bound, including the FME.

The trial was scheduled to begin on December 7th and on December 6th the FME was warned that she would not be required to attend on the first day of trial but would be needed some time after that. The trial commenced on December 7th and the accused pleaded not guilty. On December 8th, a Friday, the FME was told that she would not be needed that day but would be required the following week. She did not state that this would cause any problem. However, on December 11th the FME left the country for a prearranged vacation. On December 14th the police officer in charge of the case spoke by telephone with the FME. She said she could not return to give evidence before December 19th. The remainder of the prosecution case was finished on December 14th. The trial judge refused to adjourn the case until December 19th. On December 20th the judge accepted a defense submission of no case to answer and directed the jury to return a verdict of not guilty. A few weeks later the FME was convicted of contempt of court for failing to attend court to give evidence, and she was fined.

The female victim commenced civil proceedings against the FME, alleging negligent conduct in failing to attend, as warned, to give evidence. In her claim she asserted that if the FME had given evidence (presumably in accordance with her witness statement) the trial judge would have refused the defense submission of no case to answer. The claimant also contended that, on the balance of probability, the accused would have been convicted since the FME's evidence would have undermined the credibility of the accused's defense that no anal interference had occurred. The claimant claimed that the FME owed her a duty of care to take all reasonable steps to provide evidence of the FME's examination in furtherance of the contemplated prosecution and to attend the trial of the accused as a prosecution witness when required. She claimed to suffer persistent stress and other psychological sequelae from failing to secure the conviction of her alleged assailant and knowing that he is still at large in the vicinity.

The claimant did not contend that there was any general duty of care on the part of a witness actionable in damages at the suit of another witness who may suffer loss and damage through the failure of the first witness to attend and give evidence in accordance with his or her witness statement.

When the case came before the Court of Appeal Lord Justice Stuart-Smith stated that the attempt to formulate a duty of care as pleaded "is wholly misconceived. If a duty of care exists at all, it is a duty to prevent the plaintiff from suffering injury, loss or damage of the type in question, in this case psychiatric injury. A failure to attend to give evidence could be a breach of such duty, but it is not the duty itself." Later, Stuart-Smith LJ stated "it is quite plain in my judgment that the defendant, in carrying out an examination at the behest of the police of Crown Prosecution Service, did not assume any responsibility for the plaintiff's psychiatric welfare; the doctor/patient relationship did not arise." He concluded his judgment "it is of no assistance to the plaintiff here in trying to construct a duty of care to attend court to give evidence which, as I have already pointed out, could amount to breach of a wider duty which is not alleged and could not be supported." The other two Lords Justice of Appeal agreed.

The plaintiff's claim against the FME for damages was dismissed and it was confirmed that there was no duty of care owed by the FME to the victim to attend the trial as a prosecution witness when required.

References

1. *St George's Healthcare NHS Trust v S* 3WLR 936, 950E (1998) per Judge LJ.
2. *Airedale NHS Trust v Bland* AC789, 857 (1993) per Lord Keith of Kinkel.
3. Ibid. per Lord Goff of Chieveley, 864.
4. Ibid. per Lord Browne-Wilkinson, 882.
5. Ibid. per Lord Mustill, 891.
6. *S. v McC* and M; *W v W* AC 24 (1972) per Lord Reid, 43.
7. St George's Healthcare NHS Trust case [ibid.], 951G.
8. General Medical Council (1998) *Seeking Patients' Consent: the Ethical Considerations*.The General Medical Council, London.
9. St George's Healthcare NHS Trust case [ibid], 969C.
10. In re C 1WLR 290 (1994).
11. *Sidaway v Board of Governors of the Bethlem Royal and Maudsley Hospitals* AC 871(1985); 1 AllER 643 (1985).
12. *Rogers v Whitaker* 175 CLR 479 (1992); AMLD 6993 (1992); 16 BMLR, 148 (Australian High Court).
13. *Canterbury v Spence* 464 F2d 772 (US App DC, 1972).
14. *Reibl v Hughes* 114 DLR 3d 1 (Canadian Supreme Court 1980); 2 SCR 880 (1980).
15. *Bolitho v City & Hackney Health Authority* AC 232 (1998); 1Lloyd's Rep. Med. 26 (1998).
16. In re F [1990] 2.AC 1.
17. *Bolam v Friern Hospital Management Committee* 2 AllER 118 (1957); 1 WLR 582 (1957).
18. *Gillick v West Norfolk & Wisbech Area Health Authority* AC 112 (1984).
19. General Medical Council (1997) *Making and Using Visual and Audio Recordings of Patients*. General Medical Council, London.
20. Extract from the Hippocratic Oath, 5th century BC.
21. Extract from The Declaration of Geneva; World Medical Association, 1948, re-stated 1983.
22. Extract from The International Code of Medical Ethics, World Medical Association, Geneva, 1983.
23. General Medical Council (1998) *Good Medical Practice*. General Medical Council, London.
24. General Medical Council (1995) *Confidentiality*. General Medical Council, London.
25. Association of Police Surgeons and British Medical Association (1998) *Revised Interim Guidelines on Confidentiality for Police Surgeons in England, Wales and Northern Ireland*. Association of Police Surgeons, Harrogate. British Medical Association, London.

26. *Tarasoff v Regents of the University of California* P 551 2d 334 (Cal. Sup. Ct. 1976).
27. *W v Egdell* Ch. 359 (1990); 1 All ER 835 (1990).
28. *National Justice Compania Naviera SA v Prudential Assurance Co. Ltd.* ('The Ikarian Reefer'); (*The Times*, March 5, 1993); 2 Lloyd's Rep. 68 (High Court 1993); 1 Lloyd's Rep. 455 (CA 1995).
29. Expert Witness Institute. (1998) Newsletter. EWI, London.
30. *Whitehouse v Jordan* 1WLR 246, 256 (1981) per Lord Wilberforce.
31. *Polivitte Ltd v Commercial Union Assurance Co. plc* 1 Lloyd's Rep. 379, 386 (1987) per Garland J.
32. *Derby & Co. Ltd. and Others v Weldon and Others* (No. 9) *The Times,* November 9, 1990 per Staughton LJ.
33. Expert Witness Institute; Newspaper House, 8-16 Great New Street, London EC4A 3BN. Tel: +44 171 583 5454.
34. Civil Procedure Rules (1999) London: The Stationery Office; and on the Lord Chancellor's Department website: www.open.gov.uk/lcd.
35. *Nunes v Agrawal* (1999) Court of Appeal case number CCRTI 98/1516; (1999) MLC 0100.

Chapter 3

Sexual Assault Examination

Deborah Rogers and Mary Newton

1. Introduction

Sexual assaults create significant health and legislative problems for every society. All health professionals who have the potential to encounter victims of sexual assaults should have some understanding of the acute and chronic health problems that may ensue from an assault(s). However, the primary clinical forensic assessment of complainants and suspects of sexual assault should only be conducted by doctors and nurses who have acquired specialist knowledge, skills, and attitudes during theoretical and practical training.

There are many types of sexual assault, only some of which will involve penetration of a body cavity. Although it may be tempting to follow dogmatically a standardized proforma for these assessments, this has the potential to prolong unduly the medical examination by subjecting the patient to unnecessary, often invasive, examinations. This chapter endeavours to encourage the practitioner to adapt the medical examination to the specific allegation by dividing the text into sections covering the relevant body areas.

The chapter commences by addressing the basic principles of the medical examination for both complainants and suspects of sexual assault. Although the first concern of the forensic practitioner is always the medical care of the patient, thereafter the retrieval and preservation of forensic evidence is paramount as this material may be critical for the elimination of a suspect, identification of the assailant, and the prosecution of the case. Thus it is imperative that all forensic practitioners understand the basic principles of the forensic analysis.

From: *Forensic Science: A Physician's Guide to Clinical Forensic Medicine*
Edited by: M. M. Stark © Humana Press, Inc., Totowa, NJ

Each body cavity section commences with information regarding the range and frequency of normal sexual practices and the relevant anatomy, development, and physiology. This specialist knowledge is mandatory for the reliable documentation and interpretation of any medical findings. The practical aspects (which samples to obtain, how to obtain them, and the clinical details required by the forensic scientist) are then addressed, as this takes priority over the clinical forensic assessment.

The medical findings in cases of sexual assault should always be addressed in the context of the injuries and other medical problems associated with consensual sexual practices. Therefore each section summarizes the information that is available in the literature with regard to the noninfectious medical complications of consensual sexual practices and possible nonsexual explanations for the findings. The type, site, and frequency of the injuries described in association with sexual assaults that relate to each body area are then discussed. Unfortunately, space has not allowed for a critical appraisal of all the chronic medical findings purported to be associated with child sexual abuse, and the reader should refer to more substantive texts and review papers for this information *(1–3)*.

Throughout all the stages of the clinical forensic assessment the forensic practitioner must avoid partisanship while remaining sensitive to the immense psychological and physical trauma that a complainant may have incurred. The continuing care of the complainant, although presented at the end of the chapter, is essentially an ongoing process throughout and beyond the primary clinical forensic assessment.

2. Basic Principles of the Medical Examination

2.1. Immediate Care

The first health care professional to encounter the patient must give urgent attention to any immediate medical needs that are apparent, e.g., substance overdose, head injury, serious wounds. This care takes precedence over any forensic concerns. Nonetheless, it may be possible to task a health care worker with the retention of any clothing or sanitary wear that is removed from a complainant until this can be handed to someone with specialist knowledge of forensic packaging.

2.2. Timing of the Examination

Although in general terms the clinical forensic assessment should take place as soon as possible, reference to the persistence data given under the relevant sections will help the forensic practitioner determine whether the examination of a complainant should be conducted out of office hours or could be deferred until the next day. Even when the nature of the assault suggests there is unlikely to be any forensic evidence, the timing of the examination should be influenced by the speed with which clinical signs such as reddening will fade.

2.3. *Place of the Examination*

Specially designed facilities used exclusively for the examination of complainants of sexual offenses are available in many countries. The complainant may wish to have a friend or relative present for whole or part of the examination and this should be accommodated. Suspects are usually examined in the medical room of the police station and may wish to have a legal representative present. During the examinations of both complainants and suspects the local guidance regarding the conduct of intimate examinations should be followed *(4)*.

2.4. *Consent*

Informed consent must be sought for each stage of the clinical forensic assessment including the use of any specialist techniques or equipment (e.g., colposcope) and the obtaining of the relevant forensic samples. When obtaining this consent the patient and/or parent should be advised that the practitioner is unable to guarantee confidentiality of the material gleaned during the medical as a judge (or other presiding officer of a court) can rule that the practitioner should breach medical confidentiality. If photo-documentation is to form part of the medical examination the patient should be advised in advance of the means of storage and its potential uses (*see* below); specific written consent should then be sought for this procedure. The patient must be advised that they can stop the examination at any time.

2.5. *Details of the Allegation*

If the complainant has already provided the details of the allegation to another professional, e.g., police officer, it is not necessary for them to repeat the details to the forensic practitioner. Indeed, Hicks *(5)* notes that attempts to obtain too detailed a history of the incident from the complainant may jeopardize the case at trial because at the time of the medical examination the patient may be disturbed and, consequently, the details of the incident might be confused and conflict with subsequent statements. The details of the allegation can be provided to the forensic practitioner by the third party and then clarified, if necessary, with the complainant. It may be difficult for the complainant to describe oral and anal penetrative sexual assaults, and the forensic practitioner may need to ask direct questions sensitively regarding these acts *(6)*.

2.6. Medical and Sexual History

The purpose of obtaining the medical and sexual history is essentially twofold: first, to identify any behavior or medical conditions that might cause the doctor to misinterpret the clinical findings, e.g., menstrual bleeding, and second, to identify any medical problems that may be attributable to the sexual assault, e.g., bleeding, pain, discharge. Other specific details may be required if postcoital contraception is being considered.

When children are examined, comprehensive details of the past medical history should be provided by the parent or caregiver. When adults are examined, only relevant medical and sexual history should be sought since confidentiality cannot be guaranteed. What constitutes relevant medical history will need to be determined on a case by case basis by taking into account the differential causes for any medical findings and the persistence data for the different sexual acts (*see* below). Suspects should be reminded of their legal rights before they are questioned regarding relevant medical or sexual history.

2.7. Nature of the Examination

2.7.1. General Examination

In all cases a complete general medical examination should be conducted to document injuries and to note any disease that may affect the interpretation of the medical findings.

2.7.2. Anogenital Examination

The anogenital examination should be tailored to the individual case, e.g., if the complainant only describes being made to perform fellatio there is no indication to examine the external genitalia.

2.8. Ownership and Handling of Photo-Documentation

Any video/photographic material should be retained as part of the practitioner's confidential medical notes and stored in a locked cabinet in locked premises. To preserve anonymity the material should be labeled both on the casing and within the video/photograph itself (by holding a card within the frame) using either a unique identification code or the patient's initials and the date of the examination. With the specific consent of the patient, the video/photograph can be shown to other colleagues for second opinions, viewed by a named doctor providing expert testimony for the defense, and used for teaching purposes. The material should not be released to nonmedical parties except on the directions of the court.

3. Basic Principles of the Forensic Analysis

The scientific examination at the forensic laboratory can provide information regarding:

- which sexual acts have taken place
- the gender and possible identification of the assailant
- potential links with any other offenses

3.1. Collection of Forensic Samples

To ensure that there is no accidental transfer of body fluids or fibers between the parties who have been involved in a sexual act, each complainant and each suspect should be transported in separate vehicles and examined in different locations by different forensic practitioners.

The swabs and containers used to collect forensic evidence differ from those used in clinical tests. The swabs should be made of fibers that readily release absorbed material *(7)*. The quality and integrity of any swab or container used to obtain a forensic sample must be ensured. The provision of sealed, standardized clinical forensic examination kits or modules ensures that these requirements can be guaranteed *(8,9)*.

Forensic swabs should be placed in plastic sheaths that do not contain transport media. Blood and urine samples for drugs and alcohol analysis should be placed in containers with a preservative that prevents decomposition and fermentation of the sample (e.g. sodium fluoride), and the container for the blood sample should also contain an anticoagulant (e.g., potassium oxalate). The blood sample for DNA analysis and/or conventional grouping should be placed in a container with the appropriate preservative [e.g., ethylene diamine tetraacetic acid (EDTA)]. As many of the samples are subsequently frozen, all the containers should be shatterproof.

Only sealed, disposable instruments (e.g., proctoscopes, specula, scissors, forceps) should be used to retrieve forensic samples. Visible, dry stains on the skin should be retrieved using a swab dampened with fresh sterile water. A further swab should be dampened with water from the same ampoule and rubbed over an area of skin adjacent to the stain to act as a control sample for the skin. If any water remains in the ampoule it should be sealed and submitted to the laboratory as a control sample for the water. Sterile water may also be used to moisten the proctoscope/speculum to facilitate its insertion into a body orifice. Other lubricants should not be used when body fluid analysis or lubricant identification may be pertinent to the case (*see* Lubricants later).

3.2. Packaging and Continuity

Any retrieved items must be packaged quickly and efficiently to prevent accidental loss of material and minimize decomposition of the sample. The use of bags with integral tamper-evident seals is to be encouraged as proof that the sample has not been contaminated with exogenous substances since it was sealed. The exhibit should be labeled with the site of the sample, the date and time (24-hour clock) it was obtained, and the name of the examinee. Again, the use of bags with integral labels will prevent accidental detachment of this vital information (Fig. 1). Each exhibit is also labeled with an exhibit identification code, usually formed by the forensic practitioner's initials, and a number reflecting the order in which the samples were obtained. The latter is particularly important when more than one sample has been obtained from the same site *(7)*. Every exhibit should be signed by the person who first handled the sample and by the person who sealed the package (this may be the same person). It is good practice for everyone who subsequently handles the exhibit to sign the label also so that if necessary they can be called to court to explain their part in collection, transport, and storage *(10)*.

The clothing worn by the complainant during or subsequent to the incident may be an invaluable source of information in terms of the nature of the assault (e.g., damage to clothing and body fluid stains) and the identification of the assailant. Even stains on clothing that has been washed have been found to contain sufficient spermatozoa to produce a DNA profile (*see* later) *(11)*. Clothing should be placed in bags made of material (such as paper) that prevents the accumulation of condensation, which could accelerate decomposition of body fluids. Submitted clothing should be sealed and labeled as described above. When the clothing is overtly wet the forensic science laboratory should be asked for advice on packaging and storage. The following additional information should then be recorded on the appropriate label:

- which items were worn during the offense
- which items were removed and not replaced
- which items were removed and replaced
- which new items were worn after the offense

The forensic scientist must be provided with salient information regarding the incident and subsequent actions of the complainant in order to determine the order and type of forensic analysis required. A useful means of transmitting this information is via a proforma (Fig. 2).

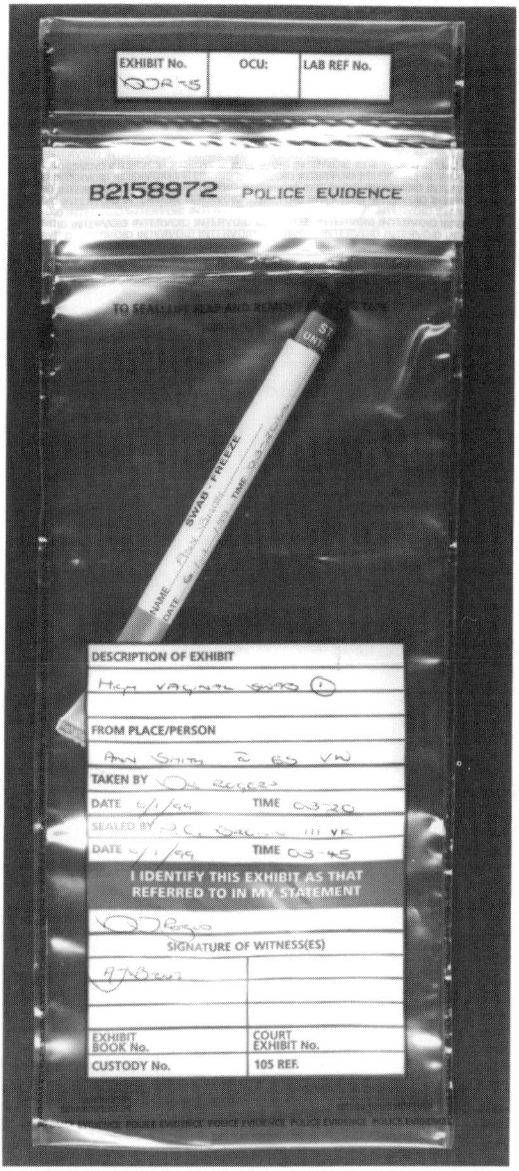

Fig. 1. Exhibit bag with integral label and tamper-evident seal.

All sections of this form must be completed and a copy forwarded to the Laboratory
Please print in capitals using biro and tick the appropriate boxes

INFORMATION FORM

For submission with Sexual Offences samples (1 Per Person)

GENERAL INFORMATION — Your Case Reference:

Name of Medical Examiner (BLOCK).
Contact Number.

Name of Subject. | (Tick the appropriate boxes)
| Age. Sex. [M] [F] [Suspect] [Complainant]

Date & Time of incident. | Date & Time of examination.
(Please use 24 hour clock)
Date & Time of other relevant intercourse within previous 10 days.

Items used in previous Intercourse. [Sheath] [Spermicide] [Lubricant] [Other (Specify)]

SPECIFIC INFORMATION RELATING TO THE ALLEGED OFFENCE

Penile/Oral penetration	No	Yes	
Penile/Vaginal penetration	No	Yes	
Penile/Anal penetration	No	Yes	
Object penetration	No	Yes	(Specify)
Ejaculation onto Skin/Hair	No	Yes	(Site)
Kissed /Licked /Bitten (circle relevant action)	No	Yes	(Site)
Condom / Lubricant /Spermicide used?	No	Yes	(Specify)
Menstrual bleeding	No	Yes	
Bleeding due to genital/anal injury	No	Yes	(Specify)
Other relevant injuries	No	Yes	(Specify)
Shower/washed/bathed/douched	No	Yes	(Specify)
Genital/Anal/relevant skin area wiped	No	Yes	(How)
Anal Intercourse: defaecated since offence	No	Yes	
Oral Intercourse: mouth cleansed since offence	No	Yes	

(Tick the appropriate box) [Drink] [Mouth wash] [Toothbrush]

TOXICOLOGY INFORMATION

Was alcohol consumed? [No] [Yes]
[prior] [during] [after] offence

Start time of drinking — End time of drinking
Quantity of alcohol consumed (Specify)

Are medicinal drugs (prescribed or otherwise) relevant ? [No] [Yes]
If Yes please specify
Have other substances used by subject within 96 hours of examination ? [No] [Yes]
If Yes please specify
Are other drugs suspected as being relevant to the offence? [No] [Yes]
If Yes please specify

ANY OTHER INFORMATION (Continue on a separate sheet if necessary)
Damp patches on clothing should be noted as their position could be important if they are subsequently found to be semen

Signature of Medical Examiner | Date

Fig. 2. Proforma used to relay relevant information to forensic scientist. (Reproduced with permission of the members of the Joint Working Party (A.C.P.O., A.P.S., F.S.S., and M.P.S.) for the design of an examination kit for sexual offences.)

3.3. Analysis

Identification microscopy (e.g., spermatozoa), comparison microscopy (e.g., hairs, fibers), serological analyses (e.g., conventional ABO grouping, species identification), and biochemical analyses (e.g., phosphoglucomutase) have played a fundamental role in the investigation of crime for many years and are still utilized today in some circumstances (*see* relevant sections). However, discovery of the specificity of an individual's DNA profile has considerably enhanced the information that can be provided by a forensic science service in terms of connecting a person to an offense and linking offenses to each other. Although a detailed consideration of DNA analysis is beyond the scope of this chapter, a general understanding of the terms and techniques will benefit the forensic practitioner.

Except for identical twins, each person's nuclear DNA is unique. An individual's gender and DNA profile may be obtained from any of their body fluids or tissues, e.g., blood, semen, and bones. The current technical process employed for DNA profiling is termed short tandem repeat (STR) analysis. STR loci are a class of polymorphic markers consisting of simple repeated sequences of 1–6 base pairs in length. STRs are present throughout the human genome (DNA), occurring, on average, every 6–10 kb along the DNA and may exhibit a high degree of length variation due to differences in the number of repeat units displayed by individuals. Their abundance and hypervariability make them ideal markers for the identification of an individual. When a DNA STR analysis is performed, the specific areas of interest on the molecule are initially targeted. Multiple copies of these areas are then produced using polymerase chain reaction (PCR) techniques, which amplify minute amounts of DNA. The pieces of DNA are then sorted according to their size, producing the individual's DNA STR profile *(12)*.

DNA STR analysis, incorporating a DNA sex test *(12a)*, is now part of the routine forensic assessment of biologic samples in Europe and is replacing both traditional serologic analysis of blood groups and classical multilocus and single locus DNA fingerprinting *(12)*. The formation of the European DNA Profiling Group has led to standardization of DNA analysis procedures used in the European community and associated Western European countries. The current standard technique is the second-generation multiplex (SGM), which analyzes six STR areas on the DNA molecule and has proved to be an invaluable tool for scientifically linking offenses. However, the forensic science laboratory must be notified when it is alleged that people who are closely related have been involved in a sexual offense as their profiles will have greater similarity than profiles from individuals picked at random, and further differentiating tests may need to be performed.

As DNA is physically much more resistant to degradation than proteins it is even possible to analyze degraded samples *(13)*. When DNA profiling was first applied to forensic science, relatively large amounts of nucleated material were required. However, the use of PCR technology has enabled much smaller amounts of material to be analyzed.

Recently, analysis of mitochondrial DNA has been used in forensic casework. This new technique examines the DNA contained within mitochondria and obviates the need for nuclear material. Since mitochondrial DNA is only passed from mother to child (unlike nuclear DNA there is no contribution from the father), all the descendants along the maternal line will have the same mitochondrial DNA. At present, the technique is best suited to discrete samples, such as hairs without roots and fecal material, and is not ideal for mixtures of body fluids, particularly when the complainant's body fluid is likely to be present in larger quantities than that of the assailant *(14)*. Therefore, in sexual offenses the selection of material to be analyzed by this technique needs to be carefully considered.

4. Skin

The comments in this section refer to nongenital skin. For genital and perianal skin, *see* the relevant sections.

4.1. Forensic Evidence

4.1.1. Method of Sampling

All areas of unwashed skin that have been licked, kissed, sucked, bitten, or ejaculated on, by either assailant or complainant, must be sampled. Although several techniques, including the use of surgical gauze pads *(15)* and cigarette papers *(16)* have been employed to recover saliva and other trace evidence from the skin with variable success, the use of sterile swabs, moistened if necessary with sterile water, is the most widely used technique, which has received international endorsement *(17)*.

Some authors comment that ultra violet (UV) light causes fluorescence of semen and saliva *(18–20)* and advocate its use in determining the areas of skin to be swabbed. However, so many commonly encountered substances, (e.g., detergents, lubricants—particularly those that contain petroleum jelly and milk) also fluoresce that most forensic science laboratories now consider the use of UV light obsolete *(21)*. Certainly, no conclusion should be reached with regard to the nature of a fluorescent stain without laboratory analysis.

4.1.2. Forensic Analysis

The commonest reason for forensic analysis of skin swabs is following licking, kissing, or biting of the skin. Forensic analysis for other body fluids or exogenous substances is considered elsewhere in the chapter.

4.1.2.1. Detection of Saliva

The only means of confirming the presence of saliva on the skin is by detecting the enzyme amylase. However, in practice this enzyme is not usually found in high enough concentrations in samples removed from the skin *(22)*.

4.1.2.2. Identification of the Assailant

It may be possible to determine the ABO-secretor status of the sample submitted. However, this test is only relevant if the saliva originates from one of the 80% of the population who secrete their ABO blood group in their body fluids. The preferred method for the forensic assessment of a possible saliva sample is the use of DNA STR analysis.

4.1.3. Persistence Data

No data are available regarding the persistence of body fluids and, in particular, the time that DNA analysis is successful on unwashed skin. Inevitably, the amount of recoverable material will diminish with time, and it is prudent to sample the relevant body areas as soon as possible after the offense.

4.2. Medical Evidence

On average 60% of complainants of sexual assaults will have no general injuries *(23–25)*. Of those who are injured, most will have only minor injuries, which will fade rapidly or heal without trace *(23,24)*. Nonetheless, the whole body must be thoroughly inspected for stains (e.g., dirt, blood), injuries (including signs of substance use), skin disease, and scars (including self-inflicted injuries). All injuries must be described using the recognized nomenclature described in Chapter 4 and recorded in terms of site (measured if possible from a fixed bony point), two-dimensional size, covering surface (e.g., scabbing, bleeding, swelling), and color. The body surfaces should then be palpated and a note made of the site and approximate size of any tender areas. More credence will be given to a finding of tenderness if it is verified later in the consultation (ideally while the patient is distracted) or at a follow-up assessment, particularly if a bruise becomes apparent. All negative observations should also be recorded.

If the person can identify an injury that they believe was caused by a true bite (as opposed to a suction or “love-bite”) or if the examination reveals an injury that has features suggesting it was caused by biting *(26)*, arrangements must be made for the area to be professionally photographed so that the injury can be considered by a forensic odontologist. Several studies have reported that the female breasts are bitten in 7–19% of sexual offenses *(27,28)*.

5. Hair: Head and Pubic

5.1. Forensic Evidence

Hair is most commonly sampled to detect body fluids or retrieve foreign hairs or particles. In addition, it may be utilized as a reference sample for DNA analysis.

5.1.1. Method of Sampling

5.1.1.1. Cutting

Hairs should be sampled by cutting if they appear to be contaminated by material that has the potential to have forensic significance (e.g., semen). If the patient does not consent to having the contaminated hairs cut, or if it is not practical to cut them due to the extent of foreign material contamination, then the relevant areas can be swabbed (follow method of sampling given in the Skin section). Whenever the hair is sampled in these circumstances, some hairs that appear to be uncontaminated should also be cut or swabbed and submitted as a control sample.

5.1.1.2. Combing

Any foreign particles or hairs identified on the head or pubic hair should be collected with forceps and submitted for analysis. It is no longer considered necessary to comb the head hair routinely as these samples are infrequently examined by forensic scientists *(29)* or are rarely pivotal to the case *(30,31)*. However, if a balaclava or other article was worn on the head during the assault, the hair should be combed with a primed comb and any debris or fibers collected onto an A4 size piece of paper, which can be folded and submitted with the comb *(32,33)*; cut control hairs should also be collected.

Pubic hairs may be transferred between individuals during sexual intercourse. Exline et al. *(34)* studied volunteer heterosexual couples who combed their pubic hairs immediately following sexual intercourse in the "missionary" position; even under such optimum collection conditions, pubic hair transfers were only observed 17.3% of the time using macroscopic and microscopic comparisons. Pubic hair transfer to males (23.6%) was more common than transfer to females (10.9%).

Some studies on sexual offense case material have shown lower rates of pubic hair transfer between complainant and assailant. Mann *(35)* reported that only 4% of female complainants and no male complainants were identified as having pubic hairs consistent with the assailant isolated from combings of their pubic hair, and Stone *(36)* identified foreign pubic hairs among the pubic hair combings of 2% of the complainants studied. However, a survey of sexual offense case material submitted to laboratories throughout the United States *(37)* found pubic hairs that associated the complainant and the assailant in 15% of cases. Therefore, we advocate that the complainant's/suspect's pubic hairs should routinely be combed onto a piece of uncontaminated paper (A4 size) with the complainant lying on the side; the paper enclosing the comb should be folded inward and submitted for analysis. Other loose pubic hairs on the complainant that are macroscopically different from their own pubic hairs can be collected with sterile forceps and submitted for forensic analysis.

5.1.1.3. Reference Sample for DNA Analysis

If it is not possible to obtain a blood sample or buccal cells, then one can seek the examinee's consent to obtain 10–25 head hairs with attached roots (plucked individually while wearing gloves) for use as the reference sample. It is never necessary to pluck pubic hair.

5.1.2. Forensic Analysis

5.1.2.1. Chemical Analysis

Chemical analysis may be relevant if the hair has been dyed or contaminated with exogenous substances e.g., lubricant, hairspray.

5.1.2.2. Comparison Microscopy

Although this was the standard method of hair analysis, discrimination of hairs by microscopic means alone yields limited information in terms of assailant identification. Therefore, although retrieved foreign hairs and pubic hair combings should be saved, it is no longer necessary to obtain control samples routinely from the defendant or complainant. In the rare circumstance that it should become necessary to perform comparison microscopy, a control sample can be obtained later.

5.1.2.3. DNA Analysis

Because of the improved sensitivity provided by PCR techniques and the development of mitochondrial DNA analysis, stronger, more objective conclusions in terms of assailant identification can be reached from hairs both with and without roots *(38)*. Buccal cells, obtained by scraping, are used as controls samples for mitochondrial DNA.

5.1.3. Persistence Data

There are no data on how long after the assault foreign pubic hairs have been retrieved from a complainant. Although spermatozoa have been recovered from head hair that was washed *(39)*, there are no detailed data regarding the persistence of spermatozoa on the hair in terms of time since assault.

5.2. Medical Evidence

On occasions head or pubic hairs may have been accidentally or deliberately pulled out during a sexual assault; the identification of bleeding hair follicles and/or broken hairs would support this complaint.

6. Nails

6.1. Forensic Evidence

Unfortunately, there is little information regarding the forensic significance of fingernail samples in terms of the material that has been recovered, the timing of the sample in relation to the offense, and the subsequent success in relating the recovered material to the assailant. However, a number of cases submitted to the Forensic Science Service, London, have produced a DNA match between the complainant and the assailant from the material recovered from the fingernails *(40,41)*. Therefore, fingernail samples should be obtained from the complainant if the circumstances of the offense suggest that blood or skin from the assailant may be present, for example, if the complainant has scratched the assailant, or if the details of the assault are not known and the forensic practitioner, in observing the complainant's hands, notices material of interest under or on the surface of the nails. They should also be considered if a fingernail broke during the offense and the broken section may be retrieved later. Samples should be obtained from the suspect if it is alleged that his hands had direct contact with the female genitalia or if he scratched the complainant.

6.1.1. Method of Sampling

The optimal sample is clippings of the whole fingernail as these are more practical to handle. However, in some cases the fingernails may be too short to cut or the complainant may withhold consent for the sample; complainants who cherish their well-manicured nails may find the proposal distressing, and the examiner must be sensitive to this. In such cases scrapings of the material under the nails should be taken using a tapered stick. Each hand should be sampled and packaged separately enclosing the stick (enveloped in a piece of folded paper) if used.

On the rare occasions when a nail is known to have broken during the incident and the broken fragment of nail is recovered, the residual nail on the relevant finger should be clipped within 24 hours to enable comparison of nail striations *(42)*. If it is not clear which finger the broken nail came from, then it may be necessary to clip and submit all the macroscopically broken nails, as the fingernail striations are individual to a particular finger.

6.1.2. Forensic Analysis

The fingernail samples may be examined microscopically for any visible staining. The nails would then be swabbed to remove any possible body fluids and the material submitted for DNA analysis.

7. Oral Cavity

Although the oral cavity may be injured in a variety of ways during a sexual assault, the specific sexual acts that may result in forensic or medical evidence are fellatio, cunnilingus, and anilingus.

7.1. Fellatio

7.1.1. Definition

Fellatio (also referred to as irrumation) is a sexual activity in which the penis is placed in the mouth; sexual stimulation is achieved by sucking on the penis while it moves in and out of the oral cavity. Ejaculation may or may not take place.

7.1.2. Frequency

7.1.2.1. Consensual

Fellatio is part of the sexual repertoire of heterosexual and male homosexual couples. A study of 1025 women attending a genitourinary clinic found that 55% practiced fellatio occasionally and 15% practiced fellatio often *(43)*.

7.1.2.2. Nonconsensual

Fellatio is a not infrequent component of a sexual assault sometimes occurring in isolation but more frequently in conjunction with other sexual acts *(6)*. Among the 1507 (1403 females, 104 males) sexual assault cases submitted to the Metropolitan Police Laboratory, London, during 1988 and 1989, 17% of the females and 14% of the males described performing fellatio, and 31% of the males had fellatio performed on them during the sexual assault *(44)*.

7.1.3. Legal Implications

The legal definitions of some jurisdictions (South Carolina, Rhode Island), consider nonconsensual fellatio to be analogous to nonconsensual penile/object penetration of the vagina and anus *(45,46)*. The law in England and other jurisdictions considers nonconsensual fellatio to amount to only an indecent assault.

7.1.4. Forensic Evidence

7.1.4.1. Method of Sampling

1. *Following oral-penile contact:* The oral cavity should be sampled when fellatio was performed during the sexual assault or in circumstances in which the details of the incident are unknown. There is no current world-wide consensus as to which is the best sampling method.

Possible techniques include saliva collection (ideally 10 mL), application of swabs, gauze pads *(47)*, or filter paper *(48)*, and oral rinses using 10 mL of distilled water *(49)*. Willott and Crosse *(50)* report that spermatozoa are found more often in the saliva sample compared with mouth swabs but also highlight several cases in which spermatozoa were recovered from swabs taken from specific areas of the oral cavity, e.g., under the tongue, the roof of the mouth, and the lips.

Although no studies have investigated the order in which the samples should be taken, our practice is to obtain 10 mL of saliva as the first sample. Then two swabs in sequence are rubbed over the inner and outer gum margins (with particular attention to the margins around the teeth), over the hard and, where tolerated, soft palate, on the inside of the cheeks and lips, and over both surfaces of the tongue. The mouth is then rinsed with 10 mL of sterile water, which is retained in a bottle as the final sample. The samples can be obtained by the patient themselves under direction of a police officer or other attending professional prior to the arrival of the forensic practitioner, minimizing any delay.

Spermatozoa have also been recovered from dentures and other fixtures that have remained in situ during fellatio. Although the optimum exhibit for the forensic scientist would be the dental fixture itself, understandably, this may not be acceptable to the complainant. A compromise would be to swab the dental fixture. Interestingly, sufficient spermatozoa for a DNA profile have also been recovered using standard extraction techniques from chewing gum that was retained in the mouth during nonconsensual fellatio *(47)*. In this case the gauze pad obtained at the scene of the incident and the oral swabs obtained subsequently during the medical were negative.

2. *DNA reference sample:* If a blood sample is not available, buccal cells can be used for the DNA reference sample from both suspect and complainant. The buccal cells are obtained by firmly rubbing a swab over the inside of the cheek.

3. *Determination of the secretor status:* A sample of saliva is used as the reference sample for the secretor status. This sample is no longer a routine requirement in the United Kingdom.

7.1.4.2. Forensic Analysis

Following actual or possible oral ejaculation the sample is initially examined microscopically to identify spermatozoa (*see* Female genitalia section) followed by DNA analysis.

7.1.4.3. Persistence Data

Rapid retrieval of the forensic samples from the oral cavity is of paramount importance due to the limited period that spermatozoa remain in this orifice. Even though the maximum persistence of spermatozoa in the oral cavity is recorded as 28–31 hours, only a few spermatozoa are detected unless the sample is taken within a few hours of ejaculation *(51)*. Consequently, the forensic exhibits must be collected as soon as an allegation of nonconsensual fellatio is made, and law enforcement agencies should be instructed accordingly.

Although rinsing of the mouth, drinking, and brushing of teeth do not necessarily remove all traces of spermatozoa *(52)*, such activities should be discouraged until the samples have been obtained. Spermatozoa have also been recovered from tooth brushes used by complainants to cleanse the mouth after fellatio *(53)*. The use of interdental tooth brushes may enhance the retrieval of spermatozoa from the interdental spaces, and research in this area is currently taking place in the United Kingdom.

In acts of fellatio it is common for the semen to be spat or vomited on to clothing where it will remain until washed. Therefore, any potentially contaminated clothing should be submitted for forensic examination.

7.1.5. Medical Evidence

Given that a significant proportion of the population perform consensual fellatio, anecdotal accounts from oral surgeons suggest that palatal lesions consequent to such acts are rarely identified during routine casework, although this may be due to the rapid resolution of the injuries. Nevertheless, several case reports have documented palatal lesions following fellatio. Areas of petechial hemorrhage and confluent bruising have been described on the soft palate and at the junction between the hard and soft palates following consensual fellatio *(54–56)*. These areas of bruising vary from discrete single or bilateral lesions of 1.0–1.5 cm in diameter, located on or either side of the midline *(55)* to larger bands of bruising that cross the midline *(54,56)*. The bruises are painless and resolve in 7–10 days *(54,55)*, although they may reappear with repeated fellatio *(55)*.

A forensic practitioner may be asked to explain to the court why these bruises occur. Although the precise mechanism is unknown, the following hypotheses have been proffered:

1. *Repeated contraction of the palatal muscles:* As the penis touches the palatal mucosa, the gag reflex is activated, with resultant contraction of the soft palate and other constrictor muscles of the pharynx. It is suggested that the combination of retching and repeated palatal movements causes rupture of the blood vessels in the highly vascular palatal mucosa *(54)*.
2. *Sucking:* Sucking on the penis produces a negative intraoral pressure, which is postulated to cause rupture of the blood vessels in the palatal mucosa. This theory is supported by the anecdotal accounts of oral surgeons who found petechial hemorrhages on the palates of children who "made a habit of forceful sucking into a drinking glass" *(55)*.
3. *Blunt trauma:* Case reports describe palatal bruises subsequent to sexual assaults wherein a digit or digits have been forced into the mouth *(57)*. However, there is no specific evidence to support the hypothesis that direct blunt trauma from a penis can cause palatal bruising.

Erythema and an erosion of the hard palate have also been described following fellatio *(55,56)* but the reliability of such findings is questionable. Indeed, in one such case the mucositis was eventually diagnosed as oral candidiasis contracted from direct contact with an infected penis *(56)*.

Other nonsexual causes for similar palatal lesions include infectious mononucleosis, local trauma (e.g., hard food stuffs, ill-fitting dentures), paroxysms of vomiting, coughing, or sneezing, playing a wind instrument, tumors, and bleeding diatheses *(58)*. Therefore, whenever palatal bruising, erythema, or erosions are identified during the examination of a complainant who may have been subjected to fellatio, alternative explanations should be excluded by taking a detailed medical, dental, and social history, conducting a comprehensive general examination, and, where necessary, undertaking relevant special investigations.

Whenever a complaint of nonconsensual fellatio is made, the head and face must be carefully examined as there may be other injuries around the oral cavity that support the allegation, such as bruises on the face and neck or lacerations of the frenula *(59)*.

7.2. Cunnilingus and Anilingus

7.2.1. Definitions

Cunnilingus (cunnilinctus) is the sexual activity in which the female genitalia are licked, sucked, or rubbed by the lips and/or tongue.

Anilingus (analingus, "rimming") is the sexual activity in which the anus is licked, sucked, or rubbed by the lips and/or tongue.

7.2.2. Frequency

7.2.2.1. Consensual

Interviews with 18,876 individuals (44% male) aged 16–59 years in the United Kingdom revealed that 66–72% had experienced cunnilingus *(60)*. Although it is not known how many heterosexual and homosexual couples engage in consensual anilingus, 15% of the women questioned in one study acknowledged erotic feelings with anal stimulation, which for the majority included anilingus *(61)*.

7.2.2.2. Nonconsensual

Cunnilingus is alleged to have taken place in only 3–9% of reported sexual assaults *(6,62)*. There are no published reports regarding the number of incidents involving anilingus; anecdotal case material suggests that it is rare.

7.2.3. Legal Implications

Penetration of the vagina or anus with the tongue during nonconsensual cunnilingus or anilingus is considered in some jurisdictions to be legally analogous to nonconsensual penile penetration of the vagina and anus (South Carolina, Rhode Island) *(45,46)*. Other jurisdictions, e.g., England, consider cunnilingus and anilingus to be lesser offenses, which attract correspondingly lower maximum sentences *(63)*.

7.2.4. Forensic Evidence

7.2.4.1. Method of Sampling

See Sections 8. and 9. for more detailed information.

7.2.4.2. Forensic Analysis and Persistence Data

Traditionally, the detection of the enzyme amylase on vulval and vaginal swabs was considered confirmatory evidence of the presence of saliva. However, in 1992 a study conducted at the Metropolitan Police Laboratory, London, using vaginal swabs from volunteer female donors who had not participated in cunnilingus revealed high levels of endogenous amylase *(64)*. Furthermore, amylase has been specifically isolated from cervical mucus *(65)*. Therefore, the Forensic Science Service, London, no longer routinely tests for amylase in such cases. Instead, DNA analysis is undertaken on the vulval and/or vaginal swabs. If the assailant's DNA profile is obtained, this can be used to support an allegation of cunnilingus, although, obviously, the precise interpretation will depend on whether the complainant was subjected to other sexual acts that could account for the presence of the DNA (e.g., ejaculation). There are no published persistence data with regard to the maximum time it is possible to obtain the assailant's DNA pattern from the female genitalia following cunnilingus/anilingus.

There are no published data regarding the possibility of obtaining the complainant's DNA STR profile from a swab or saliva sample taken from the assailant's oral cavity or lips following an allegation of cunnilingus or anilingus. Correspondence with a number of forensic biologists has not revealed any cases in which this has been undertaken, and the general consensus among these experts is that it is unlikely that such samples would isolate sufficient material for forensic analysis due to the usual time delay between the sexual act and the obtaining of the samples from the suspect and the limited number of vaginal cells that are likely to be present. Indeed, this presumption appears to be supported by the work of Banaschak et al. *(66)*, who found mixed DNA STR patterns in five samples obtained from five couples who had kissed for 2 minutes. However, in all cases the kissing partner's DNA STR pattern was only identifiable in the samples immediately after kissing (maximum 60 seconds), and no mixed DNA STR patterns were identified when the volunteers were retested at 5 minutes.

7.2.5. Medical Evidence

Repeated thrusting of the tongue over the edges of the mandibular incisors during cunnilingus or anilingus may cause ulceration of the lingual frenulum, which completely heals within 7 days *(67)*. Such lesions should be specifically sought during the examination of the suspect's oral cavity when such an act has been described by the complainant or when the precise details of the assault are unknown.

8. Female Genitalia

8.1. Frequency

Penile-vaginal intercourse is the most common sexual act performed between heterosexuals. A UK survey of the sexual practices of 10,492 females aged between 16 and 59 years found that only 5.7% of them had never experienced heterosexual penile-vaginal intercourse. By comparing the different age cohorts, the survey revealed that there has been a progressive reduction in the age at which first intercourse occurred in the past 30 years. The median age of the first act of sexual intercourse was 17 years among the 16–24-year-old females questioned. There has also been an increase in the proportion of young women who have experienced sexual intercourse before the legal age of consent (16 years in the United Kingdom). Of the women aged 16–19 years when surveyed, 18.7% had experienced sexual intercourse before the age of 16, and 0.4% of the total female respondents reported sexual intercourse before the age of 13 years *(68)*.

8.2. Legal Implications

English law has retained the term "rape" to describe nonconsensual vaginal or anal penetration with a penis. Penetration of the vagina by an object, however degrading and traumatic, is defined under English law as an indecent assault. In Scotland, nonconsensual penile vaginal penetration is defined by common law as "carnal knowledge of a female by a male against her will" *(69)*. Other jurisdictions, such as some American states, have abandoned such antiquated and emotive terms and define all penetrative acts as sexual assaults subcategorized by the degree of force and coercion used. In many jurisdictions the legal interpretation of "vaginal penetration" refers to penetration of the labia and does not require that the penis actually enter the vagina *(70)*.

The age at which a female can legally give consent for penile-vaginal intercourse varies from country to country; for example, in England the "age of consent" is 16 years, whereas in California, it is 18 years *(71)*.

8.3. Anatomy

The external female genitalia (vulva) includes the mons pubis, the labia majora, the labia minora, the clitoris, and the vestibule (which incorporates the openings of the urethra and the vagina).

The hymen is the tissue that partially or completely surrounds the opening of the vagina. It appears that all females have hymenal tissue present at birth *(72)*. The hymen may be annular, crescentic, fimbriated, or, usually following childbirth, present only as interrupted tags or remnants. It is important that the reader refer to atlases that illustrate these variations *(2,73)*. There is usually a single opening in the hymen. Uncommon congenital variants include two or more hymenal openings, referred to as septate or cribrifrom, respectively, and, rarely, complete absence of an opening (imperforate hymen).

A recent critique of the literature regarding the significance of the various hymenal appearances concluded that complete and partial (not extending to the hymenal base) transections (deficits, clefts) of the upper (anterior) hymen and partial transections of the lateral aspects of the hymen are commonly detected in both prepubertal and postpubertal females who have no history of sexual activity *(74)*. Complete transections of the lateral hymen have also been documented in postpubertal females with no history of sexual activity *(75)*, but it remains unclear whether they are natural phenomena in prepubertal females. In contrast, both complete and partial deficits of the lower (posterior) hymen do not appear to be normal variations at any age *(74,76)*.

The other pertinent anatomic landmarks in this area are the posterior fourchette (where the labia minora unite posteriorly), the fossa navicularis (a relatively concave area of the vestibule bounded anteriorly by the vaginal opening, posteriorly by the posterior fourchette, and laterally by the labia minora), and the anterior fourchette (where the labia minora meet anteriorly and form the clitoral hood).

The skin of the labia majora and the outer aspects of the labia minora is keratinized squamous epithelium, but only the outer aspects of the labia majora are hair bearing. The skin of the inner aspects of the labia minora and the vestibule (including the hymen) is nonkeratinized. This area is usually pink but in the nonestrogenized child it may appear red because the skin is thinner and consequently the blood vessels beneath its surface are more apparent *(77)*.

The forensically relevant areas of the internal female genitalia are the vagina and the cervix. The pertinent landmarks are the vaginal fornices (anterior, posterior, right, and left) and the cervical os (opening of the cervical canal).

The vagina and cervix are covered by nonkeratinized squamous epithelium that normally appears pink in the estrogenized female. On occasions the columnar endocervical epithelium (which appears red) may be visible around the cervical os due to a physiologic or iatrogenic (e.g., exogenous estrogens) eversion of the endocervical canal; these are sometimes erroneously referred to as cervical "erosions."

8.4. Development

The female hypothalamic-pituitary-gonadal axis is developed at the time of birth. During the first 5 days of life, the level of gonadotrophin-releasing hormone (GnRH) rises, with a consequent transient rise in gonadal estrogen, attributable to the withdrawal of placental estrogen *(78)*. The estrogen causes prominence of the labia and clitoris and thickening and redundancy of the hymen. The neonatal vagina is purported to measure 4 cm in length *(77)*. Although after 3 months the GnRH levels gradually fall, the estrogenized appearance of the genitalia may persist for the first 2–4 years of life *(76)*. During this period the external genitalia gradually become less prominent; eventually, the hymen becomes thin and translucent and the tissues appear atrophic; on occasions the hymen remains thick and fimbriated throughout childhood *(79)*. The noestrogenized vagina has relatively few rugae and lengthens by only 0.5–1.0 cm in early childhood *(77,78)*.

The hypothalamic-pituitary-gonadal axis is reactivated in late childhood, and the breasts and external genitalia alter accordingly. These changes are classically described in terms of their Tanner stage *(80)*. Under the influence of estrogens the vagina lengthens to 7.0–8.5 cm in late childhood, eventually reaching its adult length of 10–12 cm *(77,78)*.

The estrogenized vagina is moist due to physiologic secretions. This endogenous lubrication is enhanced with ovulation and with sexual stimulation *(81)*. When the endogenous estrogen levels fall due to the menopause, the vulva and vagina atrophy.

8.5. Forensic Evidence

Although legally it is not necessary to have evidence of ejaculation to prove that vaginal intercourse has occurred, forensic science laboratories are frequently requested to determine whether or not semen is present on the swabs taken from the female genitalia because semen evidence can play a central role in identification of the assailant. The female genitalia should also be sampled if a condom was used during the sexual act (*see* Section 11.) and if cunnilingus is alleged to have occurred (*see* Section 7.).

It is also important to sample the vagina, vulva, and perineum separately when only anal intercourse is alleged, to exclude the possibility of leakage from the vagina to account for semen in the anal canal (*see* Section 9.).

8.5.1. Method of Sampling

The scientist is able to provide objective evidence in terms of the quantity (determined crudely) and quality of the spermatozoa present and may be asked to interpret the results in the context of the case. When providing expert evidence as to whether vaginal penetration has occurred, the scientist must be able to rely on the forensic practitioner to obtain the samples in a manner that will refute any later suggestions by the defense that significant quantities of spermatozoa, which were only deposited on the outside of the vulva, could have been accidentally transferred to the high vaginal area during the medical *(7)*. It is worth noting that there has been no research to support or refute this hypothesis.

At present there is no internationally agreed method for obtaining the samples from the female genital area. The following method has recently (October 1998) been formulated by experienced forensic practitioners and forensic scientists in England to maximize the recovery of spermatozoa while taking into account these potential problems:

1. Any external (sanitary napkins or pads) or internal (tampons) sanitary wear is collected and submitted for analysis with a note about whether the item was in place during the sexual act and whether other sanitary wear has been in place but discarded since the incident.
2. Two dry swabs are rubbed sequentially over the inner aspects of the labia majora, the labia minora, and the vestibule.
3. The labia are separated and an appropriately sized transparent speculum is gently passed approximately two-thirds of the way into the vagina; the speculum is opened and any foreign bodies, e.g., tampons, condoms, are removed and submitted for analysis. Then two dry swabs are taken by comprehensively sampling the vagina beyond the end of the speculum (particularly the posterior fornix where any fluid may collect). These are labeled "high vaginal swabs."
4. When relevant (*see* below), a single endocervical sample is then obtained. At this point the speculum may be manipulated within the vagina to locate the cervix.
5. Two further sequential swabs are then obtained by comprehensively swabbing the lower vagina as the speculum is removed. These are labeled "low vaginal swabs."

In some centers additional methods of semen collection are employed *(5,45,82)* in the form of aspiration of any pools of fluid in the high vagina and/or placing 2–10 mL of saline or sterile water in the vagina and then aspirating the vaginal washings. However, vaginal aspirates should not be necessary if dry swabs are used to sample the vagina in the manner described above. Furthermore, there are no data to confirm that vaginal washings retrieve spermatozoa more effectively than vaginal swabs.

In exceptional circumstances, e.g., due to severe vaginal injuries, it may not be possible to pass a speculum to obtain the "high vaginal" and endocervical swabs. On these occasions the swabs should be inserted into the vagina under direct vision, taking care to avoid contact with the vestibule and hymen. Unfortunately, in such circumstances it is impossible to be certain that the high vaginal swab was not contaminated from semen in the low vagina (which could be there because of drainage from external ejaculation).

8.5.2. Forensic Analysis

8.5.2.1. Spermatozoa

Some guidelines recommend that the forensic practitioner perform an immediate microscopic examination of a wet mount of the material obtained from the vaginal fornices to identify motile spermatozoa on the basis that the presence and motility of spermatozoa may help determine whether recent vaginal ejaculation had occurred. However, a considerable body of opinion does not commend this practice *(83)*. Forensic science laboratories have specialist extraction procedures, staining techniques, and microscopic equipment to maximize spermatozoa recovery and facilitate identification. A survey of 300 cases in which spermatozoa were eventually identified found that they were only detected in four of the cases in the native preparation (prior to the application of specialist stains) *(84)*.

When nonconsensual penile-vaginal penetration is alleged, the samples are examined microscopically by the forensic scientist to identify spermatozoa, and a DNA analysis is performed on any spermatozoa found.

8.5.2.2. Seminal Fluid

If no spermatozoa are detected, an attempt is made to corroborate the allegation by the microscopic identification of seminal choline crystals. Seminal choline is present in high concentrations in seminal fluid, and the choline crystals can be precipitated by the addition of reagents *(85)*. There are also electrophoretic techniques by which seminal fluid can be identified *(86)*. If the assailant is a secretor, his semen, whether or not spermatozoa are present, will contain his ABO group antigens. However, serologic analysis has been superceded by DNA STR analysis in many countries.

8.5.2.3. Blood

A retrospective survey carried out at the Metropolitan Police Forensic Science Laboratory (MPFSL) found that nearly a third of the vaginal swabs received at the laboratory were blood stained. Whenever bleeding is noted during the medical examination, the forensic practitioner should communicate to the scientist any possible source for the bleeding. In the MPFSL study 22% of the blood-stained swabs were considered by the examining doctors to be due to menstruation, and 10% were attributed to female genital trauma. In the remaining cases no explanation for the bleeding was given. In these cases the presence of blood must be interpreted with caution, particularly if in small quantity, since traces of uterine blood may be present at any time of the cycle *(7)* and, at present, there is no accepted method of differentiating between traumatic or uterine blood *(87)*. Furthermore, even traumatic bleeding may result from consensual sexual acts (*see* Section 8.6.). On rare occasions assailants injure their penises during a sexual act, and this may be the source of blood found in the vagina.

8.5.2.4. Lubricant

See Section 11. for detailed information.

8.5.3. Persistence Data

Research carried out at the MPFSL has found that following vaginal intercourse spermatozoa *should* be found in the vagina for 24 hours, that they are *likely* to be found up to 3 days later, and that *occasionally* they are found 7 days later *(88,89)*. Longer times for persistence are the exception rather than the rule.

The quantity of semen in the vagina will diminish progressively with time, usually as a result of drainage. The posture and activity of the complainant subsequent to the act is likely to affect this. Similarly, washing, douching, or bathing may accelerate the loss of semen. Drainage of semen from the vagina may also result in soiling of intimate clothing items worn at the time, and these can prove valuble sources of body fluids.

It has been observed that spermatozoa can be isolated for longer periods in the endocervix. Graves et al. *(90)* report that spermatozoa were isolated from the endocervix 17 days after intercourse. Studies that compared paired swabs from the vagina and cervix have found that 2 days or more after vaginal ejaculation there is a larger quantity of spermatozoa on endocervical swabs compared with the vaginal swabs *(91)*. Therefore, it is recommended that if a complainant presents 48 hours or more after alleged vaginal intercourse, an endocervical swab be taken in addition to the swabs from the vagina.

Seminal choline has only been found on vaginal swabs up to 24 hours after vaginal ejaculation *(92)*.

There is interest in the possibility of determining the timing of intercourse by changes in spermatozoa. Spermatozoa may remain motile in the vagina for up to 24 hours and longer in the cervical mucosa *(31,93,94)*, but the periods for persistence are extremely variable. For example Rupp *(95)* observed that motile spermatozoa persisted longer in menstruating women (but added that identification is hindered by the presence of red blood cells), and Paul *(96)* reported that the period of spermatozoa motility ranged from 1–2 hours at the end of the menstrual cycle to as long as 72 hours at the time of ovulation.

However, the morphology of the spermatozoa does show more consistent temporal changes. In particular, the presence of large numbers of spermatozoa with tails is indicative of recent intercourse. The longest time after intercourse that spermatozoa with tails have been found on external vaginal swabs is 33 hours, and 120 hours on internal vaginal swabs *(97)*.

Although it should be possible to detect the assailant's DNA STR profile from semen on the genital swabs for 3–4 days after vaginal ejaculation *(88)*, the current recorded maximum for DNA STR profiling (from Forensic Science Service case reports) is 40 hours *(98)*. There are no published persistence data regarding the possibility of obtaining a DNA STR profile from an assailant if no spermatozoa are present in the seminal fluid.

8.6. Medical Evidence

8.6.1. Examination Methods

When an allegation of nonconsensual vaginal penetration is made, the vulval area must be carefully inspected prior to the insertion of a speculum, as even apparently gentle traction on the posterior fourchette or fossa navicularis during a medical can cause a superficial laceration at these sites. Whenever possible the vagina and cervix should be inspected via the transparent speculum after the high vaginal samples have been obtained. Colposcopy and the application of toluidine blue dye are two specialist techniques used by some forensic practitioners during examinations of the female genitalia.

8.6.1.1. Colposcopy

A colposcope is a free-standing, binocular microscope on wheels that is most commonly used for direct visualization of the cervix (using a bivalve speculum) following the detection of abnormal cervical cytology. Many centers, particularly those in the United States, advocate the use of the colposcope for external and, where relevant, internal genital and/or anal assessments of complainants of sexual assault.

The colposcope undoubtedly provides considerable advantages over gross visualization. First, it provides magnification (5–30 times) and greater illumination, enabling detection of more abnormalities. Slaughter and Brown *(99)* demonstrated positive colposcopic findings in 87% of female complainants of nonconsensual penile penetration within the previous 48 hours, whereas gross visualization has historically identified positive genital findings in only 10–40% of cases *(23–25,100,101)*.

Second, with attachment of a still or video camera it allows for a truly contemporaneous, permanent video/photographic record of the genital/anal findings without having to resort to simultaneous dictation, which has the potential to distress the complainant. If a video is used, this will document the entire genital examination and will show any dynamic changes such as reflex anal dilatation. If appropriate, the medical findings can be demonstrated to the complainant and carer; some teenagers have apparently appreciated the opportunity to have any fears of genital disfigurement allayed by the use of this equipment.

Finally, if a remote monitor is used, the whole examination can be viewed by another doctor for corroboration or teaching purposes without additional parties having to be present during the intimate examination. This facility is obviously more pertinent when video recording is not available.

On the other hand, some practitioners consider that colposcopy may be perceived as a "stressful invasion of a woman who is already at risk of the rape trauma syndrome" and that its routine use is "a regressive step in the management of rape victims whose histories may not be believed unless demonstrable colposcopic injuries are seen" *(102)*. Nonetheless, if a colposcope with photo-documentation improves the quality and quantity of the medical evidence while not increasing the duration or invasiveness of the genital/anal assessment *(103)*, then the courts may demand to know why the instrument was not used.

Obviously, it is important that in all cases the colposcopic evidence be interpreted in the context of the limited information that is currently available regarding colposcopic assessments following consensual sexual acts *(71,104)*.

8.6.1.2. Toluidine Blue

Toluidine blue stains nuclei and has been used on the posterior fourchette to identify lacerations of the keratinized squamous epithelium that were not apparent on gross visualization *(105,106)*. Use of toluidine blue increased the detection rate of posterior fourchette lacerations from 4 to 58% in adult (older than 19 years) complainants of nonconsenual vaginal intercourse, from 4 to 28% in sexually abused adolescents (11–18 years old), and from 16.5 to 33% in pediatric sexually abused patients (0–10 years old) *(106,107)*.

The same frequency of posterior fourchette lacerations has been identified by use of the stain in adolescents following consensual penile penetration and nonconsensual sexual acts *(106)*. In contrast, adult complainants of nonconsensual vaginal intercourse and sexually abused children had significantly more lacerations demonstrable by toluidine blue staining than control groups *(107)*, although such staining does not identify lacerations that cannot be detected using a colposcope *(99)*. Therefore, if a colposcope is not available, toluidine blue may be an adjunct to the genital assessment of prepubertal and adult complainants of vaginal penetration *(106,107)*. Furthermore, some centers use the stain during colposcopy to provide a clear pictorial presentation of the injuries for later presentation to juries *(99)*.

Vulval swabs for forensic analysis must be taken before the stain is applied. Toluidine blue (1%) is then painted on the posterior fourchette, using a swab, prior to any instrumentation. After a few seconds the residual stain is removed with lubricating jelly and gauze *(105)*. The patient may experience some stinging at the site of application. The time parameters within which the use of toluidine blue is beneficial in highlighting injuries have not been identified.

8.6.2. Injuries

Very little information is available regarding the incidence and type of genital injuries that result from consensual sexual acts involving the female genitalia. Considering that penile-vaginal pentration is the most frequent sexual act performed by heterosexual couples, anecdotal reports from doctors who regularly conduct nonforensic assessments of the female genitalia (general practitioners, gynecologists, genitourinary physicians) suggest that injuries resultant from sexual activity are rarely identified. However, this might be explained by the nature of routine assessments, which are usually limited to naked eye inspection, or because of the rapid and complete resolution of minor injuries *(71)*. On the other hand, there are reports describing genital injuries in complainants of sexual assault although, unfortunately, very few have matched the findings with the specific complaint or the subsequent outcome in court. To date, no case control study has compared the genital findings in complainants of sexual assault with those in a sexually active control population.

8.6.2.1. External Genitalia

For penile penetration of the vagina to take place the penis must first pass between the labia minora and through the hymenal opening. The apposition of the penis and the posterior fourchette in the majority of sexual positions means that this area may be stretched, rubbed, or receive blunt trauma as vaginal penetration is achieved. Lacerations, abrasions, or bruises at the posterior fourchette have all been described following consensual sexual activity, although in all these cases the examinations were enhanced by the use of toludine blue or a colposcope *(71,105,106)*. Wilson *(108)* has also described macroscopically visible hematomata of the labia with consensual sexual activity. These injuries usually heal completely without residual scarring *(71)*.

Among 313 postpubertal females (age range 11–85 years) who made a "valid" (defined as "police investigation corroborated the victim's history and the victim did not recant") complaint of sexual assault, 200 had colposcopically detected injuries at one or more of the following sites on the external genitalia: posterior fourchette, labia minora, hymen, and fossa navicularis. Although all categories of injuries ("tears," bruises, abrasions, redness, and swelling) were described at all sites, the predominant injuries described were site dependent, for example, "tears" were most frequently described on the posterior fourchette ($n = 83$) and fossa navicularis ($n = 28$) whereas abrasions were most frequently described on the labia minora (n = 66) and bruises were the most frequent injuries seen on the hymen (n = 28). The studies of macroscopic findings among complainants of sexual assault have also found that most of the injuries detected are located on the external genitalia *(109,110)*.

Healing of lacerations of the posterior fourchette is predominantly by first intention with no residual scarring being detected at follow-up assessments *(71)*. Nonetheless, scarring may occur occasionally in these areas, but it is important not to mistake a linear vestibularis, a congenital white line identified in the fossa navicularis (present in 25% of neonates), for a scar *(111)*.

Accidental injuries of the external genitalia of female childern are well documented in the literature. The site and nature of the injury will depend on the type of trauma and the conformation of any object involved *(112,113)*.

8.6.2.2. Hymen

The hymen must be examined in detail following an allegation of a nonconsensual penetrative act. When the hymen is fimbriated this assessment may be facilitated by the gentle use of a moistened swab to visualize the hymenal edges. When the hymenal opening cannot be seen at all, application of 2–3 mL of warm sterile water or saline onto the hymen will often reveal the hymenal edges. Some authors recommend using Foley catheters to aid hymenal visualization *(114)*. Obviously, in the acute setting none of these maneuvers should be attempted until the relevant forensic samples have been retrieved.

There is very little specific information available regarding the type and frequency of acute hymenal injuries following consensual sexual acts, particularly with regard to the first act of sexual intercourse. Slaughter et al *(71)* conducted colposcopic examinations of the genitalia of 75 women who had experienced "consensual" vaginal intercourse in the preceding 24 hours. They found lacerations (tears) with associated bruising at the 3 o'clock and 9 o'clock positions on the hymen of a 14-year-old and bruises at the 6 o'clock and 7 o'clock positions on the hymens of two other females (aged 13 and 33 years). No other hymenal injuries were detected. Unfortunately, no details regarding previous sexual experience are recorded on their proforma.

In the same paper the hymen was noted to be one of the four most commonly injured genital sites among 311 postpubertal complainants of nonconsensual sexual acts. The hymenal injuries detected colposcopically were bruises (n = 28), lacerations (n = 22), abrasions (n = 13), swelling (n = 10), and redness (n = 4). The hymenal lacerations were either single (n = 12), 9 of which were at the 6 o'clock position, or paired around the 6 o'clock position (n = 10). They found that hymenal lacerations were four times more common in the younger age groups. Again, there was no information regarding previous sexual experience. Bowyer and Dalton *(109)* described 3 women with hymenal lacerations (detected with the naked eye) among 83 complainants of rape who were examined within 11 days of the incident; 2 of these 3 women had not previously experienced sexual intercourse. There is no information in either paper regarding whether the lacerations were partial or complete.

Bruises, abrasions, reddening, and swelling will completely disappear within a few days or weeks of the trauma *(71,115)*. Conversely, hymenal lacerations do not appear to reunite and thus will always remain apparent as partial or complete transections *(99)*, although they may be partially concealed by the effects of estrogenization *(116)*. There is one case report of a 5-year-old who was subjected to penile penetration and acquired an imperforate hymen due to obliterative scarring *(117)*.

Once the acute injuries have disappeared, the interpretation of the hymenal findings becomes even more contentious and has been the subject of a recent review paper *(74)*. On the basis of the current literature, partial and complete transections in the lower margin of the hymen are considered to provide confirmatory evidence of previous penetration of the hymen. However, it is not possible to determine whether it was a penis, finger, or other object that caused the injury, and there is an urgent need for comprehensive research to determine whether sporting activities or tampon use can effect hymenal configuration. Although partial or complete transections of the upper hymen may represent healed partial or complete lacerations beyond the acute stage, there is no method of distinguishing them from naturally occurring anatomical variations.

Goodyear and Laidlaw *(74)* conclude that "it is unlikely that a normal-looking hymen of less than 10 mm in diameter, even in the case of an elastic hymen, has previously accommodated full penetration of an adult finger, let alone a penis." However, there is no objective evidence on which to base this conjecture, and it is not known whether measuring the hymenal opening using a digit, or other previously measured object, in the clinical setting, when the practitioner is particularly anxious not to cause the patient any distress, accurately reflects what the hymen could have accommodated during a sexual assault.

On the other hand, it is now generally accepted that postpubertal females can experience penile vaginal penetration without sustaining any hymenal deficits, which is attributed to hymenal elasticity *(74,118)*. Furthermore, the similarity between the dimensions of the hymenal opening among sexually active and non-sexually active postpubertal females *(75)* makes it impossible for the physician to state categorically that a person has ever had prior sexual intercourse unless there is other supportive evidence (pregnancy, spermatozoa on a high vaginal swab; *see* Forensic Evidence) *(74,75,119)*.

8.6.2.3. Vagina

Lacerations and ruptures (full-thickness lacerations) of the vagina have been described in the medical literature following consensual sexual acts *(120–122)*. They are most commonly located in the right fornix or extending across the posterior fornix; this configuration is attributed to the normal vaginal asymmetry whereby the cervix lies toward the left fornix, causing the penis to enter the right fornix during vaginal penetration *(122)*. Factors that predispose to such injuries include previous vaginal surgery, pregnancy and the puerperium, post-menopause, intoxication of the female, first act of sexual intercourse, and congenital genital abnormalities (e.g., septate vagina) *(120)*. Although most vaginal lacerations are associated with penile penetration, they have also been documented following brachiovaginal intercourse (fisting) *(122)*, vaginal instrumentation during the process of a medical assessment *(122)*, and the use of plastic tampon inserters *(123)*.

Vaginal lacerations have been documented without any direct intravaginal trauma following a fall or a sudden increase of intraabdominal pressure (e.g., lifting a heavy object) *(122)*.

Injuries of the vagina have been noted during the examinations of complainants of sexual assault. Slaughter et al. *(71)* describe 26 colposcopically detected vaginal injuries among the 213 complainants who had genital trauma identified. These were described as "tears" (n = 10), bruises (n = 12), and abrasions (n = 4). Other papers that only considered macroscopically detectable lesions found vaginal "injuries" in 2–16% of complainants of nonconsensual penile vaginal penetration *(109,110)*. However, one study included "redness" as a vaginal injury when in fact this is a nonspecific finding with a number of causes.

When a vaginal laceration may have been caused by an object that has the potential to fragment or splinter, a careful search should be made for foreign bodies in the wound *(120)* (this may necessitate a general anesthetic), and X-rays should be taken of the pelvis (anterioposterior and lateral), including the vagina, to help localize foreign particles *(124)*. Any retrieved foreign bodies should be appropriately packaged and submitted for forensic analysis.

8.6.2.4. Cervix

Bruises and lacerations of the cervix have been described as infrequent findings following nonconsensual sexual acts *(71,125,126)*. In one paper the injuries related to penetration by a digit and by a "knife-like" object. There are no reports of cervical trauma following consensual sexual acts.

8.6.2.5. NONSPECIFIC

Norvell et al. *(104)* have also documented areas of increased vascularity/ telangiectasia (*n* = 7), broken blood vessels (*n* = 2), and microabrasions (*n* = 2) during colposcopic assessment of the introitus, hymen, and lower 2 cm of the vagina of 18 volunteers who had participated in consensual sexual activity within the preceeding six hours. However, it appears that the areas of increased vascularity may have been normal variants *(71)*, and the precise location of the other findings was not described.

9. MALE GENITALIA

During examination of the male genitalia, the forensic practitioner is expected to document any features that could assist with subsequent identification of the assailant, to note any acquired or congenital conditions that could make an alleged sexual act impossible, to describe in detail any injuries that could relate to a sexual act, and to retrieve any forensic evidence. Although the specifics of the medicolegal assessment of the male genitalia will be case dependent, the principles of the examination, be it of the complainant or the defendant, are the same.

9.1 Anatomy and Physiology

9.1.1. Penile Size

Forensic practitioners may be asked to provide evidence on the size of a defendant's penis in the flaccid state in order to support a hypothesis that a certain sexual act could not have occurred due to intergenital disproportion between the complainant and the defendant. However, such measurements are unhelpful as it is not possible to predict the maximum erectile size from the flaccid length, and there is "no statistical support for the "phallic fallacy" that the larger penis increases in size with full erection to a significantly greater degree than does the smaller penis" *(127)*. Furthermore, even when the erect penis is measured during automanipulation or active coition, the measurements are recognized to be unreliable *(127)*.

9.1.2. Erections

Forensic practitioners may also be asked to comment on a person's ability to achieve a penile erection, particularly if the male is young or elderly. Masters and Johnson *(127)* note that during their research "penile erection has been observed in males of all ages ranging from baby boys immediately after delivery to men in their late eighties"; they report that one 89-year-old study subject was able to achieve a full penile erection and ejaculate. Therefore, it is not possible to reach a conclusion regarding erectile efficiency based on age alone. When a defendant reports erectile dysfunction the expert opinion of a urologist should be sought.

Penile erection may result from visual stimulation (including fantasy) or tactile stimulation. The penis, scrotum, and rectum are all sensitive to tactile stimulation *(127)* which may explain why involuntary penile erections can be experienced by a male subjected to nonconsensual anal intercourse.

9.1.3. Production of Semen

Semen is not produced until the male experiences puberty, which usually begins between 9 and 14 years of age *(128)*. Semen consists of seminal fluid (produced by the prostate) and spermatozoa. The normal volume of a single ejaculate is between 2 and 7 mL, and it will contain around 50–120 million spermatozoa/mL. There are numerous congenital and acquired causes for impaired spermatogenesis *(129)*, resulting in either decreased numbers (oligozoospermia) or absence of (azoospermia) spermatozoa. Both conditions may be permanent or transitory depending on the underlying cause. Permanent azoospermia (e.g., following a successful vasectomy) would be of particular forensic significance as it could lead to the elimination of a suspect from an inquiry if spermatozoa had been identified that were known to relate to the offence. It is not possible to determine whether spermatozoa are present in the ejaculate without microscopic assessment. However, analysis of a defendant's semen is not a routine part of the forensic assessment.

9.2. Forensic Evidence

Following an allegation of fellatio, swabs from the complainant's penis can be examined for saliva, but, as discussed earlier, the likelihood of definitive identification of saliva by amylase estimation is low. Nonetheless, enough material may be obtained for DNA analysis. When an allegation of vaginal or anal intercourse is made, penile swabs from the suspect can be examined for cells, feces, hairs, fibers, blood, and lubricants.

It should be noted that vaginal fluid from recent previous intercourse, unrelated to the allegation, may be detected by DNA analysis of swabs taken from the unwashed penis *(41)*.

9.2.1. Method of Sampling

Data collected by the MPFSL between 1987 and 1995 *(97)* have shown that, following vaginal intercourse, cellular material from the complainant can be recovered from the coronal sulcus (groove around the penis just below the glans) even if the suspect has washed/bathed since the offence. Swabs taken from the meatus and urethra are not suitable for microscopic assessment as some male urethral cells can be very similar to vaginal cells *(7)*. Therefore, when vaginal intercourse is alleged, two moistened swabs should be obtained sequentially from the coronal sulcus, and a further two moistened swabs should be taken sequentially from the glans and the shaft together. The swabs must be labeled accordingly, and the order in which the samples were obtained must be relayed to the scientist. The same samples are also taken if it is believed that a lubricant or condom have been used during a sexual act or if the assault has involved fellatio or anal intercourse.

9.2.2. Forensic Analysis

9.2.2.1. Microscopic and Biochemical Analyses

Such analyses of the penile swabs may be undertaken to identify cellular material, blood, or amylase. When the complaint is of anal intercourse, swabs that appear to be discolored by fecal material can be analyzed for urobilinogen and examined microscopically for vegetable matter.

9.2.2.2. Assailant Identification

DNA STR profiling of body fluids on the penis is now the method of choice used to provide evidence of penile-vaginal/oral/anal contact. It has proved particularly useful when multiple assailants have had intercourse with a single complainant *(53)*, as DNA STR profiles matching the other assailants may also be found on the penile swabs taken from one assailant.

Certain forensic science laboratories are now able to extract mitochondrial DNA from the degraded cellular material present in feces, although the value of this method of analysis in relation to sexual offences needs to be considered in relation to the other sexual acts that are alleged to have occurred during the assault.

9.2.3. Persistence Data

Cells matching the complainant have only been identified on penile swabs for up to 19 hours following sexual intercourse *(7)*. No published data are available on whether vaginal material can be detected for longer using DNA STR analysis.

Blood and feces have been recovered from penile swabs taken 15 and 18 hours, respectively, after the incident *(7)*. Again, no data are available on whether these body fluids can be detected later using DNA STR analysis (for saliva, *see* Section 7.1.).

9.3. Medical Evidence

When obtaining the relevant forensic samples, the forensic practitioner should inspect the male genitalia with particular reference to the following points:

1. Pubic hair should be described in terms of its coarseness, distribution (Tanner stages 1–5), and color. A note should be made if the pubic hair appears to have been plucked (including bleeding hair follicles), shaved, cut, or dyed.
2. Congenital abnormalities such as microphallus and cryptorchidism. Penile length in the flaccid state is said to vary from 8.5 to 10.5 cm (measured from the anterior border of the symphysis along the dorsal surface to the distal tip of the penis) with a documented range of 6.0–14.0 cm *(127)*.
3. Acquired abnormalities such as circumcision, Peyronie's disease, balanitis xerotica obliterans, vasectomy scars, phimosis, tattoos, and piercing.
4. Signs of infection such as warts, discharge, erythema, and vesicles.
5. Foreign bodies may be worn around the base of the penis, sometimes also encircling the scrotum, in an attempt to increase and sustain penile tumescence. Such devices may result in local and distal genital trauma (penile tourniquet syndrome) *(130)*. In a number of case reports children have been found to have human hairs wrapped around the penis; these hairs may be virtually invisible due to edema or epithelialization *(131)*. Kerry and Chapman *(132)* have described the deliberate application of such a ligature by parents who were attempting to prevent enuresis.
6. Assessment of injuries. Following consensual sexual intercourse lacerations of the foreskin and frenulum, meatitis, traumatic urethritis, penile edema, traumatic lymphangitis, paraphimosis, and penile 'fractures' have all been described *(133–136)*. Accidental trauma is more common when there is a preexisting abnormality such as phimosis *(133)*. Skin injury may be incurred if the genitals are deliberately bitten during fellatio *(133)*. Although the precise incidence of male genital trauma following sexual activity is unknown, anecdotal accounts suggest that it is rare to find any genital injuries when examining suspects of serious sexual assaults *(137)*.

In children the genitalia may be accidentally or deliberately injured, and the latter may be associated with sexual abuse *(138)*. Bruises, abrasions, lacerations, swelling, and burns of the genitalia of prepubescent males have all been described *(138,139)*.

10. Perianal Area and Anal Canal

10.1. Definitions

Buggery is a lay term used to refer to penile penetration of the anus (anal intercourse) of a man, a woman, or an animal (also known as bestiality). Sodomy relates to anal intercourse between humans only.

10.2. Frequency

10.2.1. Consensual

Although anal intercourse among heterosexuals is the least common component of the sexual repertoire, it has been experienced on at least one occasion by 13–25% of heterosexual females surveyed *(43,61,140)*, and it was described as a regular means of sexual gratification for 8% of women attending one gynecologist *(61)*. Among 508 men who reported having had, at some stage in their lives, a same-gender sexual experience, 33.7% reported insertive anal intercourse, and 35.4% had experienced receptive anal intercourse. Interestingly, in contrast to a common perception, more men had experienced both practices than had been in exclusively receptive or insertive roles *(141)*.

10.2.2. Nonconsensual

Anal intercourse was reported by 5–16% of females who described having been sexually assaulted *(6,109,142)*. Although it may be the only sexual act performed, it is more frequently combined with vaginal and oral penetration *(6,142)*. Fewer data are available regarding sexual assaults on males, although Hillman et al. *(143,144)* report that penetrative anal intercourse was described by 75–89% of the male complainants they studied.

10.3. Legal Implications

Under English common law the term buggery is defined as anal intercourse by a man with another man or a woman, and anal or vaginal intercourse by a man or a woman with an animal (bestiality). Although the 1967 Sexual Offences Act provided that it was not an offence for two consenting men who had attained the age of 21 to commit buggery in private, until 1994 it remained an offence for a man to commit buggery with a woman, even if both parties consented.

The Criminal Justice and Public Order Act (CJPOA) 1994 expanded the definition of rape (which had previously only related to vaginal intercourse) to include nonconsensual penile penetration of the anus independent of the gender of the recipient. The CJPOA 1994 also states that buggery between males, or between a male and a female, is not an offence provided that "the act takes place in private and both parties have sustained the age of 18."

Although in English law the insertion of an object or part of the human body other than a penis into the anus is characterized only as an indecent assault, rape definitions in other jurisdictions, such as Australia, have been extended to include it *(145)*.

10.4. Anatomy and Physiology

An understanding of the normal anatomy and physiology of the perianal area and anal canal is important for the reliable description and interpretation of the medical findings following allegations of anal penetrative acts. Unfortunately, varying definitions have resulted in considerable confusion, such that there is no consensus among forensic practitioners about the nomenclature that should be used in describing injuries to this area. Therefore, a brief overview of the relevant information is given below together with references to more substantive texts.

10.4.1. Anus

The anus refers not to an actual anatomical structure but to the external opening of the anal canal. The skin that immediately surrounds the anus is variously referred to as the anal verge or anal margin *(146)*. Because the anal canal can evert and invert as the anal sphincters and pelvic floor muscles relax and contract, the anal verge/margin is not a fixed, identifiable landmark.

10.4.2. Perianal Area

The perianal area is a poorly defined, approximately circular area that includes the folds of skin encircling the anus. It is covered by skin that is often hyperpigmented when compared with the skin on the buttocks, although this varies with age and ethnicity *(147)*.

10.4.3. Anal Canal

Although the anal canal has been variously defined, the definition that has practical clinical forensic value is that of the anatomical anal canal, which extends from the anus to the "dentate line." The "dentate line" refers to the line formed either by the bases of the anal columns (most distinct in children) or, when these are not apparent, by the lowest visible anal sinuses *(148)*. The average length of the anatomical anal canal in adults (age range 18–90 years) is only 2.1 cm, with a range of 1.4–3.8 cm in males and 1.0–3.2 cm in females *(149)*. Between the epithelial zones of the anal canal and the rectum is the anal transitional zone, which is usually located in the region of the anal columns and is purple in color *(150)*.

The anal canal, as defined above, is lined by nonkeratinized squamous epithelium and appears salmon pink in the living *(147)*. It is sensitive to touch, pain, heat, and cold to just above the dentate line *(148)*. The anus and lumen of the anal canal usually appears as an asymmetric Y-shaped slit when viewed via an proctoscope (anoscope). The folds of mucosa and subcutaneous tissue (containing small convulated blood vessels surrounded by connective tissue) between the indentations of the Y are referred to as the anal cushions. Although this appearance is usually obscured externally by the folds of skin on the perianal area, it may become apparent if the patient is anesthetized or as the anus dilates.

10.4.4. Rectum

The rectum extends from the anal transitionary zone to the sigmoid colon and is 8–15 cm long. It is lined by typical intestinal mucosa and appears red in the living. The rectum has only poorly defined dull sensation *(148)*.

10.4.5. Anal Sphincters and Fecal Incontinence

Although a number of muscles encircle the anal canal, the two that have particular forensic significance are the internal and the external anal sphincters.

10.4.5.1. Internal Anal Sphincter

This sphincter is a continuation of the circular muscle coat of the rectum and extends 8–12 mm below the dentate line. In the normal living subject it is tonically contracted so that the anal canal is closed. The internal sphincter is supplied by autonomic nerve fibers and is not considered to be under voluntary control *(3)*. Thus, although it appears to contract during a digital assessment of voluntary anal contraction, this is presumed to be due to its compression by the surrounding external sphincter fibers *(150)*.

10.4.5.2. External Anal Sphincter

This encircles the internal sphincter but extends below it, ending subcutaneously. The lower edges of the external and internal sphincters can be distinguished on digital palpation. Although this sphincter is tonically contracted in the resting state this contraction can be overcome with firm pressure *(150)*. If the patient is asked to contract the anus during a digital assessment, the external sphincter can be felt to contract and close the anus tightly. However, as the muscle fibers are predominantly of the slow twitch type, a maximal contraction of the external sphincter can only be maintained for about 1 minute *(151)*.

Fecal continence is maintained by a number of factors, the relative importance of which has not been fully elucidated. At present, the most important factor appears to be the angulation between the rectum and the anal canal, which is maintained at a mean of 92 degrees by continuous contraction of the puborectalis muscles, located above the external sphincter. Both sphincters have supportive roles in maintaining fecal continence *(148)*, and their disruption can result in incontinence (*see* below).

10.5 Forensic Evidence

The presence of semen in the anus or rectum of a male complainant can be corroborative evidence of alleged anal intercourse in conjunction with the presented history and possible physical findings.

The same is only true for a female complainant if no semen is detected in the vagina because semen has been found on rectal and anal swabs taken from women who described vaginal intercourse only. It is postulated that the presence of semen in these cases is due to drainage from the vagina *(52,152)*.

Swabs should also be taken if a condom or lubricant was used during the sexual assault and if anilingus is alleged (*see* Sections 7.2. and 11.).

10.5.1. Method of Sampling

Two samples must first be obtained from the perianal area using a dampened swab (traditionally this has been labeled "external anal swab"). The proctoscope (anoscope) is then passed 2–3 cm into the anal canal, and the lower rectum is sampled using a dry swab. As the proctoscope is withdrawn, the anal canal can be sampled, again with a dry swab. As discussed above, when examining female complainants of anal intercourse alone, swabs should also be obtained from the vagina.

Stool samples and toilet paper should not be collected since retrieval of such samples is degrading and may contribute to the distress of the complainant. The other samples, described above, should be adequate for laboratory requirements.

10.5.2. Forensic Analysis

Microscopic examination for spermatozoa (or analysis for seminal choline if no spermatozoa are present) is initially undertaken, followed by DNA analysis if any body fluids are identified. ABO grouping is not successful with anal swabs as the complainant's own group predominates *(153)*.

Lubricant and saliva analysis are discussed in Sections 11. and 7.2., respectively.

10.5.3. Persistence Data

In normal circumstances the maximum recorded interval between the act of anal intercourse and the identification of spermatozoa on a rectal swab is 65 hours *(154)*. However, in one exceptional case in which a female remained prone in hospital for several days because of injuries sustained during a sexual assault, semen was detected on anal swabs taken 113 hours after the act of anal intercourse *(154)*.

Swabs should be taken even if the complainant has defecated since the assault. An unpublished review of 36 MPFSL cases of alleged anal intercourse in which the complainant had defecated prior to the examination found that in six cases (four female and two male) the internal/external anal swabs were still positive for spermatozoa (although only a few were present); one of these subjects, a male, had a positive external anal swab 52 hours after the anal intercourse *(155)*. There are no data available regarding the periods within which DNA STR analysis will be successful.

10.6. Medical Evidence

When an allegation of anal penetration is made, the perianal skin, anal canal mucosa, and, when tolerated, the lower portion of the rectum should be examined with the aid of a proctoscope/anoscope. This can be done simultaneously with the retrieval of the forensic evidence.

It is generally accepted that with gradual dilatation and lubrication, consensual penile anal intercourse can be performed without any resultant injury *(61,156)*. Furthermore, it is important to emphasize that nonconsensual anal penetration can also occur in both children and adults without producing acute or chronic injury *(3)*.

Although anecdotal accounts have detailed the anal and rectal injuries that result from consensual penile/object anal penetration *(96,148)*, very few peer-reviewed articles have addressed this subject. Similarly, many studies have documented the presence of anal symptoms or signs among complainants of sexual assault *(109,143)*, but very few of these have described the acute injuries in any detail or related these injuries to the specific complaint and its subsequent outcome.

10.6.1. Anal Fissures, Tears, and Lacerations

The most frequent injuries that are documented following allegations of nonconsensual anal penetration are anal fissures, tears, and lacerations. Use of these different terminologies is confusing and makes comparison of the different data impossible. A consensus should be reached among forensic practitioners worldwide as to what terms should be used and what they mean.

Clinically an anal fissure refers to a longitudinal laceration in the perianal skin and/or mucosa of the anal canal. Anal fissures may be acute (usually healing within 2–3 weeks) or chronic and single or multiple. Most fissures will heal by first intention and not leave a scar. However, after healing, the site of some fissures may be apparent as a fibrous skin tag *(157)*. Manser *(110)* described the medical findings in only 16 of 51 complainants (15 males and

36 females) of anal intercourse (21 were categorized as Child Sexual Abuse). The majority (61%) of this study population were examined at least 72 hours after the sexual contact. Fissures were found in 8 cases (16%).

A major problem in the forensic interpretation of anal fissures is that there are numerous causes for them unrelated to penetrative trauma including passage of hard stools, diarrhea, inflammatory bowel disease, sexually transmitted diseases, and skin diseases *(157,158)*.

In the study by Manser *(110)*, lacerations were documented as being present in only 1 of the 51 complainants of anal intercourse and 5 of 103 females complainants of nonconsensual vaginal penetration aged between 12 and 69 years, some of whom complained of concurrent nonconsensual anal penetration with either an object or a penis (the majority of whom were examined within 24 hours of the sexual assault). It may be that these "lacerations" were in fact long or deep anal fissures, but as the parameters in terms of length or depth of an anal fissure have not been clinically defined, the distinction may be arbitrary. Conversely, these "lacerations" may have been horizontally or obliquely directed breaches in the epithelium *(159)*, which would immediately differentiate them from anal fissures and render them highly forensically significant due to the limited differential diagnoses of such injuries compared with fissures.

Slaughter et al. *(71)* described the gross and colposcopic findings in 311 females aged between 11 and 85 years who reported nonconsensual sexual acts, 55 of whom described anal contact. The majority (81%) of their population was examined within 72 hours of the sexual assault. They found "anal findings" in 56% of the 55 patients who reported anal contact. The anal injuries were categorized as tears in 19 of the cases. Although elsewhere Slaughter has qualified the term "tear" to mean "laceration" *(160)*, this was not done in this paper and again means that interpretation of the forensic significance of these injuries may limited.

Given that a significant percentage of the heterosexual and male homosexual population have engaged in consensual anal penetration, anecdotal accounts suggest that resultant injuries such as fissures are rare. This could be because the injuries do not warrant medical attention or because patients are not specifically questioned about anal intercourse when the causative factors for anal abnormalities/complaints are considered. However, one study that specifically attempted to address this issue documented that among 129 women who gave a history of anal intercourse only one patient described anal complications, namely, proctitis and an anal fissure; in fact both these signs related to a gonococccal infection *(61)*. However, as this study was limited to the medical history it is not possible to rule out the presence of minor asymptomatic conditions or injuries in this study population.

Whether an injury heals by first or secondary intention, the latter resulting in scar formation, depends on a number of factors including the width and depth of the breach in the epithelium. Manser *(110)* reported scarring in 14% of the people examined because of possible anal intercourse. The Royal College of Physicians working party stated that in children: "The only specific indicator of abuse is a fresh laceration or healed scar extending beyond the anal margin onto the perianal skin in the absence of reasonable alternative explanation, e.g. major trauma" *(146)*. Disappointingly, this report does not clarify how they differentiate between lacerations and fissures.

10.6.2. Anal Sphincter Tone

The forensic practitioner may be asked about the effects that a single episode, or repeated episodes, of anal penetration have on anal sphincter tone and subsequent continence of feces. In terms of single anal penetrative acts, partial tears and complete disruptions of the anal sphincters have been described following a single traumatic sexual act *(161,162)*; one case was caused by pliers and the others by brachioproctic intercourse (fisting). However, it is not clear from these case reports whether the sexual practices were consensual or nonconsensual. The two patients who were described as having complete disruption of the sphincters both developed fecal incontinence. There is a case report of "multiple ruptures" of the internal anal sphincter with resultant fecal incontinence following nonconsensual anal penetration with a penis and fist *(163)*.

With regard to repeated acts of anal penetration, the studies are conflicting. A study of 129 heterosexual women who gave a history of anal intercourse found no reports of "gross fecal incontinence" *(43)*. Similarly, Chun et al. *(164)* found that although the 14 anoreceptive homosexual males studied had significantly lower resting anal canal pressures when compared with the control group (10 non-anoreceptive heterosexual males), there were no complaints of fecal incontinence by the study subjects. In contrast, Miles et al. *(165)* found that a significant increase in fecal incontinence or urgency (requiring immediate defecation to avoid incontinence) in anoreceptive individuals. In addition, they found an inverse relationship between the maximum resting sphincter pressure and the estimated number of acts of anal intercourse. Not surprisingly, they also found that the more traumatic forms of anoreceptive practices such as brachioproctic intercourse (fisting) were more likely to result in objective sphincter dysfunction. Both the Chun and Miles studies used special equipment to measure the sphincter tone, and neither comments on whether sphincter laxity was apparent clinically in any of the subjects.

Interestingly, reflex anal dilatation (that is, dilatation of the external and internal anal sphincters when the buttocks are gently separated for 30 seconds), which has been said by many authors to be associated with anal intercourse, was not seen in any of the anoreceptive subjects in the Miles study group *(165)*.

10.6.3. Rectal Lacerations

Other, apparently rare, major complications that have been reported in adult males following penile anal intercourse are nonperforating and, less frequently, perforating lacerations of the rectal mucosa *(161,162)*. Mucosal lacerations are also seen in association with brachioproctic intercourse and the insertion of inanimate foreign bodies *(161,162)*. On occasions the injury may be fatal *(161,162)*. Slaughter et al. *(71)* described five rectal lacerations among eight women who underwent proctoscopy following "anal contact" during a sexual assault. The relation between the precise sexual act and the medical findings is not described.

10.6.4. Other Injuries

The other anal injuries that have been described in complainants of anal penetration are bruises (2–4%), abrasions (4–5%), erythema (2–8%), and swelling/edema (2–6%) *(71,110)*. Slaughter et al. *(71)* have described a high number of rectal injuries, in addition to the lacerations described above (ecchymosis, $n = 1$; abrasions, $n = 2$; redness, $n = 1$; swelling $n = 6$) detectable among eight sexual assaults complainants who described "anal contact" *(71)*. Although bruises are indicative of blunt trauma, the other findings may have innocent explanations, for example, a superficial abrasion of the anal verge has been identified on a child who interrupted the medical to pass a motion (observation of D. Rogers). Although erythema and swelling/edema are also nonspecific findings, if they have completely resolved at a follow-up examination it may be possible to relate them to the allegation. All these minor injuries would be expected to heal within 2 weeks of the incident without any residual scarring.

11. Lubricants

Traces of lubricant found on vaginal or internal anal swabs can provide confirmatory evidence of recent penetration of a body orifice. This has particular relevance if a condom is worn during a penetrative act. Consequently, the forensic practitioner must never use lubricant (other than sterile water) on specula, proctoscopes, or gloved digits when forensic swabs are to be taken from the anogenital areas.

In terms of lubricant analysis, the most frequent request received by the Forensic Science Service is to check vaginal swabs for the presence of condom lubricant. A review of cases at the Las Vegas Metropolitan Police Department found that 19 of 80 complainants reported that either the assailant had worn a condom during the incident or that they had experienced consensual intercourse with a partner wearing a condom within the 72 hours preceeding the assault *(166)*. The most commonly encountered lubricants applied directly to the penis to aid penetration are Vaseline (petroleum-based product) and KY Jelly (water-based product) *(167)*. However, various other substances have been used to facilitate penetration during a sexual assault including hand cream, cooking oil, and margarine, the diversity of the products apparently reflecting what is immediately at hand. Saliva is also used as a lubricant (*see* Sections 4. and 7.2.) *(168)*.

To maximize the possibility of lubricant detection, the necessary swabs should be obtained as soon as possible after the incident. The forensic science laboratory must then be told that lubricant analysis may be relevant as this potentially requires scientists from more than one discipline to examine the same sample, e.g., when both body fluids and lubricant analysis are requested. If the forensic science laboratory is not made aware of this requirement, potential evidence could be inadvertently destroyed during laboratory processes.

Many factors may affect the length of time that lubricant will persist on skin or in a body orifice. Condom lubricant has been detected on a swab taken from an unwashed penis 50 hours after intercourse and, in a different case, on a vaginal swab (also when the complainant had not washed or douched) taken 24 hours after intercourse, but detection after such prolonged periods would appear to be exceptional; water-based lubricants (e.g., those containing polyethylene glycol) have only been detected within 8 hours of the sexual act *(167,169)*.

12. Blood and Urine Analysis

12.1. Reason for Analysis

A sample of blood for analysis of the complainant's/suspect's DNA pattern should be taken whenever body fluid or tissue DNA typing may be relevant to the investigation.

When drugs or alcohol have been consumed, or possibly administered, prior to or during a sexual assault, consideration should be given to the need to obtain samples of blood and urine for toxicologic analysis. The length of time that a drug or its metabolites remain detectable in blood or urine will depend on a number of factors including the quantity taken, the metabolism of the individual, and the sensitivity and specificity of the analytical methods employed by the laboratory *(170)*. The metabolites of some substances may be excreted for up to 168 hours in the urine *(170)*. However, it cannot be presumed that the substances can be routinely detected for that length of time. In general, drugs and their metabolites will be identifiable for longer in urine than in blood. New methods of analysis may enable substances to be detectable for longer periods *(171)*, and the forensic practitioner must be aware of the capabilities of the local forensic science laboratory.

12.2. Method of Sampling

12.2.1. Blood

When both DNA and drug/alcohol analysis are potentially relevant to the sexual assault, a single sample of 10 mL of venous blood should be obtained. Approximately one-third of the sample (3 mL) is then placed in a container with EDTA or a similar preservative for DNA analysis. The remainder of the sample (7 mL) is placed in a container with an anticoagulant (e.g., potassium oxalate) and a preservative that prevents decomposition and fermentation (e.g., sodium fluoride) for drug and alcohol analysis. If it is not possible to obtain 10 ml of blood, e.g., from a young child, advice should be sought from the forensic science laboratory with regard to the minimum volumes that can be analyzed.

12.2.2. Urine

Ideally 20 mL of urine should be placed in a container with a preservative that prevents decomposition and fermentation (e.g., sodium fluoride), although samples in plain bottles can be analyzed.

12.3. Forensic Analysis

Forensic science laboratories have the capability of detecting a wide range of prescribed and illicit substances, but the persistence of different substances or their metabolites in the blood and urine of an individual depends on a number of factors. In some circumstances the forensic science laboratory may undertake back-calculations to estimate the blood alcohol concentration of the individual at the time of the sexual assault *(172)*.

Certain information is required to assist the forensic scientist with interpretation of the toxicologic results.

- Sex and body weight of the individual
- The time that any drugs/alcohol were consumed or believed to have been administered. Was it a single dose or more?
- The exact time that the blood and urine samples were taken
- Details of any prescribed medication or other substances normally consumed by the individual including quantity and the date and time of most recent use

13. Care of the Complainant

13.1. Medical Treatment

The medical facilities should be stocked with the necessary provisions to enable minor injuries to be cleaned and dressed. Analgesia may be required. On rare occasions a tetanus booster will be advisable.

13.2. Practical

The examination facilities should incorporate a shower or bath for the complainant to use after the medical is complete and a change of clothing should be available (preferably the patient's own garments). Complainants should have access to a telephone so that they can contact friends or relatives and should be encouraged to spend the next few days in the company of someone that they trust. On occasions, emergency alternative accommodation will need to be organized.

13.3. Pregnancy

Consideration must be given to the patient's risk of becoming pregnant. Whenever any risk is identified the patient should be counseled regarding the availability of hormonal and intrauterine methods of postcoital (emergency) contraception; the most suitable method will depend on the patient profile and the time since the assault *(173)*. When patients elect for insertion of an intrauterine contraceptive, they should be given prophylactic antibiotics (*see* below) either in advance of, or at the time of, the fitting. Follow-up appointments should be made at a convenient venue where pregnancy tests are available. Should the patient become pregnant because of the assault she must be referred for sympathetic counseling. If the pregnancy is terminated it may be relevant to seek permission from the patient for the products of conception to be retained for DNA analysis.

13.4. Sexually Transmitted Infections

Adult female complainants of sexual assault are at risk of acquiring a sexually transmitted infection (STI) as result of the assault *(174,175)*. Some male complainants have also described STI acquisition following the sexual assault *(143,144)*. In children who may have been sexually abused there is a low prevalence of infections that are definitely sexually transmitted, although other organisms possibly associated with sexual activity may be identified *(176)*.

As the relative risk of acquiring a particular STI will depend on the prevalence of that STI in the population, it would seem appropriate to apply the guidelines compiled by the American Academy of Pediatrics Committee on Child Abuse and Neglect with regard to STI testing in children to adults also. These guidelines state that STI testing should be done "when epidemiologically indicated or when the history and/or physical findings suggest the possibility of oral, genital or rectal contact" *(177)*.

Murphy *(178)* advocates STI screening for all adults at the time of presentation, presumably in recognition of the high default rate for follow-up consultations *(174,179)*. However, disclosure in court of preexisting STI can be detrimental to the complainant *(180)*. Consequently, it is recommended that the first tests be done 7–14 days after the assault. When interpreting the results of STI tests in young children, consideration must be given to the possibility that the sexually transmitted organisms could have been acquired perinatally *(176,181)*.

Some centers prescribe antibiotic prophylaxis for all complainants of penile penetrative sexual assaults at the time they present *(6,182,183)*, whereas others only prescribe prophylactic antibiotics when the assailant is known to have an infection, when the complainant has symptoms of infection, or if the complainant requests it *(178,184)*. Antibiotic prophylaxis should cover the prevalent, treatable, organisms in the local population, and advice should be sought from the local center for disease control regarding an appropriate regime.

No internationally accepted guidelines exist regarding whether hepatitis B virus (HBV) vaccination and/or hepatitis B immunoglobulin (HBIG) should be offered to all complainants of penile penetrative sexual assaults or only given when the assailant is at high risk of having been infected with HBV *(185)*. HBV vaccine has some efficiency in preventing HBV infection when given after HBV exposure. However, it is not known how soon after the sexual assault the HBV needs to be given to have an effect. Crowe et al. *(185)* suggest that an accelerated course of the vaccine (0 and 2 weeks, 3 months) commenced within 3 weeks of the exposure could be protective.

Similarly, there are no specific data regarding the effectiveness of HBIG following a sexual exposure to HBV. Some authors recommend that HBIG be given ". . . within 14 days of exposure to HBV through sexual contact with a person who has acute or chronic HBV infection" *(182)*, whereas other guidelines suggest that ideally it should be given within 48 hours of the exposure and certainly no later than 1 week *(186)*.

There is a continuing debate regarding the provision of preventive antiretroviral treatment [post-exposure prophylaxis (PEP)] following possible sexual exposure to human immunodeficiency virus (HIV). Desmond and Coker *(187)* propose that PEP should be offered following sexual assault if the assailant is known or strongly suspected to be seropositive for HIV. They suggest that if the HIV status of the assailant or the contact is unknown, then initiating PEP should be decided on a case by case basis, depending on the likelihood of HIV transmission in the sexual contact. Evans and colleagues *(188)* take a somewhat contrary view, stating that PEP "will seldom, if ever, be justified in heterosexual exposures where the HIV infection status of the partner is unknown." They also state that although the highest risk of sexual transmission of HIV is from unprotected receptive anal intercourse (transmission risk per sex act of 0.01), "It would be difficult to justify the use of potentially toxic drugs for any exposure involving a sexual partner of unknown HIV status when the benefit-risk ratios are so low" *(188)*. However, they do acknowledge that "Risks (of contracting HIV following a sexual exposure) will depend on the background prevalence of HIV in the population and knowledge of this will be crucial if PEP is considered without the knowledge of the HIV status of the partner." Furthermore, there is no information regarding the maximum time between sexual exposure and prophylaxis for which the PEP is likely to be effective. Animal studies suggest that the sooner it is given the greater the chance of preventing seroconversion, although it still may be effective up to 14 days after exposure *(189)*.

Whether prophylaxis is given or not, complainants should be counseled and offered baseline serologic tests for syphilis, hepatitis B, and HIV, which will be repeated at the relevant periods after assault.

13.5. Psychological

Complainants of sexual assault must be offered immediate and ongoing counseling to help them cope with the recognized immediate and long-term psychological sequelae of a sexual assault *(190)*. Some examination facilities have 24-hour access to trained counselors *(191)*.

References

1. Bays, J. and Chadwick, D. (1993) Medical diagnosis of the sexually abused child. *Child Abuse Negl.* **17,** 91–110.
2. Heger, A. H. and Emans, S. J., eds. (1992) *Evaluation of the Sexually Abused Child.* Oxford University Press, New York.
3. Royal College of Physicians (1997) *Physical Signs of Sexual Abuse in Children*, RCP, London.
4. General Medical Council (1996) *Intimate Examinations*. GMC, London.
5. Hicks, D. J. (1980) Rape: sexual assault. *Am J Obstet Gynecol.* **137,** 931–935.
6. Evrard, J. R. and Gold, G. M. (1979) Epidemiology and management of sexual assault victims. *Obstet Gynecol.* **53,** 381–387.

7. Keating, S. M. and Allard, J. E. (1994) What's in a name? Medical samples and scientific evidence in sexual assaults. *Med Sci Law.* **34,** 187–201.
8. Keating, S. M. (1988) The laboratory's approach to sexual asssault cases. Part 1: Sources of information and acts of intercourse. *J Forensic Sci Soc.* **28,** 35–47.
9. Clark, M. D. B. (1979) Metropolitan Police Laboratory Examination Kit for Sexual Offences. *Police Surg.* **15,** 447–452.
10. Ranson, D. (1996) The forensic medical examination, in *Forensic Medicine and the Law*, Melbourne University Press, Victoria, pp. 119–127.
11. Kafarowski, E., Lyon, A. M., and Sloan, M. M. (1996) The retention and transfer of spermatozoa in clothing by machine washing. *Can Soc Forensic Sci J.* **29,** 7–11.
12. Benecke, M. (1997) DNA typing in forensic medicine and in criminal investigations: a current survey. *Naturwissenschaften.* **84,** 181–188.
12a. Mannucci, A., Sullivan, K. M., Ivanov, P. L., and Gill, P. (1994) Forensic application of a rapid and quantitative DNA sex test by amplification of the X-Y homologous gene amelogenin. *Int J Leg Med.* **106,** 190–193.
13. Monckton, D. G. and Jeffreys, A.J. (1993) DNA profiling. *Curr Opin Biotechnol.* **4,** 660–664.
14. Tully, G. (1998) *Personal communication.* Manager of mitochondrial DNA Unit, Metropolitan Laboratory Forensic Science Service.
15. Sweet, D. J. (1995) Human bite marks—examination, recovery and analysis, in *Manual of Forensic Odontology* (Bowers, C. M. and Bell, G. L., eds.), American Society of Forensic Odontology, Colorado Springs, CO.
16. Clift, A. and Lamont, C. M. (1974) Saliva in forensic odontology. *J Forensic Sci Soc.* **14,** 241–245.
17. Bowers, C. M. and Bell, G. L., eds. (1995) *Manual of Forensic Odontology.* American Society of Forensic Odontology, Colorado Springs, CO.
18. Morrison, K. J. (1983) Selected cases in forensic medicine. *Police Surg.* **24,** 63–64.
19. Girardin, B. W., Faugno, D. K., Seneski, P. C., Slaughter, L., and Whelan, M. (1997) Care of the sexually assaulted patient, in *Color Atlas of Sexual Assault.* Mosby, St. Louis, p. 96.
20. Lynnerup, N. and Hjalgrim, H. (1995) Routine use of ultraviolet light in medicolegal examinations to evaluate stains and skin trauma. *Med Sci Law.* **35,** 165–168.
21. Jones, D. N. (1963) The task of the Forensic Science Laboratory in the investigation of sexual offences. *J Forensic Sci Soc.* **3,** 88–93.
22. Sweet, D., Lorente, J. A., Lorente, M., and Villanueva, E. (1997) PCR-based DNA typing of saliva stains recovered from human skin. *J Forensic Sci Soc.* **42,** 447–451.
23. Cartwright, P. S. (1986) Reported sexual assault in Nashville-Davidson County, Tennessee, 1980–1982. *Am J Obstet Gynecol.* **154,** 1064–1068.
24. Everett, R. B. and Jimerson, G. K. (1977) The rape victim: a review of 117 consecutive cases. *Obstet Gynecol.* **50,** 88–90.
25. Soules, M. R., Stewart, S. K., Brown, K. M., and Pollard, A. A. (1978) The spectrum of alleged rape. *J Reprod Med.* **20,** 33–39.

26. Clark, D. (1996) Forensic odontology, in *Cinical Forensic Medicine* (McLay, W. D. S., ed.), Greenwich Medical Media, Hong Kong, pp. 287–295.
27. Vale, G. L. and Noguchi, T. T. (1983) Anatomical distribution of human bite marks in a series of 67 cases. *J Forensic Sci Soc.* **28,** 61–69.
28. Wright, R. and West, D. J. (1981) Rape—a comparison of group offences and lone assaults. *Med Sci Law.* **21,** 25–30.
29. Lewington, F. (1994) *Personal communication.* Metropolitan Police Forensic Science Laboratory.
30. Ledray, L. (1993) Evidence collection: an update. *J Sexual Abuse.* **2,** 113–115.
31. Young, W., Bracken, A. C., Goddard, M. A. A., and Matheson, S. (1992) The New Hampshire sexual assault medical examination protocol project committee sexual assault: review of a national model protocol for forensic and medical evaluation. *Obstet Gynecol.* **80,** 878–883.
32. Cooke, R., Webb-Salter, M. T., and Marshall, L. (1997) The significance of fibres found in head hair. *Forensic Sci Int.* **87,** 155–160.
33. McKenna, F. J. and Sherwin, J. C. (1975) A simple and effective method for collecting contact evidence. *J. Forensic Sci Soc.* **15,** 277–280.
34. Exline, D. L., Smith, F. P., and Drexler, S. G. (1998) Frequency of pubic hair transfer during sexual intercourse. *J Forensic Sci.* **43,** 505–508.
35. Mann, M. J. (1990) Hair transfers in sexual assault: a six year case study. *J Forensic Sci Soc.* **35,** 951–955.
36. Stone, I. C. (1982) Hair and its probative value as evidence. *Texas Bar J.* **45,** 275–279.
37. Riis, R. (1990) Sexual assault combing evidence. Presented at the NWAFS Meeting, Jackson Hole, WY.
38. Higuchi, R., Von Beroldingen, C. H., Sensabaugh, G. F., and Erlich, H. A. (1988) DNA typing from single hairs. *Nature.* **332,** 543–546.
39. Enos, W. F. and Beyer, J. C. (1981) The importance of examining skin and hair for semen in sexual assault cases. *J Forensic Sci Soc.* **26,** 605–607.
40. Moore, E. (1998) *Personal communication.* Chorley Laboratory FSS.
41. Harris, E. (1998) *Personal communication.* Metropolitan Laboratory Forensic Science Service.
42. Thomas, F. and Baert, H. (1965) A new means of identification of the human being: the longitudinal striation of the nails. *Med Sci Law.* **5,** 39–40.
43. Evans, B. A., Bond, R. A., and Macrae, K. D. (1988) Sexual behaviour in women attending a genitourinary medicine clinic. *Genitourin Med.* **64,** 43–48.
44. Keating, S. M. and Higgs, D. F. (1992) Oral sex—further information from sexual assault cases. *J Forensic Sci Soc.* **32,** 327–331.
45. Bradham, G. B. (1981) The establishment of a treatment center for victims of rape. *JSC Med Assoc.* **June,** 283–286.
46. Girardin, B. W., Faugno, D. K., Seneski, P. C., Slaughter, L., and Whelan, M. (1997) Findings in sexual assault and consensual intercourse, in *Color Atlas of Sexual Assault*, Mosby, St. Louis, p. 19.
47. Lind, W. and Carlson, D. (1995) Recovery of semen from chewing gum in an oral sexual assault. *J Forensic Identification.* **45,** 280–282.

48. Hampton, H. L. (1995) Care of the woman who has been raped. *N Engl J Med.* **332,** 234–237.
49. Newman, J. (1998) *Personal communication.* Centre of Forensic Sciences, Toronto.
50. Willott, G. M. and Crosse, M. A. (1986) The detection of spermatozoa in the mouth. *J Forensic Sci Soc.* **26,** 125–128.
51. Allard, J. E. (1997) The collection of data from findings in cases of sexual assault and the significance of spermatozoa on vaginal, anal and oral swabs. *Sci Justice.* **37,** 99–108.
52. Enos, W. F. and Beyer, J. C. (1978) Spermatozoa in the anal canal and rectum and in the oral cavity of female rape victims. *J Forensic Sci Soc.* **23,** 231–233.
53. Forensic scientists (1998) *Personal communications.* Metropolitan Laboratory Forensic Science Service.
54. Schlesinger, S. L., Borbotsina, J., and O'Neill, L. (1975) Petechial hemorrhages of the soft palate secondary to fellatio. *Oral Surg.* **40,** 376–378.
55. Giansanti, J. S., Cramer, J. R., and Weathers, D. R. (1975) Palatal erythema, another etiologic factor. *Oral Surg.* **40,** 379–381.
56. Damm, D. D., White, D. K., and Brinker, C. M. (1981) Variations of palatal erythema secondary to fellatio. *Oral Surg.* **52,** 417–421.
57. Girardin, B. W., Faugno, D. K., Seneski, P. C., Slaughter, L., and Whelan, M. (1997) Findings in sexual asault and consensual intercourse, in *Color Atlas of Sexual Assault*, Mosby, St. Louis, p. 41.
58. Bellizzi, R., Krakow, A. M., and Plack, W. (1980) Soft palate trauma associated with fellatio: case report. *Mil Med.* **145,** 787–788.
59. Girardin, B. W., Faugno, D. K., Seneski, P. C., Slaughter, L., and Whelan, M. (1997) Findings in sexual asault and consensual intercourse, in *Color Atlas of Sexual Assault*, Mosby, St. Louis, p. 38.
60. Johnson, A. M., Wadsworth, J., Wellings, K., and Field, J. (1994) Heterosexual practices, in *Sexual Attitudes and Lifestyles*, Blackwell Scientific Publications, Oxford, p. 160.
61. Bolling, D. R., (1977) Prevalence, goals and complications of heterosexual anal intercourse in a gynecologic population. *J Reprod Med.* **19,** 121–124.
62. Keating, S. M. (1988) Oral sex—a review of its prevalence and proof. *J Forensic Sci Soc.* **28,** 341–355.
63. Rook, P. and Ward, R. (1997) Indecent assault, in *Rook & Ward on Sexual Offences*, 2nd ed., Sweet & Maxwell, London pp. 2,49.
64. Keating, S. M. and Higgs D. F. (1994) The detection of amylase on swabs from sexual assault cases. *J Forensic Sci Soc.* **34,** 89–93.
65. Skerlavy, M., Epstein, J. A., and Sobrero, A. J. (1968) Cervical mucus amylase levels in normal menstrual cycles. *Fertil Steril.* **19,** 726–730.
66. Banaschak, S., Moller, K., and Pfeiffer, H. (1998) Potential DNA mixtures introduced through kissing. *Int J Leg Med.* **111,** 284–285.
67. Mader, C. L. (1981) Lingual frenulum ulcer resulting from orogenital sex. *J Am Dent Assoc.* **103,** 888–890.

68. Johnson, A. M., Wadsworth, J., Wellings, K., and Field, J. (1994) Heterosexual practices, in *Sexual Attitudes and Lifestyles*, Blackwell Scientific Publications, Oxford.
69. Howitt, J. and Rogers, D. J. (1996) Adult sexual offences and related matters, in *Clinical Forensic Medicine*, McLay, W. D. S., ed., Greenwich Medical Media, Hong Kong. p. 193.
70. Lines 1844 I.C. and K. 393.
71. Slaughter, L., Brown, C. R. V., Crowley, S., and Peck, R. (1997) Patterns of genital injury in female sexual assault victims. *Am J Obstet Gynecol.* **176,** 609–616.
72. Jenny, C., Kunhs, M. L., and Fukiko, A. (1987) Presence of hymens in newborn female infants. *Pediatrics.* **80,** 399–400.
73. Chadwick, D. L., Berkowitz, C. D., Kerns, D., McCann, J., Reinhart, M. A., and Strickland, S. (1989) *Color Atlas of Child Sexual Abuse*, Year Book Medical Publishers, Chicago.
74. Goodyear-Smith, F. A. and Laidlaw, T. M. (1998) What is an "intact" hymen? A critique of the literature. *Med Sci Law.* **38,** 289–301.
75. Emans, S. J., Woods, E., Allred, E., and Grace, E. (1994) Hymenal findings in adolescent women, impact of tampon use and consensual sexual activity. *Pediatrics* **125,** 153–160.
76. Berensen, A. (1994) The prepubertal genital examination: what is normal and abnormal. *Curr Opin Obstet Gynaecol.* **6,** 526–530.
77. Muram, D. (1992) Anatomic and Physiological changes, in *Evaluation of the Sexually Abused Child*, Oxford University Press, New York, p. 72.
78. Emans, S. J. H. and Goldstein, D. P. (1990) The physiology of puberty, in *Pediatric and Adolescent Gynecology*, 3rd ed., Little, Brown, Boston, pp. 95–97.
79. Porkucny, S. F. (1987) Configuration of the prepubertal hymen. *Am J Obstet Gynecol.* **157,** 950–956.
80. Girardin, B. W., Faugno, D. K., Seneski, P. C., Slaughter, L., and Whelan, M. (1997) Care of the sexually assaulted patient, in *Color Atlas of Sexual Assault*, Mosby, St. Louis, pp. 111–118.
81. Masters, W. H. and Johnson, V. E. (1966) The vagina, in *The Human Sexual Response*, Little Brown, Boston. pp. 69–70.
82. Robinson, E. G. (1976) Management of the rape victim. *CMA J.* **115,** 520–523.
83. Reade, D. J. (1986) Early scientific investigations of sexual assault. *Police Surg.* **April,** 42–46.
84. Eungprabhanth, V. (1974) Finding of the spermatozoa in the vagina related to elapsed time of coitus. *Z Rechtamedizin.* **74,** 301–304.
85. Florence, A. (1896). Du sperme et des taches de sperme en medecine legale. *Arch d'Anthropol Criminelle d Criminolo Psychol Normale Pathol.* **11,** 146–165.
86. Laurell, C. B. (1972). Electroimmunoassay. *Scand J Clin Lab Invest.* **29,** 21.
87. Divall, G. B. (1985) Methods for the identification and menstrual blood, in *Advances in Forensic Science*, Lee, H.G. and Gaensslen, R.E., eds., Biomedical Publications, pp. 1–14.

88. Allard, J. (1996) The facts of life. *Contact-FSS Internal Publication*. 25.
89. Davis, A. and Wilson, E. (1974) The persistence of seminal constituents in the human vagina. *Forensic Sci.* **3,** 45–55.
90. Graves, H. C. B., Sensabaugh, G. F., and Blake, E. T. (1985) Postcoital detection of a male-specific semen protein: application to the investigation of rape. *N Engl J Med.* **312,** 338–340.
91. Wilson, E. M. (1982) A comparison of the persistence of seminal constituents in the human vagina and cervix. *Police Surg.* **22,** 44–45.
92. Keating, S. M. (1988) The laboratory's approach to sexual assault cases. Part 2. Demonstration of the possible offender. *J Forensic Sci Soc.* **28,** 99–110.
93. Gaensslen, R. E. (1983) Survival of spermatozoa in the vagina, in *Sourcebook in Forensic Serology, Immunology and Biochemistry*, Gaensslen, R. E., ed., United States Government Printing Office, Washington DC, pp. 144–152.
94. Silverman, E. M. and Silverman, A. G. (1978) Persistence of spermatozoa in the lower genital tracts of women. *JAMA.* **240,** 1875–1877.
95. Rupp, J. C. (1969) Sperm survival and prostatic acid phosphatase activity in victims of sexual assault. *J Forensic Sci Soc.* **14,** 177–183.
96. Paul, D. M. (1984) Examination of the living, in *Taylor's Principles and Practice of Medical Jurisprudence*, 13th ed., Mant A. K., ed., Churchill Livingstone, Edinburgh, pp. 64–105.
97. Allard, J. E. (1997) The collection of data from findings in cases of sexual assault and the significance of spermatozoa on vaginal, anal and oral swabs. *Sci Justice.* **37,** 99–108.
98. Hadkiss, C. (1998) *Personal communication*. Forensic Science Service.
99. Slaughter, L. and Brown, C. R. V. (1992) Colposcopy to establish physical findings in rape victims. *Am J Obstet Gynecol.* **166,** 83–86.
100. Cartwright, P. S., Moore, R. A., Anderson, J. R., and Brown, D. H. (1986) Genital injury and implied consent to alleged rape. *J Reprod Med.* **31,** 1043–1044.
101. Ramin, S. M., Satin, A. J., Stone, S. C., and Wendel, G. D. (1992) Sexual assault in postmenopausal women. *Obstet Gynecol.* **80,** 860–864.
102. Patel, H. C., Courtney, G. M., and Forster, G. E. (1993) Colposcopy and rape [letter]. *Am J Obstet Gynecol.* **168,** 1334.
103. Slaughter, L. and Brown, C. R. V. (1993) Colposcopy and rape [letter]. *Am J Obstet Gynecol.* **168,** 1335.
104. Norvell, M. K., Benrubi, G. I., and Thompson, R. J. (1984) Investigations of microtrauma after sexual intercourse. *J Reprod Med.* **29,** 269–271.
105. Lauber, A. A. and Souma, M. L. (1982) Use of toluidine blue for documentation of traumatic intercourse. *Obstet Gynecol.* **60,** 644–648.
106. McCauley, J., Gorman, R. L., and Guzinski, G. (1986) Toluidine blue in the detection of perineal lacerations in pediatric and adolescent sexual abuse victims. *Pediatrics.* **78,** 1039–1043.
107. McCauley, J., Guzinski, G., Welch, R., Gorman, R., and Osmers, F. (1987) Toluidine blue in the corroboration of rape in adult victim. *Am J Emerg Med.* **5,** 105–108.

108. Wilson, K. F. G. (1966) Lower genital tract trauma. *Aust NZJ Obstet Gynaecol.* **6,** 291–293.
109. Bowyer, L. and Dalton, M. E. (1997) Female victims of rape and their genital injuries. *Br J Obstet Gynecol.* **104,** 617–620.
110. Manser, T. (1991) Findings in medical examinations of victims and offenders in cases of serious sexual offences—a survey. *Police Surg.* **38,** 4–27.
111. Kellogg, N. D. and Parra, J. M. (1991) Linea vestibularis: a previously undescribed normal genital structure in female neonates. *Pediatrics.* **87,** 926–929.
112. De San Lazaro, C. and Sivaramakrishnan, S. (1998) Summer sandal genital injury. *J Clin Forensic Med.* **5,** 32–33.
113. Dowd, M. D., Fitzmaurice, L., Knapp, J. F., and Mooney, D. (1994). The interpretation of urogenital findings in children with straddle injuries. *J Pediatr Surg.* **29,** 7–10.
114. Ferrell, J. (1995) Sexual assault: clinical issues, Foley catheter balloon technique for visualizing the hymen in female adolescent sexual abuse victims. *J Emerg Nurs.* **21,** 585–586.
115. Muram, D. (1989) Child sexual abuse: relationship between sexual acts and genital findings. *Child Abuse Negl.* **13,** 211–216.
116. McCann, J., Voris, J., and Simon, M. (1993) Genital injuries resulting from sexual abuse: a longitudinal study. *Pediatrics.* **89,** 307–317.
117. Berkowitz, C., Evik, S., and Logan, M. (1993) A simulated 'acquired' imperforate hymen following the genital trauma of sexual abuse. *Clin Pediatr.* **26,** 307–309.
118. Teixera, W. (1981) Hymenal colposcopic examination in sexual offences. *Am J Forensic Med Pathol.* **3,** 201–214
119. Underhill, R. and Dewhurst, J. (1978) The doctor cannot always tell: medical examination of the 'intact' hymen. *Lancet.* **i,** 375–376
120. Wilson, F. and Swartz, D. P. (1972) Coital injuries of the vagina. *Obstet Gynecol.* **39,** 182–184.
121. Fish, S. A. (1956) Vaginal injury due to coitus. *Am J Obstet Gynecol.* **72,** 544–548.
122. Metsala, P. and Nieminen, U. (1968) Traumatic lesions of the vagina. *Acta Obstet Gynecol Scand.* **47,** 483–488.
123. Gray, M. J., Norton, P., and Treadwell, K. (1981) Tampon-induced injuries. *Obstet Gynecol.* **58,** 667–668.
124. Hakanson, E. Y. (1966) Trauma to the female genitalia. *Lancet.* **86,** 286–291.
125. Burgess, A. W. and Holmstrom, L. L. (1973) The rape victim in the emergency ward. *Am J Nurs.* **73,** 1741–1745.
126. Slaughter, L. and Brown, C. R. V. (1991) Cervical findings in rape victims. *Am J Obstet Gynecol.* **164,** 528–529.
127. Masters, W. H. and Johnson, V. E. (1966) The penis, in *The Human Sexual Response*, Little Brown, Boston, pp. 171–203.
128. Muram, D. (1992) Anatomy, in *Evaluation of the Sexually Abused Child*, Hegar, A. and Emans, S. J., eds., Oxford University Press, New York, p. 73.

129. Girardin, B. W., Faugno, D. K., Seneski, P. C., Slaughter, L., and Whelan, M. (1997) Anatomy and the human sexual response, in *Color Atlas of Sexual Asault*, Mosby, St. Louis, p. 11.
130. Farah, R. and Cerny, J. C. (1973) Penis tourniquet syndrome and penile amputation. *Urology.* **11,** 310–311.
131. Garty, B. Z., Mimouni, M., and Varsano, I. (1983) Penile tourniquet sydrome. *Cutis.* **31,** 431–432.
132. Kerry, R. L. and Chapman, D. D. (1973) Strangulation of appendages by hair and thread. *Pediatr Surg.* **8,** 23–27.
133. Wheatley, J. K. (1983) Genital injury during intercourse. *Med Aspects Hum Sex.* **17,** 24 A–J.
134. Ball, T. P. and Pickett, J. D. (1975) Traumatic lymphangitis of penis. *Urology.* **IV,** 594–597.
135. Davies, D. M. and Mitchell, I. (1978) Fracture of the penis. *Br J Urol.* **50,** 426.
136. Pryor, J. P., Hill, J. T., Packham, D. A., and Yates-Bell, A. J. (1981) Penile injuries with particular reference to injury to the erectile tissue. *Br J Urol.* **53,** 42–46.
137. Paul, D. M. (1977) The medical examination of the live rape victim and the accused. *Leg Med Ann.* 139–153.
138. Wells, D. L. (1996) Genital trauma amongst young boys. *J Clin Forensic Med.* **3,** 129–132.
139. Hobbs, C. J. and Wynne. J. M. (1996) Physical signs of child abuse. W. B. Saunders, Philadelphia.
140. Johnson, A. M., Wadsworth, J., Wellings, K., and Field, J. (1994) Heterosexual practices, in *Sexual Attitudes and Lifestyles*, Blackwell Scientific Publications, Oxford, p. 163.
141. Johnson, A. M., Wadsworth, J., Wellings, K., and Field, J. (1994) Sexual diversity and homosexual behaviour, in *Sexual Attitudes and Lifestyles*, Blackwell Scientific Publications, Oxford, pp. 183–223.
142. Bang, L. (1993) Rape victims—assaults, injuries and treatment at a medical rape trauma service at Oslo Emergency Hospital. *Scand J Primary Health Care.* **11,** 15–20.
143. Hillman, R. J., O'Mara, N., Taylor-Robinson, D., and Williams Harris, J. R. (1990) Medical and social aspects of sexual assault of males: a survey of 100 victims. *Br J Gen Pract.* **40,** 502–504.
144. Hillman, R., O'Mara, N., Tomlinson, D., and William Harris, J. R. (1991) Adult male victims of sexual assault: an underdiagnosed condition. *Int J STD AIDS.* **2,** 22–24.
145. Temkin, J. (1987) *Rape and the Legal Process.* Sweet & Maxwell, London.
146. Royal College of Physicians (1997) Glossary of terms, in *Physical Signs of Sexual Abuse in Children.* RCP, London, pp. 67,68.
147. Girardin, B. W., Faugno, D. K., Seneski, P. C., Slaughter, L., and Whelan, M. (1997) Anatomy and the human sexual response, in *Color Atlas of Sexual Assault*, Mosby, St. Louis, pp. 14–16.

148. Fenger, C. (1997) Anal canal, in *Histology for Pathologists*, 2nd ed., (Sternberg, S. S., ed.), Lippincott-Raven, Philadelphia, pp. 551–571.
149. Nivatovongs, S., Stern, H. S., and Fryd, D. S. (1981) The length of the anal canal. *Dis Colon Rectum.* **24,** 600–611.
150. Goligher, J. (1984) Surgical anatomy and physiology of the anus, rectum and colon, in *Surgery of the Anus, Rectum and Colon*, 5th ed., Baillière Tindall, London, p. 15.
151. Parks, A. G., Porter, N. H., and Melzak, J., (1962) Experimental study of the reflex mechanism controlling the muscles of the pelvic floor. *Dis Colon Rectum.* **5,** 401–414.
152. Davies, A. (1979) Discussion of spermatozoa in the anal canal and rectum and in the oral cavity of female rape victims. *J Forensic Sci Soc.* **24,** 541–542.
153. Green, R. J. and Sayce, M. D. (1985). Problems associated with the typing of semen on anal swabs. *J Forensic Sci Soc.* **25,** 55,56
154. Willott, G. M. and Allard, J. E. (1982) Spermatozoa—their persistence after sexual intercourse. *Forensic Sci Int.* **19,** 135–154.
155. Allard, J. (1998) *Personal communication.* Metropolitan Laboratory Forensic Science Service.
156. Bush, R. A. and Owen, W. F. (1986) Trauma and other noninfectious problems in homosexual men. *Med Clin North Am.* **70,** 549–566.
157. Goligher, J. (1984) Anal fissure, in *Surgery of the Anus, Rectum and Colon*, 5th ed., Baillière Tindall, London, p. 150.
158. Keighley, M. R. B. and Williams, N. S. (1993) Fissure in ano, in *Surgery of the Anus, Rectum and Colon.* Saunders, Philadelphia, pp. 364–386.
159. Girardin, B. W., Faugno, D. K., Seneski, P. C., Slaughter, L., and Whelan, M. (1997) Findings in sexual asault and consensual intercourse, in *Color Atlas of Sexual Assault*, Mosby, St. Louis, p. 50.
160. Girardin, B. W., Faugno, D. K., Seneski, P. C., Slaughter, L., and Whelan, M. (1997) Glossary, in *Color Atlas of Sexual Assault*, Mosby, St. Louis, p. 192.
161. Crass, R. A., Tranbaugh, R. F., Kudsk, K. A., and Trunkey, D. D. (1981) Colorectal foreign bodies and perforation. *Am J Surg.* **142,** 85–88.
162. Barone, J. E., Yee, J., and Nealon, T. F. (1983) Management of foreign bodies and trauma of the rectum. *Surg Gynecol Obstet.* **56,** 453–457.
163. Rakotomalala, L., de Parades, V., Parisot, C., and Atienza, P. (1996) Ruptures multiples du sphincter interne après viol anal: une cause peu connue d'incontinence anale. *Gastroenterol Clin Biol.* **20,** 1142,1143.
164. Chun, A. B., Rose, S., Mitrani, C., Silvestre, A. J., and Wald, A. (1997) Anal sphincter structure and function in homosexual males engaging in anoreceptive intercourse. *Am J Gastroenterol.* **92,** 465–468.
165. Miles, A. J. G., Allen-Mersh, T. G., and Wastell, C. (1993) Effect of anoreceptive intercourse on anorectal function. *J R Soc Med.* **86,** 144–147.
166. Cook, T. L. (1993) Personal communication with Blackledge, R.D., author of: Condom trace evidence: a new factor in sexual assault investigations (1996) *FBI Law Enforcement Bull.* **May,** 12–16.

167. Greaves, C. (1998) Safe sex?—Is it so safe? *Contact-FSS Internal Publication.* **25,** 20–21.
168. Keating, S. M. (1992) *Personal communication.* Metropolitan Laboratory Forensic Science Service.
169. Blackledge, R. D. and Vincenti, M. (1994) Identification of polydimethylsiloxane lubricant traces from latex condoms in cases of sexual assault. *J Forensic Sci Soc.* **34,** 245–256.
170. Jansen, K. (1998) Date rape drugs. *Bull Int Assoc Forensic Toxicol.* **28,** 18–20.
171. Guterman, L. (1998) Nailing the drug rapists. *New Scientist.* **December,** 4.
172. Ferner, R. E. (1996) Ethanol, in *Forensic Pharmacology*, Oxford University Press, Oxford, pp. 122–124.
173. Kubba, A. and Wilkinson, C. (1998) *Recommendations for Clinical Practice: Emergency Contraception.* FFP & RHC RCOG, London.
174. Jenny, C., Hooton, T. M., Bowers, A., Copass, M. K., Krieger, J. N., Hillier, S. L., et al. (1990) Sexually transmitted diseases in victims of rape. *N Engl J Med.* **322,** 713–716.
175. Estreich, S., Forster, G. E., and Robinson, A. (1990) Sexually transmitted diseases in rape victims. *Genitourin Med.* **66,** 433–438.
176. Robinson, A. J., Watkeys, J. E. M., and Ridgeway, G. L. (1998) Sexually transmitted organisms in sexually abused children. *Arch Dis Child.* **79,** 356–358.
177. American Academy of Pediatrics Committee on Child Abuse and Neglect (1997) Guidelines for the evaluation of sexual abuse of children. *Del Med J* **69,** 405–412.
178. Murphy, S. (1990) Rape, sexually transmited diseases and human immunodeficiency virus infection. *Int J STD AIDS.* **1,** 79–82.
179. Ross, J. D. C., Scott, G. R., and Busuttil, A. (1991) Rape and sexually transmitted diseases: patterns of referral and incidence in a department of genitourinary medicine. *J R Soc Med.* **84,** 657–659.
180. Lacey, H. B. (1991) Rape, the law and medical practitioners. *Br J Sex Med.* **Winter,** 89–92.
181. Hammerschlag, M. R. (1998) Sexually transmitted diseases in sexually abused children: medical and legal implications. *Sex Transm Inf.* **74,** 167–174.
182. Girardin, B. W., Faugno, D. K., Seneski, P. C., Slaughter, L., and Whelan, M. (1997) Care of the sexually assaulted patient, in *Color Atlas of Sexual Assault*, Mosby, St. Louis, p. 123.
183. Hochbaum, S. R. (1987) The evaluation and treatment of the sexually assaulted patient. *Emerg Med Clin North Am.* **5,** 601–622.
184. Glaser, J. B., Hammerschlag, M. R., and McCormack, W. M. (1989) Epidemiology of sexually transmitted diseases in rape victims. *Rev Infec Dis.* **11,** 246–254.
185. Crowe, C., Forster, G. E., Dinsmore, W. W., and Maw, R. D. (1996) A case of acute hepatitis B occurring four months after multiple rape. *Int J STD AIDS.* **7,** 133–134.
186. Salisbury, D. M. and Begg, N. T. (eds.) (1996) *Immunization Against Infectious Diseases*, Her Majesty's Stationery Office, London.

187. Desmond, N. M. and Coker, R. J. (1998) Should preventive antiretroviral treatment be offered following sexual exposure to HIV? *Sex Transm Inf.* **74,** 144,145.
188. Evans, B., Darbyshire, J., and Cartledge, J. (1998) Should preventive antiretroviral treatment be offered following sexual exposure to HIV? *Sex Transm Inf.* **74,** 146–148.
189. National HIV Prevention Information Service (1998) Post-exposure prophylaxis (PEP) against HIV infection following sexual and injection drug use exposure. Edward King of NAM Publications, London.
190. Burgess, A. W. and Holmstrom, L. L. (1974) Rape trauma syndrome. *Am J Psychiatry.* **131,** 981–986.
191. Duddle, M. (1991) Emotional sequelae of sexual assault. *J R Soc Med.* **84,** 26–28

Chapter 4

Injury Interpretation

Jack Crane

1. Introduction

All doctors, not just those engaged in forensic practice, should be able to describe and record injuries accurately. In most circumstances, except when the victim is dead, the doctor's first responsibility is usually the treatment of the injury, an obvious priority that may overshadow the necessity to make detailed contemporaneous notes of the findings. Also, as this initial examination has not been carried out for medicolegal purposes, the forensic significance of the injuries may not become apparent until many weeks or months later. Scrutiny of the doctor's notes at a later stage, possibly in court, may reveal serious deficiencies, which not only bring discredit on the individual practitioner and the profession as a whole but could seriously prejudice the legal proceedings.

Although the accurate description of injuries should fall within the capabilities of most doctors, their interpretation requires considerable skill and expertise and often is best left to a forensic physician or pathologist. Nevertheless, other doctors should be able to offer some advice and comment, albeit of a general nature, on how a particular injury or group of injuries was caused. Indeed, in some circumstances it is the ordinary practitioner who draws attention to the possible medicolegal significance of some injuries and initiates an investigation into their cause, e.g., pediatricians in cases of nonaccidental injury in children.

From: *Forensic Science: A Physician's Guide to Clinical Forensic Medicine*
Edited by: M. M. Stark © Humana Press, Inc., Totowa, NJ

2. Describing Injuries

When describing an injury, it is essential to comment on the nature of the wound, its size and shape, and its location. The age of the injury also needs to be considered although usually it is only possible to term it recent or nonrecent. It is extremely useful to record injuries on body charts or anatomic line drawings, which can be used in court if the practitioner is called to give evidence. In cases of serious assault or when injuries have distinctive characteristics or patterning, it is essential that the wounds be photographed with a suitable metric scale alongside. Self-adhesive tape incorporating both imperial and metric graduations is readily available for this purpose.

2.1. Nature of the Injury

In this chapter the terms wound and injury are used synonymously; however, in legal terms a "wound" requires the integrity of the skin surface to be breached and theoretically at least would exclude bruising and indeed abrasions *(1)*. Furthermore, the commonest reason why medical evidence on injuries given in court is contentious is the confusing assortment of terms used by doctors and the inappropriate or inaccurate description of a wound, e.g., using the term "laceration" to describe a clean-cut wound caused by a bladed weapon, such as a knife, when the wound was in fact an incision. It is therefore essential that for medicolegal purposes a standard nomenclature be adopted when describing injuries. The following classification is that adopted by forensic physicians and pathologists *(2)*:

- Bruises—often called contusions
- Abrasions—also known as scratches
- Lacerations—sometimes known as cuts and tears
- Incisions—colloquially called slashes
- Stab wounds—sometimes known as penetrating wounds

It must, of course, be recognized that a variety of wound types may coexist following trauma. Furthermore, a single wound may show features of different types—an abrasion within which is a laceration, a bruised abrasion, etc.

2.2. Size and Shape of the Injury

Even though the size of an injury is perhaps the easiest measurement to ascertain, it is probably the commonest omission from medical records. It should be ascertained using a ruler or a pair of callipers and recorded in centimeters or millimeters—it is not appropriate to compare the size of a wound to items such as eggs or oranges. Since measurements given in imperial units may be easier for a jury to understand, it is also acceptable to include the equivalent size of an injury in inches. The shape of the wound should also be noted; simple terms such as circular, triangular, V-shaped, or crescentic best express this characteristic, but if the wound shape is irregular or complex then it is possibly easier to record this feature on a body chart. Wounds also may have depth, but it is often not possible to determine this accurately in the living.

2.3. Position of the Injury

It might seem a simple matter to record the position of an injury accurately, yet when medical records are reviewed it is both surprising and disappointing to find only a vague indication of location. The best method of pinpointing the location of an injury is to use fixed anatomic landmarks. On the head, one can use the eyes, ears, nose, and mouth, on the neck the prominence of the thyroid cartilage and the sternocleidomastoid muscles, and on the trunk the nipples, umbilicus, and bony prominences can be used as points of reference. The advantages of using simple anatomic diagrams and body charts for locating the injury are self-evident.

2.4. Aging Injuries

This is one of the most contentious areas of forensic medicine. Injuries inflicted shortly before examination (both of the living and the dead) show no sign of healing. The healing process depends on a number of variables including the site of injury, the force applied, the severity of tissue damage, infection, treatment, etc., and these all make assessment of the age of a wound extremely difficult and inaccurate. Bruises often become more prominent some hours or even days after infliction because of diffusion of blood closer to the skin surface; on occasion a recent deep bruise may be mistaken for an older, more superficial lesion. Bruises resolve over a variable period ranging from days to weeks; the larger the bruise the longer it will take to disappear. Reddish blue, blue, or purplish black bruises are almost certainly of recent origin. As the extravasated red cells are destroyed, the aging bruise goes through variable color changes of bluish green, greenish yellow, and brown. It must be clearly understood that it is impossible to give the age of a bruise precisely *(3,4)*; if asked to do so in court, a medical witness would be prudent to state that a bruise undergoing these color changes is obviously not recent.

Abrasions sustained during life are usually purplish red in color, and exude serum and blood, which hardens to form a scab. This scab organizes over a period of days before detaching to leave a pink, usually intact surface. After death an unscabbed abrasion dries and has a parchment-like brown appearance.

Lacerations heal with scarring, usually over a period of days or weeks, whereas incisions, the edges of which are apposed, heal within a few days.

2.5. Transient Lesions

Swelling, redness, and tenderness, although frequently caused by trauma, are not specific signs of injury. Although it is important to record whether these features are present, it must be borne in mind that there may also be nontraumatic causes for these lesions, for example, irritation and infection.

Red marks outlining an apparent injury, for example, the imprint of a hand on the slapped face or buttock of a child, should be photographed immediately as such images may fade within an hour or so and leave no residual marks.

Reddening of the genital area in females cannot be attributed to trauma with any certainty. It should not be taken as unequivocal evidence of forceful intercourse in the absence of other signs such as bruising or hymenal injury. Mild vulvitis and vaginal infections (for example, thrush) may all be associated with redness often in conjunction with excoriation of the skin and mucosal surfaces due to irritation and scratching.

3. Types of Injury

3.1. Bruises

A bruise (or contusion) is due to the application of blunt force. The blow ruptures small blood vessels beneath the intact skin, and blood then escapes to infiltrate the surrounding subcutaneous tissues under the pumping action of the heart (Fig. 1). Thus, theoretically at least, bruising is not produced after death. In fact, severe blows inflicted after death may cause some degree of bruising, although this is usually only slight. Bruises may be associated with other injuries such as abrasions and lacerations, and these lesions may obscure the underlying bruise.

Bruising may need to be differentiated from purpura, which develop spontaneously in those with a hemorrhagic tendency and in the elderly and tend to be rather blotchy, less regular in outline, and usually confined to the forearms and lower legs. Bruising must not be confused with naevi or Campbell de Morgan spots. Also, innocent striae seen on the lower backs of adolescents have been mistaken for bruising caused by beating.

Bruises vary in severity according to the site and nature of the tissue struck, even when the force of the impact is the same. Where there is an underlying bony surface and the tissues are lax, as in the facial area, a relatively light

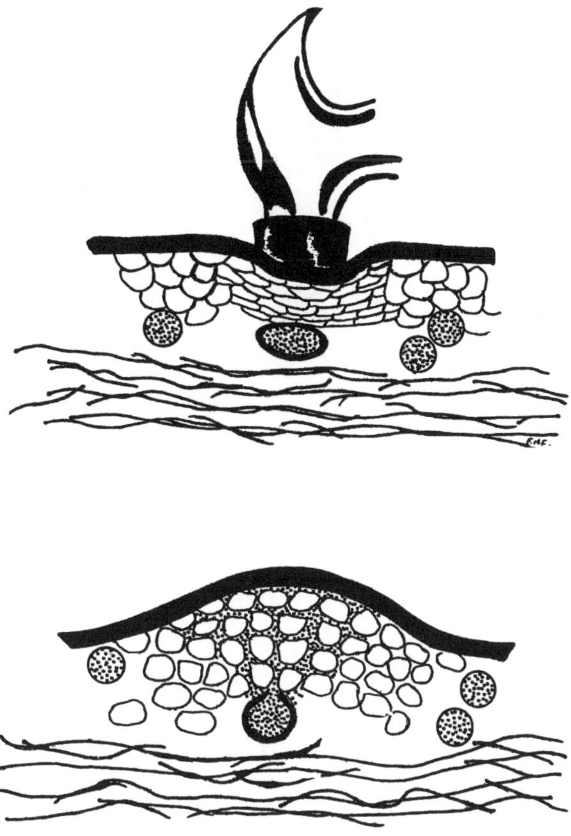

Fig. 1. Production of bruising.

blow may produce considerable puffy bruising. The orbit is the most vulnerable, giving rise to the common "black eye." Remember, however, that there are other mechanisms for the production of a black eye, such as an injury to the front of the scalp draining down over the supraorbital ridge or a fracture of the base of the skull allowing blood to escape through the roof of the orbit (Fig. 2).

Bruises tend to enlarge over a variable period of time, which can be misleading as to the actual site of injury. Since a bruise is a simple mechanical permeation of the tissues by blood, its extension may be affected by movement and gravity. Thus bruising of the face could have resulted from an injury to the scalp. Further difficulties arise if a bruise, as it extends, tracks along tissue planes from an invisible to a visible location. Bruising of this kind may not become apparent externally for some time and then at a point some distance

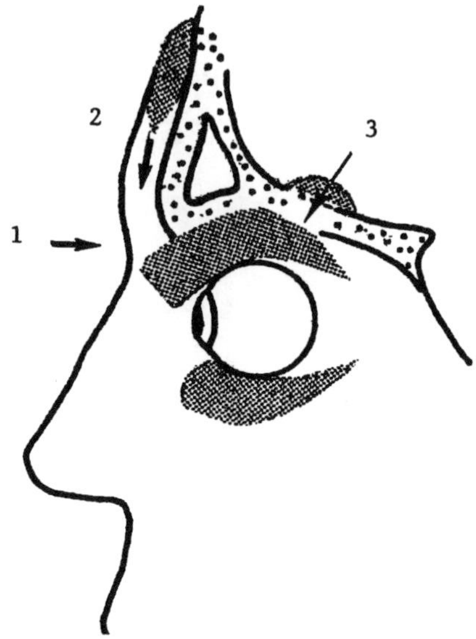

Fig. 2. Production of a black eye. 1, direct blow to the orbit; 2, injury to the front of the scalp; 3, fracture of base of skull.

from the site of the original impact. This delay in the appearance of bruising is of considerable significance since absence of apparent injury at an initial examination is not necessarily inconsistent with bruising becoming apparent 24–48 hours later. Thus, in cases of serious assault, it is often advisable to conduct a further examination a day or so later.

Generally bruises, unless superficial and of the intradermal type, tend to be nonspecific injuries, and it is usually not possible to offer any detailed opinions on the agent responsible. Some bruises, however, may have a pattern, or because of their shape or size or location, may have particular significance. Common types of patterning seen include petechial bruising reproducing the texture of clothing, the ridge pattern from the sole of a shoe or tire, or the streaky linear purple bruising seen on the neck, wrists, or ankles caused by the application of a ligature. Beating with a rod-like implement often leaves a patterned bruise consisting of an area of central pallor outlined by two narrow parallel bands of bruising, so-called tramline bruising (Fig. 3).

Other bruises of particular medicolegal significance are the small circular or oval bruises, usually about 1–2 cm in diameter, characteristic of fingertip pressure from either grasping with the hand, prodding with the fingers, or the

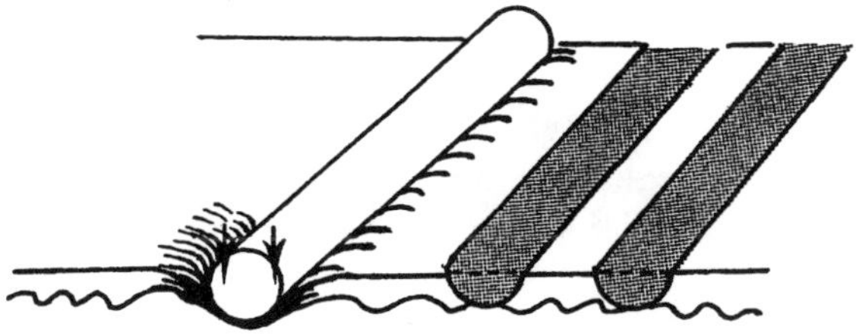

Fig. 3. Tramline bruising caused by a blow from a rod-like implement.

firm impact of a knuckle. They are often seen on the limbs in cases of child abuse when the child is forcibly gripped by the arms or legs and shaken, or on the abdomen when the victim is poked, prodded, or punched. Similar bruises may be seen on the neck in cases of manual strangulation and are then usually associated with other signs of asphyxia.

When sexual assault is alleged, the presence of bruising on the victim may help to corroborate the complaint and give an indication of how much violence was used. Also, in such cases bruising found elsewhere than about the genitalia gives some indication of how the attack was conducted. For example, grip marks or "defense" injuries may be present on the upper arms and forearms, while bruising on the thighs and the inner sides of the knees may occur as the victim's legs are forcibly pulled apart. Bruising of the mouth and lips is frequently caused when an assailant places a hand over the face to keep the victim quiet. Also "love-bites," usually in the form of discrete areas of petechial bruising, may be found on the neck and breasts.

A fresh bruise is usually red or purple depending on the amount of blood visible through the semitransluscent epidermis. However, recent but deep bruising is often more gray than reddish purple and may be mistaken for much older injuries. The progression of color changes on the bruise as the red cells (and the hemoglobin) are broken down, from purple to brown to greenish yellow, takes a variable period depending on the size of the bruise and the general physical state of the victim. In a healthy adult bruises usually resolve over a period of 1–2 weeks; in the elderly these changes may take considerably longer. Small "finger-tip" bruises seen in child abuse and sexual assault may disappear within a few days.

3.2. Abrasions

An abrasion is a superficial injury involving only the outer layers of the skin and not penetrating the full thickness of the epidermis. Abrasions exude

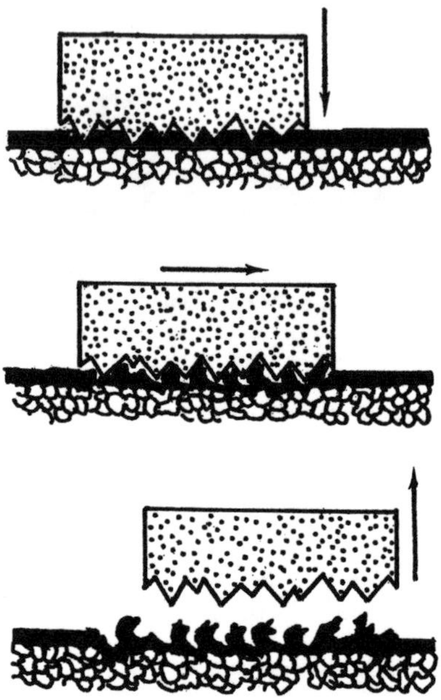

Fig. 4. Production of an abrasion.

serum, which progressively hardens to form a scab, but they may also bleed as occasionally they are deep enough to breach the vascular papillae that corrugate the undersurface of the epidermis.

Abrasions are often due to movement of the skin surface over a rough surface or vice versa (Fig. 4). Thus they may have a linear appearance, and close examination may show ruffling of the superficial epidermis to one end, indicating the direction of travel of the opposing surface. Thus a tangential blow could be shown to have been horizontal or vertical, or it may be possible to infer that the victim had been dragged over a rough surface. Multiple scratches running in an irregular criss-cross configuration may corroborate a history of being pulled through bushes.

The patterning of abrasions is clearer than that of bruises because abrasions frequently take a fairly detailed impression of the shape of the object causing them and, once inflicted, do not extend or gravitate. In manual strangulation small, crescentic abrasions, caused by the fingernails of the victim or assailant, may be the only signs visible on the neck. A victim resisting a sexual or other attack may claw at her assailant and leave linear parallel abrasions on the assailant's face. Shattered windscreen glass may leave multiple punctate and irregular abrasions, usually associated with puncture lacerations, on the faces of those sitting in the front seats of motor vehicles.

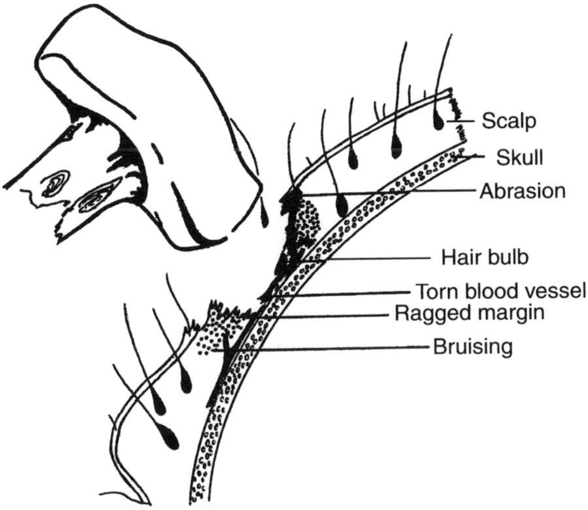

Fig. 5. Laceration of the scalp.

Some abrasions may be contaminated with foreign material such as dirt or glass, which may have important medicolegal significance. Such material should be carefully preserved for subsequent forensic analysis.

3.3. Lacerations

Lacerations occur whenever blunt force splits the full thickness of the skin (Fig. 5). They bleed, sometimes profusely, and thus when inflicted deliberately may be associated with contamination of the assailant and weapon, if one was used, with blood. In assaults they are usually caused by kicking and by the use of weapons such as sticks, bottles, or hammers. They are also features of many accidents including falls and road traffic collisions.

Lacerations have characteristic features but can occasionally mimic incised wounds, particularly where the skin is closely applied to underlying bone, for example, the scalp. Close examination of the margins of the wound, which are usually slightly inverted, normally resolves the issue. Lacerations are ragged wounds caused by crushing and tearing of the skin. They tend to gape open, and their margins are often bruised and abraded. Blood vessels, nerves, and delicate tissue bridges may be exposed in the depth of the wound, which might be soiled by grit, paint fragments, or glass.

The shape of the laceration may give some indication as to the agent responsible. For example, blows to the scalp with the circular head of a hammer or the spherical knob of a poker tend to cause crescentic lacerations. A weapon with a square or rectangular face, such as the butt of an axe, may cause a laceration with a Y-shaped split at its corners.

3.4. Incisions

These wounds are caused by sharp cutting implements, usually bladed weapons such as knives and razors, but sharp slivers of glass, the sharp edges of tin cans, and sharp tools such as chisels may also cause clean-cut incised injuries. Axes, choppers, and other similar instruments, although capable of cutting, usually cause lacerated wounds. Bottles that shatter on contact with the skin and impact with windscreen glass usually cause irregular lacerated wounds.

The features of an incision contrast with those of a laceration (Fig. 6). The margins tend to be straight, unbruised, unabraded, and not inverted. They gape, and the deeper tissues are all cut cleanly in the same plane. Hemorrhage tends to be greater than from similarly located lacerations. They are rarely soiled. If the blade of the weapon is drawn across the skin while it is lax, it may cause a notched wound if the skin creases. The direction of travel of the blade of the weapon is not always easy to decide, but usually the deeper part of the wound is near the end that was inflicted first, the weapon tending to be drawn away toward the end of the wound.

The head and neck are usual targets when incised wounds are inflicted by an assailant. In an attempt to ward off the assailant the arms are often raised in a protective gesture, and incisions are then often seen on the ulnar borders of the forearms. If the blade of the weapon is grasped, then incised wounds are apparent on the palmar surfaces of the fingers.

Incised wounds may be a feature of suicide or attempted suicide. They are usually located on the wrists, forearms, or neck although other accessible areas on the front of the body may be chosen. The incisions usually take the form of multiple parallel wounds, most of them being tentative and superficial; some may be little more than simple linear abrasions.

3.5. Stab Wounds

These are penetrating wounds having a depth greater than their width or length. They are usually caused by knives but can also be inflicted with screw-drivers, pokers, scissors, etc. Although the external injury may not appear to be particularly serious, damage to vital structures such as the heart, liver, or major blood vessels can lead to rapid death, usually from hemorrhage.

Stab wounds are rarely accidental and occasionally suicidal, but usually their infliction is as a result of criminal intent. In the case of suicide the wounds are usually located on the front of the chest or upper abdomen and, as with self-

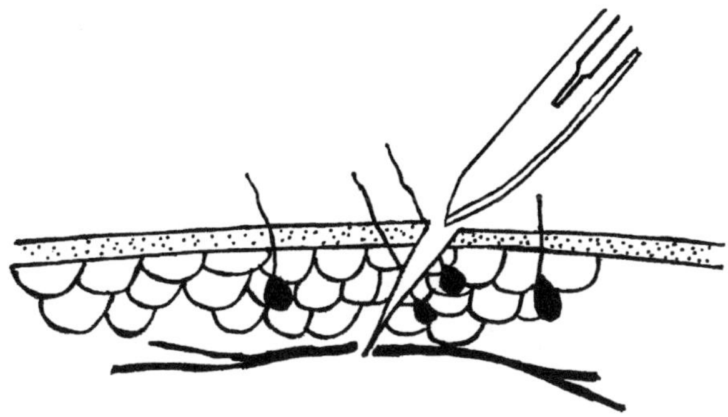

Fig. 6. Cross-section of an incision.

inflicted incisions, may be associated with a number of superficial tentative puncture wounds. When deliberately inflicted by an assailant, they may be associated with defense injuries to the arms and hands.

The appearance of the skin wound will vary depending on the weapon used and can easily be distorted by movement of the surrounding skin. Typically, when inflicted with a knife, the wound is usually elliptical in shape as the natural elasticity of the skin causes its length to shrink. If the blade was double-edged, such as that of a dagger, the extremities of the wound tend to be equally pointed. A stab wound from a single-edged blade, such as a kitchen knife, will usually have one extremity rounded, squared-off, or fish-tailed (caused by the noncutting back of the blade). When blunt weapons are used, for example, a pair of scissors, the wound tends to be more rounded or oval, with bruising of its margins (Fig. 7). Scissor wounds can sometimes have a cross-shape caused by the blade screws or rivets. Notched wounds are often caused by the blade of the weapon being partially withdrawn and then reintroduced into the wound or twisted during penetration.

It is rarely possible from an inspection of the skin wound alone to comment usefully on the width of the blade since the skin retracts and the knife is unlikely to have been introduced and removed perfectly perpendicularly. Surprisingly long skin wounds may be caused with quite narrow-width blades.

4. Firearm Injuries

The examination of fatal firearm injuries *(5)* should be left to an experienced forensic pathologist; however, it is not unusual in cases of nonfatal injuries for a hospital clinician or forensic physician to be asked to comment on the

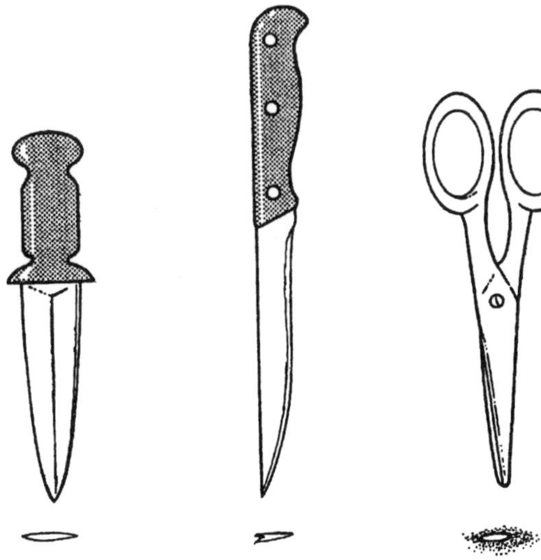

Fig. 7. Elliptical (left), fish-tailed (middle), and bruised ovoid (right) stab wounds.

nature of the wound or wounds. It is essential in these nonfatal cases that the initial appearances of the injuries be accurately described and the wounds photographed. This is particularly important since subsequent surgical treatment may distort or completely obliterate the wound characteristics. Furthermore, any fragments, bullets, or pellets found within the wounds must be carefully removed and handed over to the appropriate authorities.

Some basic knowledge of ballistics is essential for a proper understanding of wounds caused by firearms. There are essentially two types of weapon, smooth bore and rifled.

4.1. Smooth Bore Weapons

Shotguns, which fire a large number of small projectiles, such as lead shot, are the commonest type of smooth bore weapons. They are commonly used in sporting and agricultural activities and may be either single or double-barrelled. The ammunition for these weapons consists of a plastic or cardboard cartridge case with a brass base containing a percussion cap. Inside the main part of the cartridge is a layer of propellant, plastic, felt, or cardboard wads and a mass of pellets (lead shot of variable size) (Fig. 8A). It is important to appreciate that not only the pellets but also the wads and/or cards may contribute to the appearance of the wounds and may be important in estimating range and possible direction.

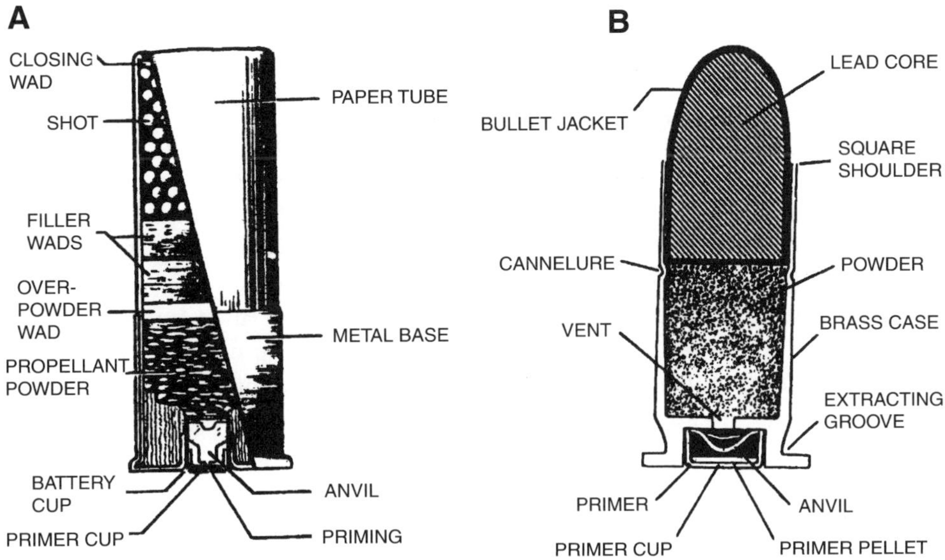

Fig. 8. Components of a shotgun cartridge **(A)** and a rifled bullet **(B)**.

4.2. Rifled Weapons

These are characterized by having parallel spiral projecting ridges (or lands) extending down the interior of the barrel from the breach to the muzzle. This rifling causes the projectile, in this case a bullet (Fig. 8B), to spin as it is ejected from the weapon and thus imparts gyroscopic stability along its flight path. The rifling also leaves characteristic scratches, rifling marks, unique to that weapon, on the bullet surface. There are three common types of rifled weapon; the revolver, the pistol and the rifle. The revolver, which tends to have a low muzzle velocity of the order of 150 m/s, is a short-barrelled weapon with its ammunition held in a metal drum, which rotates each time the trigger is released. The spent cartridge case is retained within the cylinder after firing. In the self-loading pistol, often called "semi-automatic" or erroneously "automatic," the ammunition is held in a metal clip-type magazine under the breach. Each time the trigger is pulled, the bullet in the breach is fired, the spent cartridge case is ejected from the weapon, and a spring mechanism pushes up the next live bullet into the breach ready to be fired. The muzzle velocity of pistols varies between 300 and 360 m/s. The rifle is a long-barrelled shoulder weapon capable of firing bullets with velocities up to 1500 m/s. Most military rifles are "automatic," allowing the weapon to continue to fire while the trigger is depressed until the magazine is empty. They are thus capable of discharging multiple rounds within seconds.

4.3. Shotgun Wounds

When a shotgun is discharged, the lead shot emerges from the muzzle as a solid mass and then progressively diverges in a cone shape, as the distance from the weapon increases. The pellets are often accompanied by particles of unburnt powder, flame, smoke, gases, wads, and cards, which may all affect the appearance of the entrance wound and are dependent on the range of fire. Both the estimated range and the site of the wound are crucial factors in determining whether the wound could have been self-inflicted.

If the wound has been sustained through clothing, then important residues may be found on this if it is submitted for forensic examination. When clothing is being cut off in the hospital, it is helpful for the staff to avoid cutting through any apparent holes. Once removed, the items should be separately bagged, preferably in paper bags, for collection by a Scenes of Crime Officer.

Contact wounds are caused when the muzzle of the weapon is held against the skin. The entrance wound is usually a fairly neat circular hole, the margins of which may be bruised or abraded due to impact with the muzzle. In the case of a double-barrelled weapon, the circular abraded imprint of the nonfiring muzzle may be clearly seen adjacent to the contact wound. The wound margins and the tissues within the base of the wound are usually blackened by smoke and may show signs of burning due to the effect of flame. Because the gases from the discharge are forced into the wound, there may be subsidiary lacerations at the wound margin, giving it a stellate-like shape. This is seen particularly where the muzzle contact against the skin is tight and the skin is closely applied to underlying bone, such as in the scalp. Carbon monoxide contained within the gases may cause the surrounding skin and soft tissues to turn pink due to the formation of carboxyhemoglobin. Contact wounds to the head are particularly severe, usually with bursting ruptures of the scalp and face, multiple explosive fractures of the skull, and extrusion or partial extrusion of the underlying brain. Most contact wounds of the head are suicidal in nature, with the temple, mouth, and under the chin being the sites of election. In these types of wounds, which are usually rapidly fatal, fragments of scalp, skull, and brain tissue may be dispersed over a wide area.

At close, noncontact range, with the muzzle up to about 15 cm (6 inches) from the skin, the entrance wound is still usually a single circular or oval hole with possible burning and blackening of its margins from flame, smoke, and unburnt powder. Blackening due to smoke is rarely seen beyond about 20 cm; tattooing from powder usually only extends to about 1 m. The wads and cards rarely travel more than about 2 m.

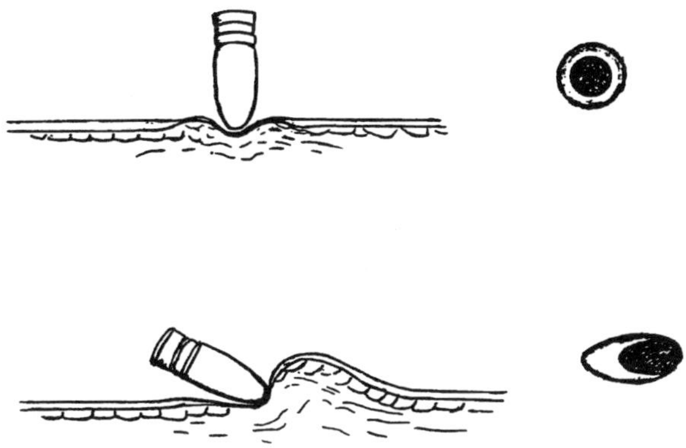

Fig. 9. Entrance wounds caused by perpendicular (top) and tangential (bottom) bullet strikes.

As distance increases the pellets begin to diverge. Up to about 1 m they are still travelling as a compact mass but between about 1–3 m the pellets start to scatter and cause variable numbers of individual satellite puncture wounds surrounding a larger central hole. At ranges greater than 8–10 m there is no large central hole, only multiple small puncture wounds, giving the skin a peppered appearance.

Exit wounds are unusual with shotgun injuries as the shot is usually dispersed in the tissues. The pellets, however, may penetrate the neck or a limb, and in close-range wounds to the head the whole cranium may be disrupted.

4.4. Rifled Weapon Wounds

Intact bullets penetrating the skin orthogonally, that is nose-on, usually cause neat round holes about 3–10 mm diameter. Close examination reveals that the wound margin is usually fairly smooth and regular and bordered by an even zone of creamy pink or pinkish red abrasion. A nonorthogonal nose-on strike is associated with an eccentric abrasion collar, widest at the side of the wound from which the bullet was directed (Fig. 9). Atypical entrance wounds are a feature of contact or near contact wounds to the head where the thick bone subjacent to the skin resists the entry of gases, which accumulate beneath the skin and cause subsidiary lacerations to the wound margins, imparting a stellate lacerated appearance. Contact wounds elsewhere may be bordered by the imprint of the muzzle and the abraded margin possibly charred and parchmented by flame. Punctate discharge abrasion and sooty soiling are usually absent from the skin surface, but the subcutaneous tissues within the depth of the wound are usually soiled. The effects of flame are rarely seen beyond 10 cm (4 inches), with sooty soiling extending to about 20 cm (8 inches). Punctate discharge abrasions, which may be particularly heavy with old revolver ammunition, are often present at ranges up to about 50 cm (20 inches). It is important to remember that sooty soiling of the skin surrounding a wound is easily removed by vigorous cleaning carried out by medical or nursing staff. Also, the soiling of contact close-range entrance wounds may be absent if clothing or other material is interposed between the skin surface and the muzzle of the weapon.

Exit bullet wounds tend to be larger than entrance wounds and usually consist of irregular lacerations or lacerated holes with everted, unabraded, and unbruised margins. When the skin at the site of an entrance wound has been supported by tight clothing, for example, eversion of the margins of the wound may be absent and the margins may even be abraded, albeit somewhat irregularly but nevertheless making differentiation from entrance wounds more difficult.

Entrance wounds caused by damaged or fragmented bullets may be so atypical that it may not be possible to offer a useful opinion as to their nature. Also, it is inappropriate to offer an opinion on the caliber of a bullet based on the size of an entrance wound nor is it possible to state from the appearance of the wound whether the bullet was fired from a revolver, pistol, or rifle.

5. Defense Injures

The natural response to an attack by an assailant is to try to defend oneself against injury, assuming of course that the victim has not been restrained or lost consciousness. Clearly some victims, particularly the very young and the very old, are rarely capable of offering much defense against the perpetrators of assault. In trying to protect the head it is usual to raise the arms in front of the face, and consequently deflected blows are received on the extensor and ulnar surfaces of the forearms and hands. The injuries sustained usually take the form of bruises if the victim is being punched or kicked, but there may also be abrasions and/or lacerations depending on the nature of any weapon used. If the victim is lying on the ground while being assaulted he or she will tend to curl up into a fetal position to protect the face and the front of the trunk, particularly from kicks. In these circumstances defensive bruising is likely to be seen on other surfaces of the trunk and limbs. If the assailant is armed with a bladed weapon, such as a knife, then defensive injuries usually take the form of incised wounds to the arms. If the blade of the weapon is grasped by the victim, then some of these wounds will be found on the palmar surfaces of the hands and fingers.

The absence of defense injuries in persons otherwise capable of defending themselves against an assault may be of particular significance if it is thought that other injuries found on the victim could have been self-inflicted.

6. Torture

The World Medical Association's Declaration of Tokyo in 1975 defined torture as "the deliberate, systematic or wanton infliction of physical or mental suffering by one or more persons acting alone or on the orders of any authority, to force another person to yield information, to make a confession, or for any other reason" (*see* Appendix 1) *(6)*. The Declaration also laid down guidelines for doctors when faced with cases of suspected torture. As far as clinicians are concerned, torture is seen in two main contexts: first, that perpetrated by criminals and terrorist organizations and second, that carried out, or allegedly carried out, by the police or other security force personnel during the detention and interrogation of prisoners and suspects. The systematic abuse of children, which theoretically could be defined as torture, is discussed elsewhere (*see* Chapter 5).

Criminal groups and paramilitary organizations may torture their captives for a variety of reasons. It may be to extract information from an opposing gang or faction, to discipline informants and others engaged in unsanctioned criminal activity, or simply to instil fear and division within a community. The methods used are fairly crude and barbaric. The victim is usually bound, blindfolded, and gagged, and the wrists and ankles may bear the pale streaky linear bruises and abrasions caused by ligatures. "Beating up" is typical, with extensive bruises and abrasions scattered on the head, trunk, and limbs. Black eyes, fractures of the nose and jaws, and dislodgment of the teeth are all fairly typical. Cigarette burns, usually seen as discrete circular areas of reddish yellow parchmented skin, are also quite common. Patterned injuries due to being struck with the butt of a gun or tramline bruising due to blows with a truncheon or baseball bat may be seen; in Northern Ireland, shooting through the lower limbs ("knee-capping") is a favored method of punishment by paramilitary organizations.

Systematic torture by security personnel, usually during interrogation of suspects, ranges from the subtle use of threats and intimidation to actual physical violence. Hooding, prolonged standing, and the use of high-pitched sound have all been used, as have attempts to disorientate prisoners by offering food at erratic times, frequent waking up after short intervals of sleep, and burning a light in the cell 24 hours a day. Physical abuse includes beating of the soles of the feet, so-called *falanga*, which although extremely painful and debilitating, does not usually cause any significant bruising. Repeated dipping of the victim's head under water, *submarining*, may prove fatal if prolonged, as can the induction of partial asphyxia by enveloping the head in a plastic bag.

Electric torture is well documented and carries the risk of local electric shocks as well as fatal electrocution. Another favorite torture is *telefono*, consisting of repeated slapping of the sides of the head by the open palms. Tympanic membrane rupture is the result.

Doctors who have access to prisoners in custody have a heavy responsibility to ensure that they are properly treated during detention and interrogation. In all cases of suspected or alleged ill-treatment of prisoners it is essential that the doctor carry out a methodical and detailed "head to toe" examination. All injuries and marks must be accurately recorded and photographed and the appropriate authorities informed immediately.

References

1. Knight, B. (1996) The pathology of wounds, in *Forensic Pathology* (Knight, B., ed.), Arnold, London, pp. 133–169
2. Crane, J. (1996) Injury, in *Clinical Forensic Medicine* (McLay, W. D. S., ed.), Greenwich Medical Media, London, pp. 143–162.
3. Langlois, N. E. I. and Gresham, G. A. (1991) The ageing of bruises: a review and study of the colour changes with time. *Forensic Sci Int.* **50,** 227–238.
4. Stephenson, T. and Bialas, Y. (1996) Estimation of the age of bruising. *Arch Dis Child.* **74,** 53–55.
5. Di Maio, V. J. M. (1985) *Gunshot Wounds*. Elsevier, New York.
6. British Medical Association—Report of a Working Party (1992) *Medicine Betrayed*. British Medical Association, London.

Chapter 5

Nonaccidental Injury in Children

Amanda Thomas

1. Introduction

Nonaccidental injury (NAI) is a common condition in children and carries a significant morbidity and mortality. Doctors have an important role in recognizing, assessing, and managing children with suspected NAI.

1.1. Definition

Child abuse is difficult to define, and although many definitions exist in the legal and scientific literature there is no consensus on an absolute definition. Issues that arise in the debate include the influence and attitudes of societies, cultural differences in child rearing, politics, and religious beliefs. In addition, there is a need to examine the factors involved in particular episodes, the context in which the episodes occurred, the opinion of the professionals who are describing or judging these episodes, the current knowledge of the long-term outcomes of particular behaviors to children, and the effectiveness of current interventions. Definitions are, however, very important as they provide a general framework for policy setting, statutory and legal interventions, gathering statistical information, and an understanding of current and future research.

In the United Kingdom, the Children Act *(1)* defines a child as:

"a person under the age of eighteen years."

From: *Forensic Science: A Physician's Guide to Clinical Forensic Medicine*
Edited by: M. M. Stark © Humana Press, Inc., Totowa, NJ

Working Together Under the Children Act 1989 *(2)* defines physical injury as:

> *"Actual or likely physical injury to a child, or failure to prevent physical injury (or suffering) to a child including deliberate poisoning, suffocation and Munchausen's syndrome by proxy."*

In the United States, legal definitions vary from state to state, and individual institutions develop their own definitions and guidelines. For example, the Child Abuse Program (CAP) at Children's Hospital, Columbus, Ohio *(3)* has defined physical child abuse as:

> *"An injury to a child caused by a caretaker—for any reason, including injury resulting from a caretaker's reaction to an unwanted behavior. Injury includes tissue damage beyond erythema or redness from a slap to any area other than the hand or buttocks. Physical discipline should not be used on children who are under 12 months of age. The child should be normal developmentally, emotionally, and physically. Tissue damage includes bruises, burns, tears, punctures, fractures, ruptures of organs, and disruption of functions. The use of an instrument on any part of the body is abuse. The injury may be caused by impact, penetration, heat, a caustic, a chemical, or a drug."*

1.2. Effects of Child Abuse

There is extensive literature on the effects of child abuse. It is generally accepted that child abuse carries a significant mortality and morbidity with consequences including:

- death or disability in severe cases
- affective and behavior disorders
- developmental delay and learning difficulties
- failure to thrive and growth retardation
- predisposition to adult psychiatric disorders
- an increased risk of the abused becoming an abuser

In a study of 170 children by Gibbons et al. *(4)*, an attempt was made to disentangle the impact of the abuse from the contributing circumstances and the results of intervention. The authors found that abused children, 10 years after diagnosis, were more likely to show behavior problems at home and at school, had greater difficulties with friendships, and scored lower on certain cognitive tests. There was evidence that persistent abuse, a combination of different kinds of abuse, or abuse and neglect together had a poorer prognosis. Isolated incidents of physical abuse in the context of a nonviolent family and in the absence of sexual abuse or neglect did not necessarily lead to poor long-term outcomes for children. What has emerged from this research has been the importance of the style of parenting in families: children exposed to a harshly punitive, less reliable, and less warm environment are the children with the poorest outcomes.

1.3. Risk Factors for Abuse

The picture of child abuse is complex, with social, psychological, economic, and environmental factors all playing a part. Often there is evidence of family stress followed by a triggering event leading to abuse. Newberger *(5)* pinpointed three categories of predisposing family stress:

Child factors	disability, learning difficulties, behavior problems, adoption
Parental factors	mental health problems, alcohol or drug abuse, domestic violence, previous abuse as a child
Socio-situational factors	single parent, young parent, new partner, poverty, unemployment

Gibbons et al. *(6)* studied children on the child protection registers in England and Wales (that is, children identified by agencies as at risk for significant harm and for whom a child protection plan had been developed) and found that domestic violence was recorded in over one-fourth of cases. A substantial minority of parents had histories of mental illness, criminal behavior, or substance abuse. Substance abuse is more common worldwide and is associated with an elevated risk of neglect in the children of substance abusing parents. Cross et al. *(7)*, in the United States, reported that disabled children are more than one and a half times as likely to be abused in any one year as other children.

The harmful effect of socioeconomic deprivation on children is well established. Poverty is associated with postnatal and infant mortality, malnutrition and ill health, low educational attainment, delinquency, teenage pregnancy, and family tension and breakdown. Parental stress leads to greater vulnerability of the children, and common stress factors include unemployment and debt, which are linked to poverty. Abuse occurs across all social classes, but children from the most disadvantaged sectors of society are brought to the attention of child protection agencies more frequently *(8)*.

1.4. Extent of Abuse

The true prevalence of child abuse is difficult to determine in all countries. Official estimates will only represent a fraction of the total number of cases, as many go unreported or unrecognized, and information systems are incomplete or track just one limited part of the picture. In the United States the referral rate for child abuse investigations is three times higher than in the United Kingdom, and twice as many children are in state care, with four times as many child abuse deaths *(9)*.

Physical injury is the second commonest reason for registration of a child on the child protection register in England (33%, including mixed categories, in 1998) *(10)* and the second most frequent type of maltreatment of children under 18 years recorded in the United States (25%, 1995) *(11)*. Neglect is the commonest category of registration or type of maltreatment in both countries *(10,11)*.

2. Nonaccidental Injury in Children

NAI in children (physical abuse, battering) includes injuries that result from deliberate actions against the child or failure to prevent injury occurring to the child. The spectrum of injury includes:

- Soft tissue injury
- Thermal injury
- Skeletal injury
- Internal injuries (brain, abdomen, eye)
- Munchausen Syndrome by Proxy (factitious illness)

The range of NAIs extends from minor (e.g., bruising) to fatal, and younger infants are at risk of more serious injuries.

Different types of abuse overlap. Physical abuse will often coexist with emotional abuse. Injury may occur in the context of neglect such as leaving a child unsupervised and exposed to dangerous situations. Physically abused children are at increased risk of sexual abuse. Hobbs and Wynne *(12)* found that 1 in 6 of 769 physically abused children and 1 in 7 of 949 sexually abused children had suffered both forms of abuse.

2.1. Role of the Physician

Physicians have a duty (a legal one in some countries, such as the United States and Australia) to recognize and report suspected abuse to the statutory, investigative agencies. Physicians need to work together with statutory agencies and have an awareness and understanding of other agencies' roles and responsibilities. Physicians should be aware of current guidance on accountability and confidentiality produced by their professional bodies.

Physicians may be involved in a wide range of child protection activities including:

- Recognition, diagnosis, and treatment of injury
- Joint interagency activity
- Court attendance
- Ongoing care and monitoring of children following suspected abuse
- Support for families and children
- Prevention
- Teaching, training, supervision, and awareness raising

2.2. Assessing the Nonaccidentally Injured Child

For the physician faced with the assessment of a child for suspected physical injury, the following points should be remembered:

- Physical abuse often overlaps with other forms of abuse.
- Abuse may involve other siblings and family members.
- Abuse may recur and escalate.
- Younger children and infants are more at risk of physical injury and death than older children.
- The aim of recognition and early intervention is to protect the child, prevent mortality and morbidity, and diagnose and improve disordered parenting.
- Early intervention in families may prevent more serious abuse and subsequent removal of children into care.
- The medical examination is important, but it is only one part of the wider assessment of the child and family.

A recommended approach to the pediatric assessment is as follows:

1. Obtaining background information from professionals, e.g., social worker or police officer, if accompanying the family, or by telephone prior to the assessment.
2. Full pediatric history from the parent/carer and child. Remember to document the responses as well as the questions asked and any spontaneous disclosures.
3. Assessment of the "whole child" including:
    - Growth plotted on a centile chart.
    - Development. Is this child developmentally capable of what has been described? Is this child's developmental delay part of a wider picture of abuse or neglect?
    - A description of the child's demeanor and behavior. Is the child's behavior normal for age?
    - Full physical examination including genitalia and anus.
    - Description of injuries: types of lesions, sites, sizes, shapes and patterns, colors, and estimate of ages.
4. Legible, signed, dated, hand-written, contemporaneous record of the assessment with drawings of injuries detailing measurements.
5. Photographs of injuries.
6. Appropriate investigations (discussed below).
7. Ask to see siblings.

8. Initial information gathering from other professionals (e.g., family doctor, health visitor, or teachers from nursery or school) already involved with the family. This does not replace the formal investigation procedures but may be helpful for the examining physician, who must consider the wider picture to formulate an opinion and guide the child protection agencies.
9. Provision of a clear, factual report detailing the findings, summarizing the assessment, and providing a medical opinion for child protection agencies and any criminal proceedings.
10. Maintenance of written records of contacts with families and professionals.

2.3. Pointers to the Diagnosis

The following factors can help with the diagnosis *(13)*:

- Delay in presentation of the injury
- Discrepant or absent history
- History incompatible with the injury
- Pattern of injury more suggestive of abuse
- Repetitive injuries
- Unusual parental behavior or mood
- Child's demeanor, behavior, or interaction with the parent/carer unusual
- Disclosure by child or witness

3. Types of Injuries

3.1. Soft Tissue Injuries

3.1.1. Bruising

A bruise is an escape of blood into the skin, subcutaneous tissue, or both, following the rupture of blood vessels by the application of blunt force *(14)*. The initial color of the bruise is the product of the child's natural skin pigmentation, the color of the pigments in the extravasated blood, and any color added by the inflammatory reaction. The color of the bruise changes as the extracellular hemoglobin breaks down into various pigments *(15)*.

Factors affecting the appearance of a bruise include *(16)*:

- The severity of the force applied to the area
- The connective tissue support at the site of injury—increased extravasation of blood occurs around lax, loose areas of skin, such as the eye
- Skin color—bruising is more visible in pale skin
- Diseases affecting coagulation, blood vessels, or connective tissues
- Drugs, e.g., steroids, salicylates
- Continued extravasation of blood and tracking between tissue planes, which may delay the appearance of the bruise or lead to a different site of bruising from the site of injury

- Bruising reduced if pressure is maintained over the area until death has occurred or when death has occurred rapidly
- The pattern of the bruise, reflecting the implement used

3.1.1.1. Clues to Distinguish NAI from Accidental Bruising

For further information, *see* ref. *17*.

1. Patterns
    - Hand marks
        - Fingertip bruises consisting of circular or oval bruises from squeezing, poking, gripping, or grabbing injuries
        - Linear petechial bruises in the shape of a hand caused by capillaries rupturing at the edge of the injury from the high-velocity impact of the hand slap
        - Pinch marks consisting of paired, crescent-shaped bruises separated by a white line
    - Implement marks
        - High-velocity impact causing a rim of petechiae outlining the pattern of the inflicting instrument, e.g., parallel sided marks from sticks—"tramline bruising"
        - Higher velocity impacts causing bruising underlying the injury in the shape of the object used, e.g., wedge-shaped bruises from kicks with shoes
        - Pressure necrosis of the skin from ligatures, causing well-demarcated bands partially or fully encircling limbs or the neck
        - Coarse speckled bruising from impact injuries through clothing
    - Petechial bruises
        - Pinprick bruises from ruptured capillaries, e.g., suction bruises, squeezing, slapping, strangulation, suffocation
2. Sites more commonly associated with NAI
    - Facial—soft tissues of the cheek, eye, mouth, ear, mastoid, lower jaw, frenulum, and neck
    - Chest wall
    - Abdomen
    - Inner thighs and genitalia strongly associated with sexual abuse
    - Buttock and outer thighs commonly associated with punishment injuries
    - Multiple sites

3.1.1.2. Dating Bruising

For further information, *see* refs. *15* and *16*.

- Bruises cannot be reliably aged.
- The development of a yellow color in a bruise has been found to be the most significant color change, occurring, at the earliest, 18 hours from the time of injury *(16)*.

- Bruises can change color at different rates, and several different colors can be present at the same time in the same bruise.
- Bruises of identical age and etiology may not show the same colors.
- Possible indicators of more recent injury include:
  - Fresh cuts and abrasions overlying a bruise
  - Swelling underlying the bruising
  - Pain or tenderness at the site of injury

3.1.1.3. Differential Diagnosis of Bruising

- Accidental injury—commonly on bony surfaces, appropriate history
- Artefact—dirt, paint, felt tip, dye from clothing or footwear
- Benign tumors—halo nevus, blue nevus, hemangiomas
- Vascular and bleeding disorders—thrombocytopenic purpura, Henoch-Schoenlein purpura, hemophilia, purpura in association with infection, e.g., meningococcal septicemia
- Disturbances of pigmentation—café-au-lait patches, Mongolian blue spots
- Erythematous lesions—erythema nodosum
- Hereditary collagen disorders—osteogenesis imperfecta, Ehlers-Danlos syndrome

3.1.1.4. Investigations

In the presence of excessive or reported spontaneous bruising, it is reasonable to exclude an underlying bleeding disorder. However, O'Hare and Eden *(18)* found abnormal tests in 16% of 50 children with suspected NAI and concluded that the two conditions can coexist.

Suggested tests include: full blood count, platelet count, prothrombin time, thrombin time, partial thromboplastin time, fibrinogen level, bleeding time (after discussion with a hematologist).

3.1.2. Bite Marks

A bite mark is a mark made by teeth alone or in combination with other mouth parts and may be considered a mirror image of the arrangement and characteristics of the dentition. Human bite marks rarely occur accidentally and are good indicators of inflicted injury. Children can be bitten in the context of punishment, as part of a physical assault, or in association with sexual abuse. Children can also be bitten by other children. (For further information, *see* refs. *19* and *20*.)

Human bite marks have a broad U-shaped arch, and broad, shallow, blunt indentation marks on the skin, compared with animal bites, which have a narrower arch size and deeper, smaller skin indentations, from sharper teeth.

Factors influencing the appearance of a bite mark include:

- The status of the skin (ante or post mortem) and the skin condition
- The time period between the bite and the examination
- The clarity of the marks and the reaction of the surrounding tissue
- The strength of the bite pressure (stronger bite pressures cause deeper skin depressions)
- The strength of the sucking pressure (stronger sucking pressures lead to reduced markings by the incisors)

3.1.2.1. Good Practice Tips

- When defined bite marks are found, advice should be sought from a forensic odontologist. Impressions and dental casts of suspects can be made that may be able to establish the identity of the perpetrator.
- Bite marks can be found on any site of the human anatomy, and when a single bite mark is found, particular care should be taken to search for other bites. Vale et al. *(21)* found that 40% of their victims had more than one bite and 22% had bite marks in more than one anatomic site.
- Documentation of the bite should include the location, contour of the skin surface, size and number of tooth marks, diameter of the mark, and intercanine distance.
- An intercanine distance of 3 cm or more indicates that the bite was inflicted by a person with a permanent dentition (an adult or a child older than 8 years) *(22)*.
- Plain sterile swabs (moistened if necessary) can be used to obtain residual saliva from the bite area, for forensic purposes. The swabs should be air dried and managed according to standard procedures for the collection of forensic evidence (*see* Chapter 3).
- Good-quality photographs, both black and white and color, should be taken. These should include a scale (rigid L-shaped measuring rule) and, when appropriate, a color standard. Serial daily photographs are useful to record the bite mark's evolution and optimum definition.

3.1.3. Other Soft Tissue Injuries

- Subgaleal hematoma—diffuse, boggy swelling on the scalp can occur following hair pulling (often associated with broken hairs and petechial hemorrhages)
- Periorbital injury—from a direct blow, e.g., a punch
- Ocular injury:
  - Subconjunctival hemorrhage from direct trauma, suffocation, strangulation, chest, or abdominal trauma
  - Direct trauma can also lead to corneal or scleral laceration or scarring, ruptured globe, vitreous or retinal hemorrhage, acute hyphema, dislocated lens, traumatic cataract, detached retina
- Perioral injuries—bruising or laceration to the lips from a direct blow to the mouth

- Intraoral injuries:
  - Ulceration to the inner lips or cheeks from a blow to the face causing impaction of the tissues against teeth, torn frenulum from a blow to the upper lip, or penetrating injury from a feeding utensil
  - Abrasions or lacerations to the palate, vestibule, or floor of the mouth from penetrating injuries, e.g., from a feeding utensil
  - Petechial injury to the palate from direct trauma to the palate or oral abuse
  - Tooth injury, e.g., breaks, fractures, avulsions caused by blunt trauma
- Abrasions—superficial areas of skin loss caused by friction injuries, scratches from fingernails, or sharp-edged objects
- Cuts or incised wounds—a superficial injury that is longer than it is deep, produced by a sharp-edged object

3.2. Thermal Injury

Burns and scalds to children can occur accidentally, be inflicted, or follow neglect. The injury can be superficial or partial or full skin thickness depending on the temperature and duration of exposure.

3.2.1. Types of Thermal Injury

For further information, *see* ref. *23*.

- Scalds—immersion, pouring or throwing a hot liquid onto a child. The affected skin is soggy, blanched, and blistered. The shape of the injury is contoured. The depth of the burn is variable.
- Contact burns—direct contact of a hot object with the child. Characteristically, the burn is shaped like the hot object with sharply defined edges and usually of uniform depth. The burn may blister.
- Fire burns—flames from fires, matches, lighters in close or direct contact with the skin, causing charring and skin loss with singeing of hairs.
- Cigarette burns—inflicted direct contact leaves a characteristically well-demarcated circular or oval mark with rolled edges and a cratered center, which may blister and tends to scar. Accidental contact with a cigarette tends to leave a more superficial, irregular area of erythema with a tail.
- Electrical burns—small, deeply penetrating burns with an entry and exit wound with possible necrosis of underlying tissues.
- Friction burns—dragging or rubbing injury causing superficial skin loss, with broken blisters, usually on bony prominences.
- Chemical burns—the chemical in liquid form is drunk, poured, or splashed onto the skin, or in solid form is rubbed on the skin. The skin may stain, may have the appearance of a scald, and may scar.
- Radiant burns—more extensive areas of erythema and blistering on exposed body parts.

3.2.2. Features of Thermal Injuries Suggestive of NAI

For further information, *see* ref. *24*.

- Those features discussed under "pointers to the diagnosis of NAI"
- Repeated burns
- Sites—backs of hands, buttocks, feet, and legs
- Types—clearly demarcated burns shaped like a particular object, immersion burns with a tide mark (clear edge) and no splash marks
- The presence of other NAIs

3.2.3. Differential Diagnosis of Thermal Injuries

- Accidental burns—appropriate history and presentation
- Infection—staphylococcal, streptococcal (impetigo, scalded skin syndrome)
- Allergy—urticaria, contact dermatitis
- Insect bites
- Bullous diseases—porphyria, erythema multiforme

3.2.4. Good Practice Tips

- Identify the type, depth, and extent of the burn.
- Accurately measure the injury and document with photographs.
- Manipulate the child's posture to reflect the position at the time of the injury.
- Assess the child's developmental skills. Can the child climb? Turn on a tap?
- Assess for other signs of abuse.
- Assessment of the home or place of injury with reenactment of the episode to include the events leading up to the injury, the child's position at the time of the incident, the length of time the child was exposed to the heat or liquid, the temperature of the appliance or liquid and measurements of suspected appliances, e.g., the height/depth of the bath, height of the work surface, and position of appliance.
- Remember that burns and infection can coexist.

3.3. Skeletal Injury

Historically, skeletal injury played a major role in the recognition of child abuse *(25,26)*. In 1946, Caffey *(27)* described six patients presenting with chronic subdural hematoma in which 23 unexplained fractures of the long bones were found. Caffey concluded that the fractures were traumatic in origin and introduced the concept of inflicted injury.

Most skeletal injuries of NAI occur in children under the age of 2 years, and some may be occult, particularly in the under 1-year-old who has other signs of physical injury. Merten et al. *(28)* found fractures in 47% of abused children under the age of 1 year who had skeletal surveys, in which 67% were occult and 60% were multiple. Fractures in infants and children resulting from falls of under 3 feet are relatively uncommon. Research evidence suggests that 1% of children falling less than 3 feet may sustain a simple linear skull fracture *(29)*.

Accidental fractures in infants and toddlers do occur, usually as a result of falls, often from a height, but they can occasionally occur in long bones of ambulant children from twisting, running, and falling. There is usually a consistent history and a prompt presentation. Fractures cause pain and distress and are often accompanied by nonuse of the affected body part and local swelling.

Any fracture can occur as a result of NAI, but some have a high specificity for abuse such as:

- Metaphyseal—a shaking, pulling, or twisting force applied at or about a joint, resulting in a fracture through the growing part of the bone
- Epiphyseal separation—resulting from torsion of a limb, particularly in children younger than 2 years old
- Rib—resulting from severe squeezing or direct trauma; posterior rib fractures virtually pathognomonic of NAI and commonly associated with shaking injury
- Scapular—resulting from direct impact
- Lateral clavicle—resulting from excessive traction or shaking of an arm
- Humerus or femur—in nonambulant children (under 1 year); transverse fractures from angulation including a direct blow; spiral fractures from axial twists with or without axial loading; oblique fractures from angulation, axial twisting with axial loading
- Vertebral—resulting from hyperflexion injuries, impact injuries, or direct trauma
- Digital—resulting from forced hyperextension or direct blows
- Skull—resulting from blunt impact injuries, particularly occipital fractures and fractures that are depressed, wide (or growing), bilateral, complex, crossing suture lines multiply, or associated with intracranial injury *(30)*.
- Periosteal injury—resulting from pulling or twisting of a limb separating the periosteum from the surface of the bone, leading to hemorrhage between the periosteum and the bone and subsequent calcification

Other features of skeletal injury suggestive of abuse include:

- Absence of an appropriate history
- Multiple fractures
- Fractures of differing ages
- Fracture in association with other features of NAI, e.g., bruising at other sites
- Unsuspected fractures (recent or old) found when X-rays taken for other reasons

Precise dating of fractures cannot be achieved, although ranges of fracture ages are available. Advice from an experienced pediatric radiologist should be sought to assist with dating injuries, to obtain further radiologic or other imaging views, and to exclude other causes of skeletal abnormality.

3.3.1. Dating Fractures

Resolution of soft tissues	2–10 days
Early periosteal new bone	4–21 days
Loss of fracture line definition	10–21 days
Soft callus	10–21 days
Hard callus	14–90 days
Remodeling	3 months–2 years

For further information *see* ref. *31*.

Detecting occult injury is particularly important in the younger child and infant and recommended indications for a skeletal survey include the following *(17,25,28)*:

- Any child less than 2 years when there is a suspicion of physical abuse
- Any child less than 2 years presenting with a fracture suggestive of abuse
- Children aged 2–4 years with severe bruising
- Older children with severe injuries
- Children dying in unusual or suspicious circumstances
- Physical abuse in an infant twin (or multiple birth sets) less than 1 year—consider skeletal survey of the other infant(s) *(32)*
- Repeat views, particularly of ribs, may be useful 2 weeks following the initial survey, as periosteal reaction may not have formed around acute injuries

3.3.2. Differential Diagnosis of Skeletal Injury

- Accidental injury—appropriate, consistent history, prompt presentation
- Normal variation—e.g., skull suture, physiologic periosteal reaction (symmetric and smooth around the long bones of children from 6 weeks to 6 months)
- Birth trauma—commonly clavicle or humerus
- Infection—e.g., osteomyelitis, congenital syphilis
- Rickets—nutritional, renal, chronic illness, prematurity
- Cancers—e.g., neuroblastoma, leukemia
- Osteogenisis imperfecta—a rare condition, incidence of 1 in 20,000, usually accompanied by a family history of fractures, fractures with minimal trauma, easy bruising, joint laxity, early-onset deafness, blue sclerae, and dentinogenesis
- Copper deficiency—low-birth-weight preterm infants, malnutrition, malabsorption

3.4. Internal Injuries

3.4.1. Intracranial Injury

There is a high incidence of mortality and morbidity following inflicted head injury, and it is the most common cause of traumatic death in infancy *(33)*. It has been generally accepted from research evidence that serious or fatal injury from accidental injury, other than that sustained in road traffic accidents or falls from major heights, is rare in children under 2 years and that simple skull fractures in accidental trauma have a low risk of intracranial sequelae *(26)*.

The major acute intracranial lesions of NAI are subdural hematoma, cerebral edema with hypoxic ischemic encephalopathy, and, more rarely, brain lacerations, intracerebral and intraventricular hemorrhage, and extradural hematomas *(26)*.

The mechanism of brain injury is considered to be a whiplash motion of acceleration and deceleration, coupled with a rotational force, during a shaking episode of an infant, where the head is unsupported. Shaking alone may lead to brain injury *(34)*, although it is more common to have an associated impact injury. Impact may be against a hard surface, leading to external injury and an associated skull fracture, or against a soft surface, with no associated external injury. Hypoxia may also lead to brain injury from impairment of ventilation during chest squeezing, suffocation, or strangulation *(26)*.

Retinal hemorrhages are strongly suggestive of abuse when accompanied by intracranial injuries and in the absence of a confirmed history of severe accidental injury. Retinal hemorrhages can be found following severe closed chest injury, asphyxia, coagulation disorders, carbon monoxide poisoning, acute hypertension, sepsis, meningitis, and normal birth (usually disappearing by 2 weeks, rarely persisting to 6 weeks). When shaking injuries are suspected, retinal examination is essential and should include direct and indirect opthalmoscopy preferably by an ophthalmologist. Subhyaloid hemorrhages and local retinal detachment occur earliest and are often peripheral, found only by indirect ophthalmology. When intraocular injury is present, subdural hemorrhage is very likely, and the presence of retinal detachment and multiple hemorrhages may indicate additional cerebral lacerations or intracerebral hemorrhages *(34)*.

Children with acute intracranial injury may present with fits, lethargy, irritability, apnea, unconsciousness and signs of shock, a tense fontanelle, increasing head circumference, and a low hemoglobin. Children with chronic subdural hematomas may present with poor feeding, failure to thrive, vomiting, increasing head circumference, and fits. The presentation may suggest sepsis, meningitis, encephalitis, or toxic or metabolic bone disease. The findings of retinal hemorrhages, other signs of abuse, and blood-stained cerebrospinal fluid may assist with the differential diagnosis.

When brain injury of abuse is suspected, a full blood count, platelet count and coagulation studies, skull X-ray, skeletal survey, and brain computed tomography (CT) are recommended. Magnetic resonance imaging (MRI) should be undertaken when CT is equivocal or normal and there are neurologic signs or symptoms *(26)*.

3.4.2. Abdominal Injuries

Visceral manifestations of NAI are uncommon and considered to contribute 2–4% of injuries in NAI *(35,36)*. However, visceral injuries carry a high morbidity and mortality (estimated mortality of 40–50%) and are the second commonest cause of fatal child abuse due to the shear force of trauma, delay in recognition of injury because of frequent lack of signs and symptoms, and delay in recognition of NAI *(36,37)*.

Injuries arise mainly from blunt trauma (punching, kicking, trampling, or stamping) or sudden acceleration/deceleration injuries (swinging or throwing a child into a solid object) and include contusion, laceration, and rupture of solid or hollow viscera. The duodenum, jejunum, pancreas, and liver are common sites of injury in abdominal NAI. Colonic or rectal injury are associated with sexual abuse *(26)*.

Vomiting, abdominal distension, pain, and shock may be presenting features. Other features of NAI and skeletal injury may provide clues to the underlying etiology. Immediate surgery may be necessary.

Suggested investigations include full blood count, blood biochemistry, pancreatic and liver enzymes plain, abdominal and chest X-ray (free air or free fluid), ultrasound, CT, and gastrointestinal contrast studies where indicated.

3.5. Munchausen Syndrome By Proxy (MSPB)

MSPB is a persistent fabrication of a child's illness either simulated or produced by the child's parent or caretaker. This form of child abuse is uncommon but severe and carries a high mortality and morbidity with a high incidence of reabuse and harm to siblings, commonly requiring separation of the child from the abusing parent *(38)*. The perpetrator is more commonly the mother. The range of fabricated illness is wide and can be complicated further by multiple medical investigations. Among the commonest presentations are fits, apnea, bleeding, diarrhea, vomiting, fever, and rash *(39)*. Suffocation, poisoning, drug administration, and lying are mechanisms of fabricating illness. Emotional abuse is associated in almost all cases with considerable overlap with other forms of abuse. Diagnosis is difficult and often delayed. Management should follow the usual child protection procedures. Covert video surveillance can play an important role in detection, offering definitive evidence, but this approach must be carefully coordinated and multidisciplinary *(40)*.

4. Summary

NAI in children is a common condition and carries with it a significant morbidity and mortality. Physicians need to be able to recognize NAI and take appropriate action to protect children. Young children and infants are at particular risk, and there is often an overlap with other forms of abuse. A multidisciplinary approach aimed at early intervention, support for families, improvements in parenting styles, and prevention of mortality and morbidity in the child is essential to safeguard the welfare of children.

References

1. Department of Health (1991) *Children Act 1989—Guidance and Regulations*. Her Majesty's Stationery Office, London.
2. Home Office, Department of Health, Department of Education and Science, Welsh Office (1991) *Working Together Under the Children Act 1989. A Guide to Arrangements for Interagency Co-operation for the Protection of Children from Abuse*. Her Majesty's Stationery Office, London.
3. Johnson, C. F. (1990) Inflicted injury versus accidental injury. *Pediatr Clin North Am.* **37,** 791–814.
4. Gibbons, J., Gallagher, B., Bell, C., and Gordon, D. (1995) *Development After Physical Abuse in Early Childhood: A Follow-up study of Children on the Child Protection Registers*. Her Majesty's Stationery Office, London.
5. Newberger, E. H. (1993) Child physical abuse. *Primary Care.* **20,** 317–327.
6. Gibbons, J., Conroy, S., and Bell, C. (1995) *Operating the Child Protection System: A Study of Child Protection Practices in English Local Authorities*. Her Majesty's Stationery Office, London.
7. Cross, S. B., Kaye, E., and Ratnofsky, A. C. (1993) *A Report on the Maltreatment of Children with Disabilities*. National Center on Child Abuse and Neglect, Washington DC.
8. National Commission of Inquiry into the Prevention of Child Abuse (1996) *Childhood Matters. Report of The National Commission of Inquiry into the Prevention of Child Abuse*. Her Majesty's Stationery Office, London.
9. (1995) *Child Protection Messages from Research*. Her Majesty's Stationery Office, London.
10. Department of Health (1998) *Children and Young People on Child Protection Registers Year Ending March 1998 England*. Government Statistical Service.
11. Department of Health and Human Services (1995) *Child Maltreatment*. Reports from the States to the National Child Abuse and Neglect Data System (NCANDS). U.S. Administration for Children and Families, Washington, DC.
12. Hobbs, C. J. and Wynne, J. M. (1990) The sexually abused battered child. *Arch Dis Child.* **65,** 423–427.
13. Speight, N. (1993) Nonaccidental injury, in *ABC of Child Abuse*, 2nd ed., BMJ Publishing Group, London.
14. Stephenson, T. and Balias, Y. (1996) Estimation of the age of bruising. *Arch Dis Child.* **74,** 53–55.
15. Stephenson, T. (1997) Ageing of bruising in children. *J R Soc Med.* **90,** 312–314.
16. Langlois, N. and Gresham, G. (1991) The ageing of bruises: a review of the study of the colour changes with time. *Forensic Sci Int.* **50,** 227–238.

17. Hobbs, C. J., Hanks, H., and Wynne, J. M. (1993) Physical abuse, in *Child Abuse and Neglect. A Clinician's Handbook*, Churchill Livingstone, Edinburgh.
18. O'Hare, A. and Eden, O. (1984) Bleeding disorders and nonaccidental injury. *Arch Dis Child.* **59,** 860–864.
19. McDonald, D. and McFarland, T. (1972) Forensic odontology—report of a case involving bite marks. *Glasgow Dent J.* **3,** 16–19.
20. Glass, R., Andrews, E., and Jones, K. (1980) Bite mark evidence: a case report using accepted and new techniques. *J Forensic Sci.* **25,** 638–645.
21. Vale, G. and Noguchi, T. (1983) Anatomical distribution of human bite marks in a series of 67 cases. *J Forensic Sci.* **28,** 61–69.
22. Scmitt, B. D. (1987) The child with non-accidental trauma, in *The Battered Child,* 4th ed. (Helfer, R. E. and Kempe, R. S., eds.), University of Chicago Press, Chicago, pp. 178–196.
23. Hobbs, C. (1993) Burns and scalds, in *ABC of Child Abuse*, 2nd ed.(Meadow, R., ed.), BMJ Publishing Group, London, pp. 20–23.
24. Hobbs, C. (1986) When are burns not accidental? *Arch Dis Child.* **61,** 357–361.
25. Feldman, K. W. (1997) Evaluation of physical abuse, in *The Battered Child*, 5th ed. (Helfer, R. E., Kempe, R. S., and Krugman, R. D., eds), University of Chicago Press, Chicago, pp. 175–220.
26. Carty, H. (1997) Non-accidental injury: a review of the radiology. *Eur Radiol.* **7,** 1365–1376.
27. Caffey, J. (1946) Multiple fractures of the long bones of infants suffering from chronic subdural haematoma. *AJR.* **56,** 163–173.
28. Merten, D., Radkowski, M., and Leonidis, J. (1983) The abused child: a radiological reappraisal. *Radiology.* **146,** 377–381.
29. Helfer, R., Slovis, T., and Black, M.(1977) Injuries resulting when small children fall out of bed. *Pediatrics.* **60,** 533–555.
30. Hobbs, C. J. (1984) Skull fracture and the diagnosis of child abuse. *Arch Dis Child.* **59,** 246–252.
31. O'Connor, J. F. and Cohen, J. (1987) *Diagnostic Imaging of Child abuse.* (Kleinman, P. K., ed.). Williams & Wilkins, Baltimore. p. 112.
32. Hansen, K. K. (1994) Twins and child abuse. *Arch Pediatr Adolesc Med.* **148,** 1345,1346.
33. Duhaime, A. C., Christain, C. W., Rorke, L. B., and Zimmerman, R. (1988) Nonaccidental head injury in infants—"the shaken baby syndrome." *N Engl J Med.* **338,** 1828,1829.
34. Green, M. A., Lieberman, G., Milroy, C. M., and Parsons, M. A. (1996) Ocular and cerebral trauma in non-accidental injury in infancy; underlying mechanisms and implications for paediatric practice. *Br J Opthalmol.* **80,** 282–287.
35. Merten, D. F. and Carpenter, B. L. M. (1990) Radiologic imaging of inflicted injury in the child abuse syndrome. *Paediatr Clin North Am.* **37,** 815–837.
36. Ng, C. S., Hall, C. M., and Shaw, D. G. (1997) The range of visceral manifestations of non-accidental injury. *Arch Dis Child.* **77,** 167–174.
37. Cooper, A., Floyd, T., Barlow, B., et al. (1988) Major blunt abdominal trauma due to child abuse. *J Trauma.* **28,** 1483–1487.

38. Davis, P., McClure, R. J., Rolfe, K., et al. (1998) Procedures, placement, and risks of further abuse after Munchausen syndrome by proxy, non-accidental poisoning, and non-accidental suffocation. *Arch Dis Child.* **78,** 217–221.
39. Rosenberg, D. A. (1987) Web of deceit: a literature review of Munchausen syndrome by proxy. *Child Abuse Negl Int J.* **11,** 547–563.
40. Southall, D. P., Plunkett, M. C., Bank, M., et al. (1997) Covert video recordings of life-threatening child abuse: lessons in child protection. *Pediatrics.* **100,** 735–760

Chapter 6

Crowd Control Agents

Kari Blaho

1. Introduction

Forms of chemical restraint were used as early as 423 BC in the Peloponnesian war. Modern chemical crowd control agents were first employed by the French in the early months of World War I when they launched tear gas grenades against the German army. In addition to chlorobenzylidene (tear gas), World War I also saw the introduction of chlorine gas and mustard gas. The Germans first used chlorine gas in the spring of 1915 against the French army at Ypres. The chlorine gas formed a cloud that was mistaken for a smoke screen behind which the German Army would advance. Instead of evacuating the area, the French Army entrenched, readying for an attack. Mustard gas was used in 1917 by the Germans against the French army. Unlike chlorine, which wafted in a cloud described as a greenish yellow smoke, mustard gas was nearly odorless, and its effects took much longer to manifest. Chlorine is an immediate choking agent resulting in severe respiratory distress and death; the full effects of mustard gas take 12–24 hours. Any surface exposed to mustard gas is affected. Mucosal membranes such as those in the eye and respiratory tract, as well as the skin, develop blisters, slough, and can fully incapacitate the individual for long periods.

World War I was the first modern forum to use chemical weapons for controlling large numbers of individuals. Since that time, agents with wider safety margins have been developed that promote crowd dispersal without significant morbidity and mortality. Modern crowd control agents such as

From: *Forensic Science: A Physician's Guide to Clinical Forensic Medicine*
Edited by: M. M. Stark © Humana Press, Inc., Totowa, NJ

chlorobenzylidene were first used by the military as training agents and then by law enforcement as alternatives to lethal force; most recently some have been available to civilians for personal self-defense. Chemical crowd control agents could also be used by terrorists to incite fear or panic in crowds; there is always the potential for accidental dispersal in a public forum or, rarely, the potential for self-abuse.

There is considerable debate concerning the use of chemical agents for crowd control. Three agents have been used to replace potentially lethal force (firearms and batons). They are capsaicin oleum [pepper spray (PS or OC)], chloracetothenon [mace (CN)], and chlorobenzylidene [tear gas (CS)].

Five major areas are of concern when these agents are used by law enforcement:

1. Possible toxicity to the offender
2. Potential for exposure to the person administering the agent
3. Potential for any ancillary exposure to health care providers and to bystanders *(1–4)*
4. Expansion of their use to nonviolent offenders such as peaceful protesters
5. Long-term effects from repeated and occupational exposure *(5)*

Some of these issues become more complicated as chemical control agents are increasingly popular with civilians as readily available, often legal, nonlethal, self-defense weapons.

Several incidents in the United States and other countries have brought into question the appropriateness of use of chemical crowd control agents *(5,6)*. In one reported U.S. incident, law enforcement officers applied oleum capsicum liquid via a cotton-tipped applicator directly to the periorbital area of protesters who were sitting and refused to disperse *(7)*. The use of oleum capsicum against these nonviolent offenders when other methods of control had failed generated negative publicity and resulted in legal action against the law enforcement officials. Ultimately, the courts decided in favor of the law enforcement officers who opted for this type of application, which would limit exposure in the enclosed space occupied by the protestors.

When used appropriately, crowd control agents have a good safety margin and generally do no permanent harm. In addition to the furious debate over the agents themselves, there has been some concern over the safety of the delivery vehicles, particularly methyl-isobutyl ketone (MIBK). Although chronic exposure to MIBK has been associated with neurologic and respiratory effects, no data support the theory that acute exposure to the low concentrations that occur with CS spray poses these same problems *(8–10)*. Despite the controversy surrounding chemical control agents, they offer a less hazardous method of restraint than other potentially lethal alternatives such as firearms.

Table 1
Examples of Chemical Restraint Products Available

Brand name	Ingredients	Delivery system
Cap-Stun	5% oleoresin capsicum	Spray
Alan's Pepper Spray	10% oleo capsicum pepper	Spray
Pepper Foam	10% oleo capsicum	Foam spray
Pepper Gard, Triple Action Spray	10% oleo capsicum and 10% CS	Spray
Mark III	5% oleo capsicum and 5% CS	Spray

2. Clinical Features and Treatment

As mentioned above, the three main chemical restraint compounds are capsaicin oleum, OC, CN, and CS. These agents are available in varying concentrations, with several vehicles, in aerosols or foams, and in particulate form with dispersal devices. Some of these are listed in Table 1.

Essentially a means of nonlethal chemical warfare, chemical crowd control products are used as defensive agents to incapacitate individuals temporarily or disperse groups without requiring more forceful means. The clinical effects are short-lived once exposure has ended. These agents share common effects that include lachrymation, ocular irritation and pain, dermal irritation, blepharospasm, conjunctivitis, transient impairment of vision, and mild to moderate respiratory distress *(11–13)*. Some corneal defects after exposure have been noted, but whether this is a direct tissue effect of the agent or a result of rubbing the ocular surface is unknown *(14)*. Contact dermatitis and periocular edema can also result. Other more severe effects such as pulmonary edema have been documented when concentrations are several hundred-fold above what produces intolerable symptoms or with trauma associated with the explosive device used to deliver the chemical agent *(6,15)*.

All these clinical effects produced by chemical crowd control agents render the recipient temporarily unable to continue violent action or resist arrest. Since they all share a high safety ratio, are effective at low concentrations, and can be used without direct forceful contact by the law enforcement officer, they are ideal agents either for control of the individual offender or for riot control. Because of their relative safety, these agents are generally excluded from international treaty provisions that address chemical weapons. The United States, England, Ireland, France, China, Korea, Israel, and Russia are a few of the countries that utilize these compounds as riot control agents. The legal availability to law enforcement and the general public differs between countries; however, most can be easily obtained through international markets or ordered on the Internet.

Chemical restraint compounds differ from most agents because some, such as CS, are solid particles with low vapor pressures. They are usually dispersed as fine particles or in a solution. For large crowds, "bombs" have been developed that can be dropped from aerial positions producing wide dispersal of the compound. They are also formulated in grenades or canisters, which can be propelled either by throwing or with a projectile device. The most common method of dispersal is by individual spray cans that deliver either a stream, spray, or foam containing the agent. These individual dispersal units were designed to render immediate incapacitation to an offender without the use of more forceful methods. Canisters containing a lower concentration of the active ingredient have been marketed to civilians for personal protection. Since there is no formal training for civilians on the use of these devices, there is a significant risk for exposure to the users as well as bystanders.

2.1. Oleum Capsicum

OC (or PS) selectively stimulates nociceptors in exposed mucous membranes that release substance P, bradykinin, histamine, and prostaglandins. The physiologic effects of these mediators result in vasodilation, increased vascular permeability, pain, and altered neurotrophic chemotaxis. Other common symptoms are listed in Table 2.

Capsicum in its pure form is a crystalline material. The oleoresin extract of capsicum contains over 100 volatile compounds that act in a similar manner to capsicum *(16)*. Because of the variability in the individual components of oleum capsicum, as well as variation in quality control, products containing this extract have differences in efficacy *(16,17)*. Most are formulated in a propylene vehicle to enhance adherence to the skin surface. PS is the most common spray marketed to civilians for nonlethal, noncontact self-defense. It can be purchased in a variety of sprays or foams, in various concentrations, or combined with other crowd control agents such as CS (Fig. 1).

In a retrospective study by Watson et al. *(11)*, patients presenting to an emergency department (ED) after PS exposure during a law enforcement action were evaluated. Most patients complained of ocular irritation as well as irritation and pain at the site of exposure. The symptoms were transient, and very few required treatment. The most significant adverse effects were corneal abrasions, which were treated with topical anesthetics and topical antibiotics.

Table 2
Common Clinical Findings with Exposure to Crowd Control Agents

Finding	CS	CN	OC
Ocular			
Lacrimation	√	√	√
Blepharospasm	√	√	
Pain and/or burning	√	√	√
Conjunctival injection	√	√	√
Conjunctival edema	√	√	
Photophobia	√	√	
Corneal abrasion	√	√	√
Impaired vision	√	√	√
Upper airway			
Pain and/or burning	√	√	
Shortness of breath	√	√	√
Increased secretion	√	√	
Congestion	√		
Coughing	√	√	√
Throat irritation	√	√	√
Wheezing	√	√	√
Irregular respiration[a]	√	√	
Dermal			
Pain	√	√	√
Contact dermatitis		√	√
Blistering	√	√	√
Miscellaneous			
Nausea/vomiting	√		
Bad taste	√		
Headache	√		
Increased blood pressure	√[a]		

[a]Initial response thought to be associated with pain.

Five of 94 patients complained of wheezing or shortness of breath. No patient required treatment for wheezing, and two of the five had a history of reactive airway disease. No patient in this study had significant morbidity or mortality, and all were discharged from the ED. There are no data to support the notion that PS exacerbates pulmonary disease or that patients with reactive airway disease are more sensitive to the effects *(8,18–20)*.

There have been a few reports of severe reactions to PS. One case report summarized respiratory distress that necessitated extracorporeal membrane

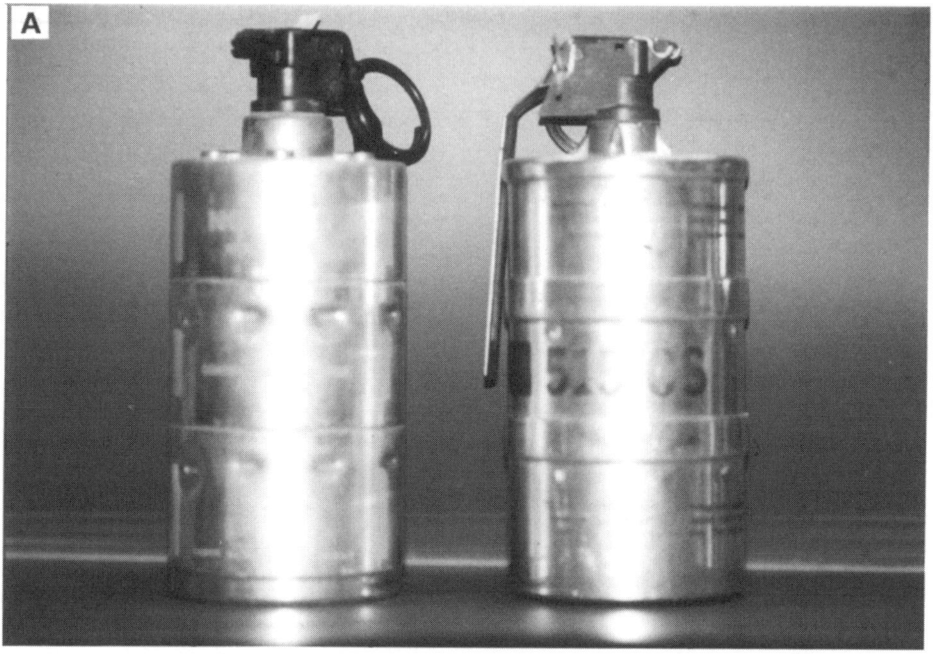

Fig. 1. (A–C) Examples of individual spray containers with crowd control agents.

oxygenation in a 4-week-old infant after 5% PS was accidentally discharged in his face *(21)*. The infant had a rocky clinical course but recovered. Another case report summarized the clinical course of an 11-year-old child who intentionally sprayed and inhaled PS from an individual canister and developed reversible wheezing *(22)*. These case reports are anecdotal in that they report symptoms temporally related to PS exposure and demonstrate that these compounds, when used improperly, can cause severe symptoms. Thus far, these adverse events have been rare.

Of concern were reports of violent prisoners who died after being sprayed with pepper spray and being restrained *(23)*. It was assumed that the police used excessive force and that the prisoners died from positional asphyxia from the restraints or that pepper spray played a role in their deaths *(23)*. There is no evidence that pepper spray causes any type of respiratory effects sufficient to cause death. All the prisoners who died exhibited characteristics consistent with excited delirium from substance abuse. Most were obese, had hyperthermia, and were violent; cocaine was also present on postmortem analysis. The cause of death can be difficult to determine, as often these patients will have

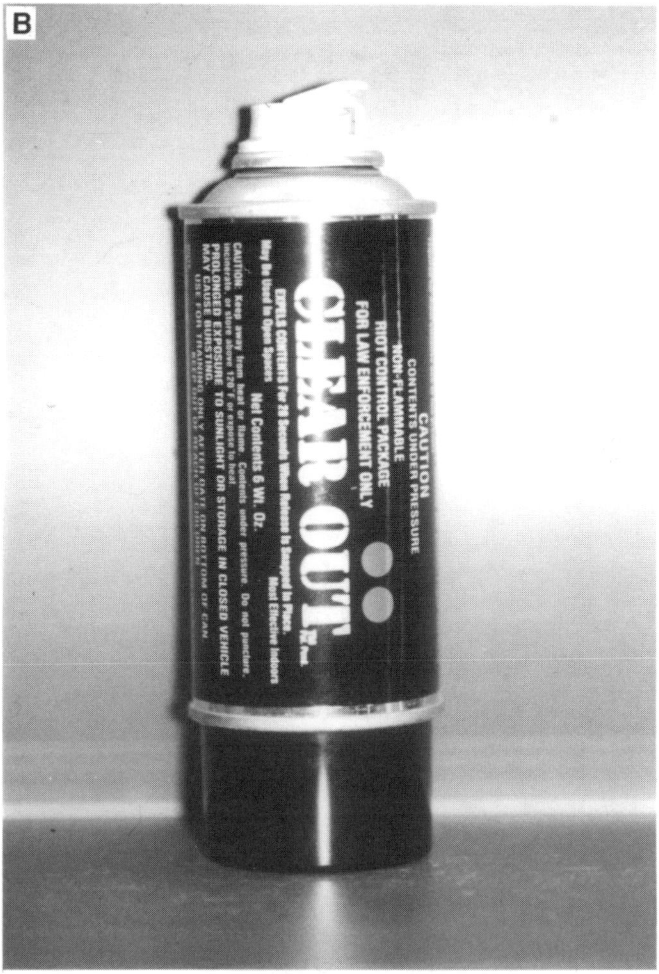

Fig. 1B.

only subtle changes consistent with stimulant abuse, and autopsy reports can be inconclusive or incomplete. The lesson should be that all violent prisoners, whether or not a chemical restraint has been used, should be evaluated and closely monitored and perhaps evaluated by health care professionals. A small population of acutely intoxicated individuals are at risk of sudden death, independent of their treatment.

Treatment of exposure to PS is based on severity of symptoms. The first order of treatment should always be the removal of contaminated clothing. Copious irrigation of affected areas will attenuate the burning sensation

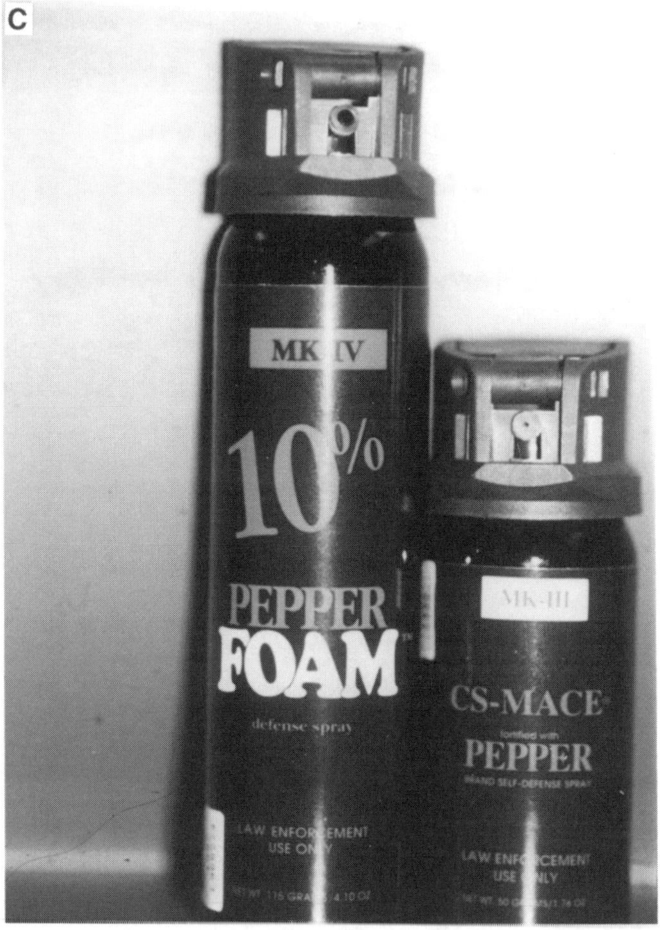

Fig. 1C.

(24,25). However, one must use caution not to contaminate other sites with the irrigant, for example, washing PS from the hair into the eyes or oral pharyngeal mucosa. A slit lamp exam of the anterior chamber is warranted to rule out corneal abrasion in patients who remain symptomatic. If present, the abrasion should be treated appropriately with topical antibiotics, cycloplegics, analgesics, and follow-up. Dermatitis associated with PS has been reported *(26,27)*. Topical corticosteroids, systemic antihistamines, and analgesics have been employed in reducing symptoms. An example of rather severe PS dermatitis and ocular swelling is shown in Fig. 2. This particular patient was sprayed during arrest by police officers and brought to an ED for evaluation. He was

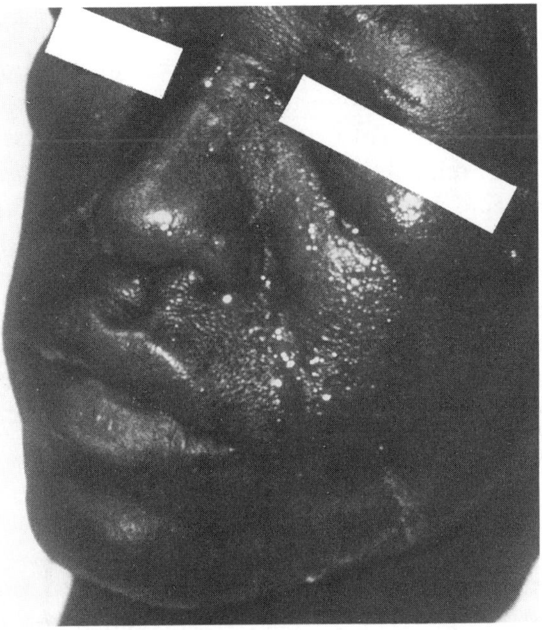

Fig. 2. Periocular swelling and facial contact dermatitis from pepper spray exposure during an arrest by law enforcement.

treated with irrigation, systemic antihistamines, and steroids with resolution of his symptoms within 4 days.

2.2. Chlorobenzylidene Malononitrile and Chloracetophenone

CS, or tear gas, is frequently used by the military and by law enforcement as a method of controlling both individuals and crowds. The military also uses it during exercises to train personnel in the use of protective equipment. CN, known by its common name Mace, is the oldest of the crowd control agents. CS was developed in the 1950s, and it has largely replaced CN.

CS and CN are both lachrymating agents. CS is usually mixed with a pyrotechnic compound for dispersal in grenades or canisters as a fine particulate, which forms the characteristic smoke. CN is usually prepared for aerosol dispersal by individual canisters. Both agents are available in individual containers or large bombs, or they can be dispersed through a hand-held aerosolizer. They are formulated with a variety of solvents such as alcohol, ether, carbon sulfide, and methylchloroform *(28)*, or they can be dispersed as solid particles. In the United States, a combination of CS (10%) and PS (10%) is used by some law enforcement agencies for chemical control.

CS and CN are highly soluble in a variety of agents. When contact with mucous membranes is made, the symptoms described in Table 2 occur. Even though there is the perception of shortness of breath, pulmonary function tests performed shortly after exposure to either agent have shown minimal alterations *(29)*. The mechanism of irritation is not fully understood. The effects of CS are thought to be related to the formation of highly irritating chlorine atoms and hydrochloric acid when it comes in contact with water *(1,30)*. CS and CN have also been described as alkylating agents that target sulfhydryl groups *(29)*. In addition, there is some controversy surrounding the production of cyanide molecules at the tissue level with exposure to high concentrations of CS *(31,32)*. Regardless, the effects of CS and CN usually manifest without permanent tissue injury. Exposure is most often limited as individuals flee the scene. Exposure can be significant if the affected person is forced into a confined space for extended periods.

Most of the dispersal methods achieve concentrations far below what is considered to be lethal *(33)*, however, there is some question as to concentrations achieved in close proximity to grenades or other delivery devices or for those who cannot or will not leave the exposure area *(6,33)*. Based on animal studies, it is generally thought that a concentration of 25,000–150,000 mg/m^3/min or 200 mg/kg body mass represents the LD_{50} for CS. A grenade can generate a concentration of 2,000–5,000 mg/m^3 at the center, with concentrations becoming significantly less within a few yards from the center of the explosion *(33)*.

Treatment of CS exposure is based largely on the severity of clinical findings. Most patients will fully recover within minutes after removal from the agent and will not require medical attention *(34)*. The most common lasting complaints are facial and ocular irritation. In contrast to other forms of chemical exposure, irrigating the affected area will only intensify and prolong the effects of CS gas or particles. For patients who require medical evaluation, the first order of treatment should always be removal of contaminated clothing, with special attention to eliminating secondary exposure by using protective equipment and not placing a contaminated patient in a confined space. Clothing should be removed outside, placed inside a plastic bag, and then bagged again. Blowing dry air directly onto the eye assists in vaporizing the dissolved CS gas *(35)*. Some clinicians have recommended copious ocular irrigation with sterile saline, although this has been thought in some cases to cause an initial acute increase in ocular irritation *(35,36)*. A careful slit lamp exam of the anterior segment of the eye, including evaluation under the lids, should be done for persistent ocular irritation. If particles have become imbedded in the cornea or under the lids, they should be removed. If corneal abrasions are present, a few days of topical broad-spectrum antibiotics, cycloplegics, and appropriate analgesics in addition to close follow-up should be prescribed.

Dermal irritation in the form of burning and blistering can be treated with irrigation, preferably with an alkaline solution other than sodium hypochlorite *(26)*. Erythema can be common in skin that has been freshly abraded but resolves 45–60 minutes after exposure. Contact dermatitis can be effectively treated with topical corticosteroids and/or antihistamines such as diphenhydramine. Typically, dermatitis associated with CS exposure resolves within a few days *(26)*.

Home remedies such as the application of cooking oils are contraindicated and pose an increase risk for irritation and infection *(36)*. Sodium hypochlorite solutions will exacerbate any dermal irritation and should not be used. Plain soap and water is effective, but in most cases, removal of clothing in a well-ventilated area is all that is needed.

There are conflicting reports about the long-term effects of CS exposure. With an exposure to high concentrations, usually for prolonged periods in a confined space, pulmonary edema, pneumonitis, heart failure, hepatocellular damage, and death have been reported *(12,37)*. There are no data to support any claims of tetratogenity, or toxicity to the pregnant woman *(12,38)*. These agents do not appear to exacerbate chronic diseases such as seizure disorders, respiratory disease, or psychiatric illnesses. Contact allergies in those previously exposed have also been reported *(39–41)*.

The possibility of secondary exposure to health care and law enforcement providers exists with the use of all chemical crowd control agents. Although published reports are few, effects can be minimized with common sense practices like decontamination before the patient is placed in a confined area such as a police car, ambulance, or an isolated room in the ED. The use of protective personal equipment such as gloves and careful washing of exposed areas prevents cross-contamination.

3. Conclusions

The most important considerations in utilizing chemical crowd control agents are that they be used judiciously, in the correct manner, and in place of more forceful means of controlling violent or potentially violent prisoners or crowds. Law enforcement officers should be educated on the common clinical effects and the appropriateness of seeking medical care. Medical care should never be withheld from those who request it or in those prisoners who have lingering effects. Treatment of exposure is summarized in Table 3. To limit

Table 3
Options for Treatment of Exposure to Chemical Crowd Control Agents

Treatment	PS	CS	CN
Removal of contaminated clothing	√	√	√
Ocular irrigation	√		√
Dermal irrigation	√	√	√
Alkaline solution irrigation of skin		√	√
Soap and water decontamination	√	√	√
Topical steroids for dermatitis	√	√	√
Systemic antihistamines for dermatitis	√	√	√
Systemic steroids for dermatitis	√	√	√
Topical antibiotics for corneal abrasion	√	√	√
Cycloplegics	√	√	√
Analgesics for pain	√	√	√

injury or potential liability, many police forces regulate the use of chemical crowd control agents by establishing policies to guide their use. One example is the "ladder of force" employed by the Berkley, California police department. Words are used first, followed by more defensive actions such as chemical agents, then batons, and finally firearms. Use of these agents is monitored and formal reports are filed when they are used. These agents afford control of violent offenders with much less risk to life and limb than do firearms, explosives, and battering.

ACKNOWLEDGMENT

The author would like to thank Lt. Ruff, Lt. R. Proctor, and Officer D. Crowe of the Memphis Police Department.

References

1. Bhattacharya, S. T. and Hayward, A. W. (1993) CS gas—implications for the anesthetist. *Anaesthesia.* **48,** 896–897.
2. Editorial (1998) "Safety" of chemical batons. *Lancet.* **352,** 159.
3. Stark, M. M. and Knight, M. (1998) "Safety" of chemical batons. *Lancet.* **352,** 1633.
4. Blaho, K. and Winbery, S. (1998) "Safety" of chemical batons. *Lancet.* **352,** 1633.
5. Gray, P. J. (1997) CS gas is not a chemical means of restraining a person. *BMJ.* **314,** 1353.
6. Hu, H., Fine, J., Epstein, P., Kelsey, K., Reynolds, P., and Walker, B. (1989) Tear gas—harassing agent or toxic chemical weapon. *JAMA.* **262,** 660–663.

7. Van Derbeken, J. (1997) Pepper spray in the eyes—protesters sue police. *San Francisco Chronicle.* 1A.
8. Spencer, P. S., Schaumburg, H. H., Raleigh, R. L., and Terhaar, C. J. (1975) Nervous system degeneration produced by the industrial solvent methyl n-butyl ketone. *Arch Neurol.* **32,** 219–222.
9. Iregren, A., Tesarz, M., and Wigaeus-Hjelm, E. (1993) Human experimental MIBK exposure: effects on heart rate, performance, and symptoms. *Environ Res.* **63,** 101–108.
10. Dick, R. B., Krieg, E. F., Setzer, J., and Taylor, B. (1992) Neurobehavioral effects from acute exposures to methyl isobutyl ketone and methyl ethyl ketone. *Fundam Appl Toxicol.* **19,** 453–473.
11. Watson, W. A., Stremel, K. R., and Westdorp, E. J. (1996) Oleoresin capsicum (Cap-Stun) toxicity from aerosol exposure. *Ann Pharmacother.* **30,** 733–735.
12. Tominack, R. L. and Spyker, D. A. (1987) Capsicum and capsaicin—a review: case report of the use of hot peppers in child abuse. *Clin Toxicol.* **25,** 591–601.
13. Weaver, W. and Jett, M. B. *Oleoresin Capsicum Training and Use.* FBI Academy Firearms Training Unit, Quantico, VA.
14. Lee, R. J., Yolton, R. L., Yolton, D. P., Schnider, C., and Janin, M. L. (1996) Personal defense sprays: effects and management of exposure. *J Am Optom Assoc.* **67,** 548–560.
15. Himsworth, H. (1971) *Report of the Inquiry into the Medical and Toxicological Aspects of CS (Ortho-chlorobenzylidene Malonitrile), II: Inquiry into Toxicological Aspects of CS and its Use for Civil Purposes.* Her Majesty's Stationery Office, London.
16. Cordell, G. A. and Araujo, O. E. (1993) Capsaicin: identification, nomenclature, and pharmacotherapy. *Ann Pharmacother.* **27,** 330–336.
17. Haas, J. S., Whipple, R. E., Grant, P. M., Andresen, B. D., Volpe, A. M., and Pelkey, G. E. (1997) Chemical and elemental comparison of two formulations of oleoresin capsicum. *Sci Justice.* **37,** 15–24.
18. Fuller, R. W. (1991) Pharmacology of inhaled capsaicin in human. *Respir Med.* **85,** 31–34.
19. Maxwell, D. L., Fuller, R. W., and Dixon, C. M. S. (1987) Ventilatory effects of inhaled capsaicin in man. *Eur J Clin Pharmacol.* **31,** 715–717.
20. Collier, J. G. and Fuller, R. W. (1984). Capsicum inhalation in man and the effects of sodium cromoglycolate. *Br J Pharmacol.* **81,** 113–117.
21. Billmire, D. F., Vinocur, C., Ginda, M., Robinson, N. B., Panitch, H., Friss, H., et al. (1996) Pepper-spray induced respiratory failure treated with extracorporeal membrane oxygenation. *Pediatrics.* **98,** 961–963.
22. Winograd, H. L. (1977) Acute croup in an older child: an unusual toxin orgin. *Clin Pediatr.* **16,** 884–887.
23. Karch, S. B. and Stephens, B. G. (1999) Drug abusers who die in custody. *J R Soc Med.* **92,** 110–113.
24. Burnet, J. (1989) Capsicum pepper dermatitis. *Cutis.* **43,** 534.
25. Jones, L. A., Tandberg, D., and Troutman, W. G. (1987) Household treatment of chili burns of the hands. *Clin Toxicol.* **25,** 483–491.

26. Holland, P. and White, R. G. (1972) The cutaneous reactions produced by CS and CN when applied directly to the skin of human subjects. *Br J Dermatol.* **86,** 150–155.
27. Penneys, N. S., Israel, R. M., and Indgin, S. M. (1969) Contact dermatitis due to 1-chloroacetophenone and chemical mace. *N Engl J Med.* **281,** 413–415.
28. Schmutz, J. L., Rigon, J. L., Mougeolle, J. M., Weber, M., and Beurey, J. (1987) Cutaneous accidents caused by self-defense sprays. *Ann Dermatol Venerol.* **114,** 1211–1216.
29. Chemical Casualty Care Office (1995) *Medical Management of Chemical Casualties Handbook*, 2nd ed. US Army Medical Research Institute of Chemical Defense, Aberdeen Proving Ground, MD.
30. Ballantyne, B. (1977) Riot control agents: biomedical and health aspects of the use of chemicals in civilian disturbances. *Med Ann.* pp. 7–14.
31. Jones, G. R. N. (1971) Verdict on CS. *BMJ.* **4,** 170.
32. Jones, G. R. N. and Israel, M. S. (1979) Mechanism of toxicity of injected CS gas. *Nature.* **228,** 1315–1316.
33. Weigand, D. A. (1969) Cutaneous reactions to the riot control agent CS. *Mil Med.* **134,** 437–440.
34. Punte, C. L., Owens, E., and Gutentag, P. J. (1963) Exposures to ortho-chlorobenzylidene malonitrile. *Arch Environ Health.* **67,** 366–374.
35. Yih, J. P. (1995) CS gas injury to the eye. *BMJ.* **311,** 276.
36. Folb, P. I. and Talmud, J. (1989) Tear gas—its toxicology and suggestions for management of its acute effects in man. *SAMJ.* **76,** 295.
37. Krapf, R. and Thalmann, H. (1981) Akute Exposition durch CS-Rauchgas und linische Beobachtungen. *Schweiz Med Wockenachr.* **11,** 2056–2060.
38. Upshall, D. G. (1973) Effects of o-chlorobenzylidene malononitrile (CS) and the stress of aerosol inhalation upon rat and rabbit embryonic development. *Toxicol Appl Pharmacol.* **24,** 45–59.
39. Maucher, O. M., Stengel, R., and Schopf, E. (1986) Chloroacetophenone allergy. *Hautarzt.* **37,** 397–401.
40. Fuchs, T. and Ippen, H. (1986) Contact allergy to CN and CS tear gas. *Derm Beruf Umwelt.* **34,** 12–14.
41. Fuchs, T. and in der Wiesche, M. (1990) Contact allergies to CN and CS (tear gas) in participants in demonstrations. *Z Hautk.* **65,** 288–292.

Chapter 7

Care of Detainees

Guy Norfolk and Margaret M. Stark

1. Introduction

Doctors may be asked by the police to assess the fitness for detention in police custody of adults and juveniles arrested in connection with an offense, detained by immigration, or requiring a place of safety (children and the mentally ill), or remanded or sentenced (convicted) prisoners. A person in police custody is referred to as a detainee in this chapter. Detainees may have to be interviewed regarding their involvement in an offense and possibly further detained overnight for court; guidance may therefore have to be given to the custodians regarding their care.

Although various laws govern the powers of the police in different jurisdictions *(1)*, the basic principles remain the same *(2)*. If an individual detained in police custody appears to be suffering from a mental or physical illness and needs medical attention or has sustained any injuries whether at arrest or prior to arrest, such attention should be sought as soon as possible. Increasingly the police have to deal with individuals who misuse alcohol and drugs or are mentally disordered; if the detainee's behavior gives rise to concern, medical advice should be sought.

Custody staff should also seek medical advice if an individual requests a doctor or requires medication or if the custody staff suspect that the detainee is suffering from an infectious disease and need advice. In some areas, when a person under arrest is discharged from the hospital and taken to a police station, a doctor will be called to review the detainee and assess whether he or she is fit to be detained and fit for interview *(3)*.

From: *Forensic Science: A Physician's Guide to Clinical Forensic Medicine*
Edited by: M. M. Stark © Humana Press, Inc., Totowa, NJ

Table 1
Briefing on Arrival

- Discuss reason called (physical or mental illness/medication/injuries)
- Obtain details from the custody records including reason for arrest (may be related to drugs)
- Ask the arresting officer for information regarding the circumstances of arrest (concerns regarding behavior/use of force)
- Other information may be obtained from relatives/friends/family doctor/ hospital/police computer
- Is request to assess fitness for detention only?
- The anticipated length of detention if known
- Is the detainee to be interviewed?
- Are any samples required?
- Whether the detainee will be in custody overnight

Medical assessments of detainees may be performed by either a doctor or nurse retained to attend the police station *(4,5)* or by staff in the local hospital accident and emergency department *(6)*. The basic principles on which doctors should base their conduct have already been outlined in Chapter 2. The health and welfare of detainees should be paramount, with any forensic considerations of secondary importance. The role of any physician in this field should be independent, professional, courteous, and nonjudgmental.

If the police bring a detainee to the accident and emergency department or if the health professional is contacted by the police to attend the police station, it is important to find out the reason why a medical assessment is required. It is essential that the doctor or nurse be properly briefed by the custody staff or investigating officer (Table 1).

Fully informed consent from the detainee should be obtained after explaining the reason for the examination. Detainees should understand that they are under no obligation to give consent and that there is no right to absolute confidentiality. Notwithstanding the latter, custody staff should only be given that information necessary for them to care for detainees while they are in police detention. Such information will include details of any medical concerns, required observations, medication, and dietary requirements.

Although those detained in police custody are usually young, there remains the potential for considerable morbidity and mortality among this group. Therefore, it is essential that a full medical assessment be performed and detailed contemporaneous notes made. Obtaining an accurate account of a detainee's drug history, including prescribed and illicit drugs, can be difficult.

Table 2
The DRUGS Mnemonic[a]

Doctor	Any medication prescribed by a registered medical or dental practitioner
Recreational	Tobacco, alcohol, illicit drugs, anabolic steroids, etc.
User	Over the counter purchases/alternative medicine/homeopathy
Gynecologic	Contraceptive or hormone replacement treatment
Sensitivities	Including the exact nature of the response

[a]Adapted from ref. *7*.

A useful aid to obtaining a better drug history has recently been described (Table 2) *(7)*.

2. Administration of Medication

The doctor should ensure that clear and detailed instructions regarding any medication to be administered while the detainee is in police custody (including the dose, times of administration, and special instructions) are given to custodians with confirmation that these instructions are understood *(8)*. A sufficient quantity of medication should be prescribed to cover the time in detention. The medication should be given to the police in appropriately labeled individual containers or sachets; alternatively, medication may be prescribed and collected from the local pharmacist.

It is most important that there be a safe regime for the administration of medication to detainees. Records should be kept showing that the prescribed medication is given at the correct time and that any unused medicines are accounted for. Medication should be stored in a locked cupboard. Ideally police should ensure that when administering medication they are accompanied by another person as a witness and the detainee should be observed taking the medication to prevent hoarding.

If detainees are arrested with medications on their persons, medical advice should be sought as to whether they should be allowed to self-administer them. It may be prudent for an assessment by a doctor to be performed either in the custody suite or in the local hospital prior to self-administration.

Medication brought with the prisoner or collected from the home address should be checked to ensure that it has the correct name and dosage and that the quantity left is consistent with the date of issue. If there is doubt, checks should be made with the pharmacist, family doctor, or hospital. If the medicine is unlabeled it is preferable to issue a new prescription, especially with liquid preparations such as methadone.

Table 3
Common Medical Problems

- Epilepsy
- Asthma
- Diabetes
- Heart disease
- Sickle cell disease
- Injuries
- Infectious diseases
- Mental health
- Self harm
- Claustrophobia
- Alcohol
- Drugs

3. Conditions of Detention

The doctor should ensure that the conditions of detention are satisfactory with regard to the temperature and ventilation of the detention cells, cleanliness of the cell, bedding, personal hygiene, dietary needs, and fluids *(9)*. The detainee should have access to food and fluids as appropriate and should also have a period of rest of 8 hours during each 24 hours.

4. Medical Problems

A number of common medical problems are encountered when the doctor is assessing fitness to be detained in police custody. These are now considered in more detail (Table 3). Alcohol and drugs are fully discussed in Chapter 8.

4.1. Epilepsy

Many detainees state that they have "fits" and there is a need to differentiate, if possible, between epilepsy and seizures related to withdrawal from alcohol or benzodiazepines; it is also important to consider hypoglycemia.

The type of seizure should be ascertained together with the frequency and date of the most recent one. Details of medication should be obtained including time of the last dose. Treatment may be given if the detainee is in possession of legitimate medication; however, if he or she is intoxicated with alcohol or other central nervous system depressant drugs, treatment should generally be deferred until the detainee is no longer intoxicated.

Table 4
Signs of Acute Asthma[a]

Parameter	Severe	Life-threatening
Pulse rate	>110/min	Bradycardia
Respiratory rate	>25/min	
Peak expiratory flow rate	33–50%	<33% predicted
Blood pressure	Pulsus paradoxus	Hypotension
Speech	Inability to complete sentences	
Chest auscultation		Silent
Mental state	Agitation Restlessness	Exhaustion Confusion Coma

[a]Adapted from ref. *11*.

The custody staff should have basic first aid skills to enable them to deal with medical emergencies such as what to do when someone has a fit. If a known epileptic has a seizure while in custody, a medical assessment is advisable, although there is probably no need for hospitalization. However, if a known epileptic has more than one fit or a detainee has a "first-ever" fit while in custody, then transfer to a hospital is recommended.

Diazepam intravenously or rectally is the treatment of choice for status epilepticus *(10)*. Any detainee requiring parenteral medication to control fits should be observed for a period in the hospital.

4.2. Asthma

Asthma is a common condition; a careful history and objective recording of simple severity markers such as pulse and respiratory rate, blood pressure, speech, chest auscultation, mental state, and peak expiratory flow rate should identify patients who require hospitalization or urgent treatment (Table 4) *(11)*. Asthmatics should be allowed to retain bronchodilators for the acute relief of bronchospasm, e.g., salbutamol or the equivalent, with instructions left with the custody sergeant on other treatment if required.

4.3. Diabetes

It is often desirable to obtain a baseline blood glucose measurement when diabetic detainees are initially assessed and for this to be repeated if necessary throughout the period of detention. All doctors should have the means to test blood glucose, using either a strip for visual estimation or a quantitative meter. A wide range of small portable meters is now available.

Oral hypoglycemics and insulin should be continued and consideration given to supervision of insulin injections. Regular meals and snacks should be provided, and all diabetic patients should have access to rapidly absorbed carbohydrate-rich food.

Hypoglycemia is easily treated: if the blood glucose is less than 4 mmol/L in a conscious person, oral carbohydrate should be given. In an unconscious or restless detainee, an intravenous bolus of 50 mL of 50% dextrose solution may be difficult to administer and may result in skin necrosis if extravasation occurs; therefore glucagon 1 mg can be given intramuscularly followed by 40% glucose gel orally or applied to the inside of the mouth. Glucagon can give an initial glycemic response even in a patient with alcoholic liver disease *(12)*; however, it should be remembered that in severe alcoholics with depleted glycogen stores, the response to glucagon may be reduced or ineffective.

4.4. Heart Disease

The main problems encountered include a history of hypertension, angina, cardiac failure, and stable dysrhythmias. Basic cardiovascular assessment may be required including examination of the pulse and blood pressure together with auscultation of the heart and lungs for evidence of murmurs or cardiac failure.

Prescribed medication should be continued, and detainees should be allowed to keep their glyceryl trinitrate (GTN) spray or tablet with them in the cell. Chest pain that does not settle with GTN will obviously require further assessment in the hospital.

4.5. Sickle Cell Disease

Most detainees with sickle cell disease are aware of their illness and the symptoms to expect during an acute sickle cell crisis. Medical management in custody should not pose a problem unless there is an acute crisis, when hospital transfer may be required. Conditions of detention should be suitable, with adequate heating and access to fluids and analgesics as appropriate.

4.6. General Injuries

Detailed documentation of injuries is an important and common request. The injuries may have occurred prior to or during the arrest, and documentation of such injuries may form part of the investigation to refute counterallegations of assault.

Table 5
Head Injuries: Indications for Hospital Assessment[a]

Problems with assessment of the patient
Age
Cognitive function
Influence of alcohol or drugs
Neurologic impairment
Impairment of conscious level
Increased risk of skull fracture or intracranial bleed
Loss of consciousness
Amnesia
Vomiting
Headache
Bruising
Laceration
Blood or cerebrospinal fluid leak
Social considerations
Patient lives alone
Lack of responsible supervision
Homelessness

[a]Adapted from ref. *16*.

A record of each injury as outlined in Chapter 4 should be made and basic first aid provided. Certain wounds may be treated with Steristrips or Histoacryl glue in the police station *(13)*, although occasionally transfer to a hospital will be required for further medical assessment, e.g., suturing, X-rays.

4.7. Head Injuries

Any suspected head injury should receive a detailed assessment *(14)*. The time, place, and nature of the injury should be ascertained from the detainee or from any witnesses who were present. The duration of any loss of consciousness and the behavior since the injury should be noted. Examination should include measurement of pulse and blood pressure, Glasgow Coma Scale *(15)*, and neurologic assessment. The indications for hospital assessment include situations in which there are problems with the assessment of the patient or an increased risk of skull fracture or an intracranial bleed (Table 5) *(16)*.

Ingestion of alcohol or drugs and relevant past medical history should be ascertained. Although deaths in police custody are rare, head injuries accounted for 10% and substance abuse, including alcohol and drugs, accounted for

25% in a survey of such deaths between 1990 and 1997 in England and Wales *(17)*. There should be a low threshold for referral to hospitals, especially if a detainee with a head injury is also under the influence of alcohol or drugs.

If the detainee is to remain in custody, then instructions regarding the management of head-injured patients should be left verbally and in writing with the custody staff and given to the patient on release *(18)*. Police should be advised particularly that when checking a detainee's conscious level they are required to rouse and speak with the detainee, obtaining a sensible response. Appendix 3 outlines the Glasgow Coma Scale, a head injury warning card for adults, and an observation checklist for custody staff responsible for the health care of detainees.

4.8. Infectious Diseases

The doctor may be called to advise the police regarding infectious diseases. As the population in police custody could be seen as high risk for blood-borne viruses such as hepatitis and the human immunodeficiency virus *(19)*, all individuals should be considered a potential risk, and observation of good clinical practice relating to body fluids to avoid contamination risks is essential *(20)*.

Concerns regarding untreated acute infections such as open tuberculosis should warrant transfer to the nearest infectious diseases unit for assessment regarding treatment. Scabies may be treated in the custodial setting; however, bedding and cells should be professionally cleaned.

5. Mental Health

5.1. General Psychiatric Problems

When a psychiatric disorder is suspected, an assessment involving background information, full psychiatric history if known, observation of the detainee, and mental state examination (Table 6) should be performed by the doctor to assess whether there is in fact any evidence of mental illness.

The doctor should then consider whether diversion from the criminal justice system is appropriate. If the detainee has committed a minor offense and there is only evidence of minor to moderate mental illness, treatment may be arranged in the community, in outpatients, or in the day hospital. If, however, the detainee is found to have an acute major mental illness but has only committed a minor or moderate offense, then admission to the hospital for further assessment and treatment will be required either informally or if necessary formally. When the offense is more serious and there is evidence of probable mental illness needing further assessment, then the detainee may need to go before the court for such an assessment to be ordered.

Table 6
Brief Mental State Examination

- Appearance—self-care, behavior
- Speech—rate, volume
- Thought—association, content (delusions)
- Perception—hallucinations, illusions
- Obsessive/compulsive behaviors
- Mood—biologic symptoms (sleep, appetite, energy, concentration, memory)
- Cognitive function—short-term memory, concentration, long-term memory
- Risk behaviors—self-harm, harm to others

Chronic stable mental health problems usually pose no specific problems for police detention but may require specific safeguards when the detainee is to be interviewed by the police (*see* Section 9). Long-term medication should be continued.

5.2. Substance Misuse and Mental Illness

A specific problem is seen with dual diagnosis—severe mental illness and substance misuse. In the Epidemiologic Catchment Area (ECA) study, 29% of individuals with a lifetime history of any mental disorder (other than substance use) had a history of substance use (22% alcohol disorder and 15% a drug disorder) *(21)*.

Substance misuse may be associated with a psychotic state through a number of mechanisms *(22)*. First, intoxication may mimic psychosis until such time as the drug is metabolized, as may occur with stimulants and cannabis. Second, an independent psychotic state may arise that persists beyond the elimination of the drug, the so-called drug-induced psychosis. Withdrawal states such as that seen with alcohol or benzodiazepines may result in vivid hallucinations and clouding of consciousness, and chronic hallucinosis induced by substance misuse such as alcohol may occur. Substance misuse may also be associated with affective symptoms such as depression that can result in acts of deliberate self-harm (DSH); this is a particular problem following stimulant withdrawal.

5.3. Deliberate Self-Harm

Research has shown that episodes of DSH typically occur soon after arrest. Particular risk factors include a previous history of DSH and a past psychiatric history *(23,24)*. Medical assessments should be requested for those detainees who give a clear intention of DSH with attention given to any visible evidence of previous acts of DSH.

If a detainee commits an act of DSH, a medical assessment should be carried out irrespective of whether there has been any physical injury, and an attempt should be made to assess the risk of suicide. When the risk is thought to be high, then referral to a hospital will be required, and the detainee should be kept under constant supervision until such transfer is arranged. When the risk is deemed to be low, clear instructions will need to be given to the police regarding care and supervision. The police may consider removal of the detainee's clothing and personal effects to prevent self-harm. Cells should be checked with respect to their structural integrity to prevent any defects being used for DSH, and bedding should be of an appropriate standard.

Liaison between agencies is essential, and when the detainee is transferred to prison, another police station, or hospital, details regarding the DSH incident should be passed to the custody or hospital staff concerned so they can take appropriate precautions.

5.4. Claustrophobia

Claustrophobia is a common complaint, and a detailed history and examination with an emphasis on the presence or absence of anxiety when faced with the problem in everyday life should be sought. Enquiry regarding behavior at home such as leaving doors and windows open, avoidance of elevators and underground trains, and a history of the original precipitant for such behavior should be noted.

Often reassurance is enough, and it is rarely necessary to give any medication. The custody staff should be advised if genuine claustrophobia is suspected as this may affect the detainee's fitness to be interviewed.

6. Personal Safety Issues

Certain health care groups are at increased risk of violence in the workplace, for example those working in clinical forensic medicine *(25)* or accident and emergency services *(26)*.

There are a number of strategies for interviewing a difficult patient *(27)*, which include being fully aware of the person's history (be prepared!), and considering how the person sees you (as uninterested or hostile?), being polite and respectful, avoiding confrontation, using appropriate eye contact, keeping calm, and showing interest. Look for signs of tension and find out why tension may be increasing. Finally, be ready to leave if necessary and consider the need to have a chaperone.

Accurate assessment regarding the possibility of violence will reduce the danger, but it should never be assumed that there is no risk, and every clinical situation should be categorized as high risk due to an obvious risk or unknown risk due to undiscovered factors *(28)*.

7. Drug Searches

Persons unlawfully in possession of illicit drugs for personal use or involved in drug supply or trafficking may ingest drugs or pack them into certain body cavities ("body packers" or "mules"). A person who is about to be arrested by the police may swallow drugs ("body swallower" or "stuffer").

Doctors may then be called by the police to carry out intimate searches of those arrested (*see* Chapter 2) *(29)*. The doctor should discuss the possible implications of the ingestion of certain drugs and obtain fully informed consent from the detainee before carrying out any search that may involve examination of the mouth, nostrils, ears, foreskin, rectum, or vagina.

Although heroin or cocaine are the drugs usually involved, cannabis and amphetamine have also been found. All searches for such drugs should be carried out in premises where there are full facilities for resuscitation *(30)* in case significant quantities of the drugs leak into the bloodstream, resulting in acute intoxication and death from overdose *(31)*. Other medical problems such as bowel obstruction may also occur.

The aim of medical management is to prevent these complications, but for ethical reasons the retrieval of packages for legal purposes alone is no indication for intervention without the patient's permission. Therefore, without such permission, the doctor can do nothing except advise the police authorities that the detainee should be observed. In most asymptomatic patients, a trial of conservative treatment, provided bowel obstruction or package perforation is not suspected, will result in the uncomplicated elimination of all ingested packages *(32)*.

In a genuine emergency, when there is no possibility of obtaining consent, the doctor has a duty to carry out treatment to safeguard the life and health of a patient in accordance with what would be accepted as appropriate treatment in the patient's best interests *(33)*.

8. Forensic Samples

Samples from a detainee such as dental impressions, blood, saliva, urine, hair, fingernail scrapings and cuttings, and swabs (e.g., mouth, penile) may be requested by police authorities in connection with the investigation of an offense. These samples should only be taken by a doctor or nurse for evidential purposes with the detainee's fully informed consent and should be packaged in accordance with local procedures to ensure the chain of evidence. For further details regarding samples *see* Chapter 3.

9. Fitness to Be Interviewed

9.1. Introduction

The custodial interrogation of suspects is an essential component of all systems of criminal investigation. The confessions and other incriminating statements that are obtained during these interrogations have always played an important role in prosecutions and continue to be relied on as evidence of guilt in a substantial number of trials. For example, in England and Wales, confessions have been found to provide the single most important piece of evidence against defendants in the Crown Court, being crucial in about 30% of cases *(34)*. Similarly, an influential American observational study found that interrogation was necessary for solving the crime in about 17% of cases *(35)*. The quest to obtain confessions from the mouths of suspects has seen a slow and uneven move away from the inquisitions aided by torture and oppression of the Middle Ages toward the doctrine that:

> *A free and voluntary confession is deserving of the highest credit, because it is presumed to flow from the strongest sense of guilt and therefore it is admitted as proof of the crime to which it refers; but a confession forced from the mind by the flattery of hope or by the torture of fear comes in so questionable a shape when it is to be considered as the evidence of guilt, that no credit ought to be given to it; and therefore it is rejected (36).*

In the years since this judgment, considerable effort has been expended on attempting to regulate the custodial interview in order to minimize the risk of false confessions while preserving the value of interrogation as a means of solving crime. In this section we will consider the important psychological aspects of interrogation and confession and then discuss the role the forensic physician can play in ensuring that suspects are fit to be interviewed.

9.2. Police Interview Techniques

A number of American manuals detail the way in which coercive and manipulative interrogation techniques can be employed by police officers to obtain a confession *(37,38)*, with similar techniques being advocated by Walkley *(39)* in the first such manual written for British officers. The authors of these manuals propound various highly effective methods for breaking down a suspect's resistance while justifying a certain amount of pressure, deception, persuasion, and manipulation as necessary in order for the "truth" to be revealed. Walkley acknowledges that "if an interviewer wrongly assesses the truth-teller as a lie-teller he may subject that suspect to questioning of a type which induces a false confession." Generally, however, the manuals pay scant attention to the fact that, in certain circumstances, the techniques they recommend may make a suspect confess to a crime he or she did not commit. Although studies in the United Kingdom have suggested that coercive interview techniques are employed less frequently than in the past, manipulative and persuasive tactics continue to be used, particularly in relation to more serious crimes *(40,41)*.

Interrogators are encouraged to look for nonverbal signs of anxiety, which are often assumed to indicate deception. However, the innocent as well as the guilty may exhibit signs of nervousness. Innocent suspects may be anxious because they are erroneously being accused of being guilty, because of worries about what is going to happen to them while in custody, and possibly because of concerns that the police may discover some previous transgression. Furthermore, there are three aspects of a police interview that are likely to be as stressful to the innocent as to the guilty: the stress caused by the physical environment in the police station, the stress of being isolated from family and friends, and the stress caused by the suspect's submission to authority. All these factors can markedly impair the performance of a suspect during interview. Indeed, American research has suggested that for most suspects interrogations are likely to be so stressful as to impair their judgment on such crucial matters as the exercise of legal rights *(42)*.

Given the interview techniques employed by the police and the stresses interrogation places on the accused, there is little wonder that false confessions are occasionally made to the police.

9.3. False Confessions

Over the last two decades, the United Kingdom has witnessed a number of well-publicized miscarriages of justice in which the convictions depended heavily on admissions and confessions made to the police that were subsequently shown to be untrue *(43–45)*. In reviewing 70 wrongful imprisonments that occurred between the years 1950–1970, Brandon and Davies *(46)* found that false confessions were second only to incorrect identification evidence as the most common cause of wrongful conviction. More recently, in 1994, Justice *(47)* identified 89 cases in which an alleged miscarriage of justice rested on a disputed confession. Thus, it is clear that people can and do make false and misleading admissions against their own interest. We need to turn to modern psychology to obtain insights into why this might happen.

9.3.1. Why Make a False Confession?

There is no single reason why people falsely confess to crimes they have not committed. Indeed, such confessions usually result from a combination of factors unique to the individual case. Nonetheless, Kassin and Wrightsman *(48)* have been able to identify three distinct types of false confession, which have been developed by Gudjonsson *(49)* and expanded in two respects by Shepherd *(50)*. These categories are voluntary, accommodating-compliant, coerced-compliant, and coerced-internalized.

9.3.2. Voluntary False Confessions

Voluntary false confessions are offered by individuals without any external pressure from the police. Commonly the individuals go voluntarily to the police to confess to a crime they may have read about in the press or seen reported on television. Often they do so out of a morbid desire for notoriety, the individual seeming to have a pathologic desire to become infamous, even at the risk of facing possible imprisonment.

Alternatively, a voluntary false confession may result from the individual's unconscious need to expiate guilt feelings through receiving punishment. The guilt may concern real or imagined past transgressions or, occasionally, may be part of the constant feeling of guilt felt by some individuals with a poor self-image and high levels of trait anxiety.

By contrast, some people making this type of confession do so because they are unable to distinguish between fact and fantasy. Such individuals are unable to differentiate between real events and events that originate in their thinking, imagination, or planning. Such a breakdown in reality monitoring is normally associated with major psychiatric illness, such as schizophrenia.

On occasions, people may volunteer a false confession to assist or protect the real culprit. Gudjonsson *(49)* highlights some evidence that confessing to crimes to protect others might be particularly common in juvenile delinquents.

Finally, Shepherd *(50)* identifies a subset of individuals who falsely confess to crimes to preempt further investigation of a more serious crime.

9.3.3. Accommodating-Compliant False Confessions

Expanding on the original three distinct categories of false confession, Shepherd recognizes a group of people for whom acquiescing with the police is more important than contradicting police assertions about what happened. In such circumstances a false confession arises from a strong need for approval and to be liked. Police conduct is noncoercive, although it does involve the use of leading questions sufficiently obvious to suggest to the suspect what answers the police want to hear. People at all intellectual levels are at risk of behaving in this manner, with those who are excessively compliant being at greatest risk.

9.3.4. Coerced-Compliant False Confessions

Coerced-compliant false confessions are typically elicited during persuasive interrogation: the person perceives that there is some immediate instrumental gain from confessing. The suspect does not confess voluntarily but comes to give in to the demands and pressures of the interrogators. He or she is fully aware of not having committed the crime of which he is accused, and the confession is usually retracted once the immediate threat is over.

Gudjonsson *(49)* suggests that the four main types of perceived immediate gain are being allowed home after confessing, bringing the interview to an end, a means of coping with the demand characteristics (including the perceived pressure) of the situation, and avoidance of being locked up in police custody.

In these circumstances the suspect may be vaguely or fully aware of the consequences of making a false self-incriminating statement, but the perceived immediate gain outweighs, in their mind, the potential long-term consequences. They may naively believe that the truth will come out later in court, perpetuating the belief shared by many police officers and legal advisers that what happens in the police station is not really that important.

9.3.5. Coerced-Internalized False Confessions

Coerced-internalized false confessions occur when suspects are gradually persuaded that they have committed a crime of which they have no memory recollection, or when they have become so confused that they begin to mistrust their own memory and accept a false scenario suggested by the police. This type of confession can happen under two distinct conditions:

1. The suspects have no memory of the alleged offense, even whether or not they committed it. This can be as a result of amnesia or alcohol-induced memory loss. In essence, the suspects have no clear recollection of what they were doing at the time the offense was committed and come to believe they must have committed the crime.
2. At the outset of the interview, the suspects have a clear recollection that they were not involved in the alleged offense. However, as a result of subtle manipulative techniques employed by the interrogator, they begin to distrust their own memory and beliefs. Interrogators attempt to undermine the suspects' confidence in their own recollection of events, which would create sufficient self-doubt and confusion to cause them to adjust their perceptions of reality.

In contrast to the makers of coerced-compliant false confessions, those who make coerced-internalized false confessions only come to retract when they realize, or suspect, that they are in fact innocent. These retractions can take considerable time and, on occasion, may never occur if the original memory of events becomes permanently distorted.

9.4. Suggestibility and Compliance

Of vital importance to an understanding of why false confessions can often prove so incriminating is an awareness of the theory of interrogative suggestibility *(51,52)*. At the heart of the theory is the way leading questions can produce distorted responses from suspects because they are phrased in such a way as to suggest the expected response. Through this process people can come to accept a piece of post-event information and incorporate it into their memory, thus appearing to have "special knowledge" about the alleged offense. This special knowledge may seriously mislead the police and the courts to assume the suspect's guilt erroneously. Suggestibility has been found to correlate with anxiety, lack of assertiveness, poor self-esteem, and low intelligence *(53)*.

Compliance refers to the tendency of people to obey the instructions of others when they don't really want to, either because they are overeager to please or are simply unable to resist the pressure *(54)*. The traits of both suggestibility and compliance have been shown to be relevant to the issue of false confessions *(55)*.

9.5. Preventing False Confessions

It is a fundamental tenet of both American and English law that reliance should only be placed on confession evidence that is given freely and voluntarily. In considering the voluntary nature of a confession, several factors will need to be considered. These include the vulnerability of the accused (through factors such as age, mental illness and handicap, physical illness or injury, intoxication), the conditions of detention (lack of access to legal advice, failure to be given legal rights, adequate rest periods during detention), and the characteristics of the interrogation (threats, physical abuse, inducements etc.).

In America the most important legal development designed to protect the rights of suspects and deter police misconduct relates to the case of *Miranda v Arizona*, which was decided in 1966 *(56)*. The effect of this judgment was to ensure that all criminal suspects in police custody must be warned against self-incrimination and made aware of their right to remain silent and to receive legal advice. These rights have to be actively waived by the accused before interrogation can commence, and any violations of the requirements render any subsequent confession inadmissible.

In the United Kingdom statutory safeguards are provided by the Police and Criminal Evidence Act 1984 (PACE) and the Codes of Practice set up under section 66 of this Act *(1)*, which regulate practice in respect to a number of matters including the detention, treatment, and questioning of persons by police officers. Confessions will generally be inadmissible if the provisions of the Codes of Practice are breached by the police *(57)*.

The role of the forensic physician when assessing a suspect's fitness for interview is seen as fitting into this overall legal framework, the doctor's primary concern being to recognize any characteristics that might render the individual vulnerable to providing a false confession so that adequate safeguards can be put in place.

10. A Definition of Fit for Interview

Until recently there has been no clear definition of what precisely is meant by the term "fit to be interviewed," which has led to confusion among those doctors called on to perform these assessments *(58)*. To address this deficiency Norfolk *(59)* proposed a definition that was used as the starting point for discussion by a subgroup set up by the Home Office Working Party on police surgeons in the United Kingdom. That working party made the following recommendation *(60)*:

"A detained person may be unfit for interview when:

(a) Conducting an interview could worsen any existing physical or mental illness to a significant degree

(b) Anything said or done by the detained person at the time of detention may be considered unreliable in subsequent court proceedings *because* of the physical or mental state of the detained person."

Thus, a suspect with known ischemic heart disease who is experiencing chest pain satisfies the criteria of (a) above and clearly needs assessment and appropriate treatment before it is safe to conduct an interrogation.

The concept of unreliability may be harder to evaluate and will require consideration of the various vulnerability factors associated with false confessions. In making an assessment, the doctor should quantify the risk of unreliability into one of the following categories:

1. Definite — Unlikely to be fit for interview at any stage (e.g., severe dementia, severe mental handicap).
2. Major risk — Unfit for interview at present. Reassessment or further review is considered necessary to establish fitness at a later stage (e.g., drunkenness, intoxication with drugs, severe drug withdrawal, severe physical illness, major mental disorders that may be amenable to treatment such as mania and acute confusional states).

3. Some risk	Precautions are advised, such as the presence of an appropriate adult (*see* Appendix 4) or referral for other medical or psychiatric advice (e.g., mental illness such as hypomania, schizophrenia and depression, mild dementia or mental handicap, significant anxiety).
4. No discernible risk	Fit for interview, in so far as the interview can proceed without any special precautions.

10.1. Scheme of Examination

When assessing a detainee's fitness for interview, the traditional medical model of taking a history and then conducting an examination should be employed. As always, informed consent should be obtained and detailed and contemporaneous notes should be taken.

10.1.1. The History

As much background information as is practicable should be obtained and, when possible, an indication of how long any interview is likely to take. The demand characteristics of a long interview about a suspected murder will be much greater than a short interview about a shoplifting offense.

A general medical history should be taken with enquiry made about significant illness and any prescribed medication. The detainee should be asked whether he or she has suffered from psychiatric illness, past or present, and specific enquiry should be made about alcohol and drug misuse. There should be questions about the person's educational background, as individuals with learning difficulties can be difficult to recognize and enquiring about schooling may aid identification.

Make sure the detainee has not been deprived of food or sleep and enquire about significant social distractions (for example, a single parent may make a false confession in order to obtain early release from custody and a speedy reunion with his or her child). Detainees should be asked whether they have been detained before and if so whether they have had unpleasant experiences while in custody in the past.

10.1.2. The Examination

The examination should include observations on the general appearance, physical examination as appropriate, and mental state examination. A functional assessment should be performed as to whether the detainee is aware of the reason for arrest, is aware of legal rights, and is capable of making a rational decision (able to choose between relevant courses of action) and of carrying out the chosen course of action.

Each examination needs to be tailored to the individual, but doctors should be able to assess the vulnerabilities of the detainees they have been asked to examine and thus ensure that any necessary safeguards are put in place before interrogation begins.

10.2. Alcohol and Fitness for Interview

It is generally accepted that severe alcohol intoxication renders a suspect unfit to be interviewed. There is much less agreement, however, when it comes to deciding when somebody with mild or moderate intoxication should be considered fit to interview *(58,61)*. The customary view that intellectual processes are impaired at lower blood alcohol levels than sensory or motor processes has been challenged. Indeed, the very opposite has been shown, with intellectual processes appearing to be more resistant to alcohol than sensory and motor skills *(62)*. Nonetheless, the effect alcohol can have on short-term memory should be borne in mind when advising the police on fitness. Research suggests that moderate quantities of alcohol impair the process of forming new memories *(63)*. Deterioration in performance of a task assessing short-term memory occurred at blood alcohol levels of 70 mg/100 mL in one study *(64)*, and a significant impairment of eyewitness memory has been demonstrated at average blood alcohol levels of 100 mg/100 mL *(65)*. When suspects mistrust their own memory of events, they are at increased risk of providing coerced-internalized false confessions *(49)*.

The ultimate decision regarding whether a suspect who has been drinking is fit for interview is best decided on the medical and functional assessment performed by the doctor rather than on arbitrarily defined "safe" blood alcohol levels *(66)*.

Alcohol withdrawal states and the complications of alcohol withdrawal can impair cognitive functioning and affect both a suspect's ability to cope with interrogative pressure and the ability to provide reliable testimony. Even the aftereffects of alcohol, or "hangover," have been shown to impair critical task performance, such as aircraft operation, and can impair judgment *(67)*.

10.3. Substance Misuse and Fitness for Interview

A substance misuser may be rendered unfit for interview by virtue of either intoxication or withdrawal. Generally speaking, intoxication is easy to recognize, and the police will usually wait until the intoxication has cleared before starting their questioning. However, problems may be encountered with hallucinogenic substances. For example, the mental state may fluctuate in the recovery stages of an LSD experience, which may not be immediately obvious to the interrogator *(68)*.

Withdrawal states can pose a bigger problem for the doctor assessing fitness for interview. Although most confessions made in these circumstances are reliable *(69)*, it should be recognized that the person suffering from drug withdrawal may be particularly vulnerable to providing a false confession. Such persons may believe that compliance will result in early release and that the risks entailed in providing a false confession may seem worthwhile in the presence of an overwhelming desire to reestablish access to their supply of drugs *(70)*.

Although symptoms of mild withdrawal from opiates, for example, is considered unlikely to be a barrier to interview *(68,71)*, the physical and mental distress occasioned by established withdrawal may seriously impair a suspect's fitness to undergo the somewhat threatening and difficult experience of police interrogation.

When faced with a suspect suffering from severe withdrawal, the doctor should consider advising that the interview be deferred until such time as the withdrawal has subsided or been adequately treated. If the doctor decides to treat the withdrawal state, consideration should be given to the risk that the therapeutic intervention may in itself have a bearing on fitness to interview. Arranging for therapy that the suspect has been receiving in the community to be continued in police custody is unlikely to influence fitness for interview *(72,73)*. However, when substitution therapy is initiated in custody, or when symptomatic treatment alone is provided, the doctor may well need to assess the impact of the treatment before an interview takes place.

10.4. The Impact of Psychiatric Illnesses

There has been a considerable amount of research into the manner in which certain functional psychiatric illnesses can affect the reliability of testimony *(74,75)*. Thus anxiety has been shown to increase a suspect's suggestibility and depression can lead to feelings of guilt and poor self-esteem that render a suspect vulnerable to providing a false confession *(49)*. Psychiatric illness may also render a person unfit for interview by virtue of its effect on cognitive processes or because of associated thought disorder *(76,77)*. However, careful questioning that avoids the use of leading questions and coercive pressures can often elicit reliable testimony. The fact that a suspect suffers from an illness such as schizophrenia does not necessarily mean that he or she is unfit for interview *(78)*; such an opinion would depend on the likely demand characteristics of the interview and the functional assessment by the doctor.

10.5. Learning Difficulties

The police rarely have difficulty recognizing moderate or severe learning difficulties, but borderline or low-normal intelligence may not be obvious even to trained observers *(79–81)*. It is important to identify people with learning difficulties—questions regarding reading and writing ability and the need for special help with education can be useful—because they will be particularly vulnerable in police custody. Such individuals may have difficulties in understanding their legal rights and in communicating with police officers. They are also more likely to be suggestible and acquiescent *(82)*.

10.6. The Effect of Physical Illnesses on Fitness for Interview

The presence of any physical illness renders an individual more vulnerable when faced with a stressful situation such as a custodial interrogation. Features such as anxiety or depression will affect a person's ability to function during the police interview, and physical illness, especially if severe, is as likely to cause anxiety and depression as any other form of stress *(83)*. The severity of the emotional response will depend on the nature of the illness itself, the personality of the individual, and social circumstances. Suspects who are already coping with physical illness are more likely to focus on the short-term consequences of their behavior than the long-term ones, thus increasing the risk that they might provide a false confession *(49)*.

As the impact of physical illness on a person's coping strategy is not disease specific, depending more on the actual or perceived severity of the illness rather than the nature of the illness itself, the actual diagnosis is unimportant. By contrast, there are many physical illnesses in which characteristic disturbances in cognitive functioning have been recognized *(84)*. With these illnesses the nature and degree of the mental disturbance produced depends entirely on the diagnosis of the underlying condition. The more common of the conditions encountered in custody are discussed below.

10.6.1. Epilepsy

It is now clear, after long historical dispute, that a predisposition to epileptic fits does not mean *per se* that there will be associated intellectual impairment, personality disorder, or mental illness. Most epileptic patients remain mentally normal, although this does depend on the presence, site, and extent of any brain damage underlying the epilepsy *(84)*.

However, those epileptics without significant brain damage do, nonetheless, remain prone to cognitive impairment, particularly memory impairment, as a result of their epilepsy and its treatment. The potential impact of this cognitive impairment has to be considered when assessing an epileptic suspect's fitness for interview.

For example, problems with concentration, memory, and intellectual functioning can be seen when anticonvulsant drugs are administered in toxic doses or unsuitable combinations *(85)*. Suspicion should be raised when a suspect complains of mental lethargy or appears to be performing below expected levels, symptoms particularly associated with toxicity.

Further problems with the reliability of testimony from epileptics may be related to their personality. Patients with epilepsy are often overprotected in childhood by concerned parents and, later in life, can be exposed to profound social and occupational discrimination *(86)*. All these factors can lead to personality problems, which include feelings of insecurity, low self-esteem, and dependency. Individuals with these personality traits are likely to be highly suggestible and may strive to please interviewing officers by giving answers that seem plausible and consistent with the external cues provided, even though the responses are known to be untrue.

The neurophysiologic consequences of an epileptic fit can in themselves seriously distort an individual's perception of events occurring around the time of the fit, thus rendering any subsequent account of that event potentially unreliable. Complex disturbances of thinking, memory, or awareness may feature as part of an aura preceding the actual seizure. These may include distortion of time sense, mental confusion, or feelings of depersonalization or déja vu. The fit may also be ushered in by distorted perceptions or actual hallucinations of sight, hearing, taste, or smell. When the ensuing fit is mild or abortive, the connection between these reported experiences and their epileptic causation may be missed *(87)*.

Typical absences (or petit mal epilepsy) is a disorder that usually starts in childhood, but the attacks can continue into adult life. Absence attacks are brief, with an abrupt onset and termination; several such absences may occur in quick succession, producing significant gaps in memory.

Further cognitive disturbances can follow in the wake of seizures, with clouding of consciousness and disorientation lasting for a few minutes or up to an hour or more, so that recollection for events occurring during the postictal period may also be unreliable *(85)*.

10.6.2. Head Injury

Head injuries may occur in a number of circumstances involving possible criminal offenses such as road traffic accidents and assaults; therefore, it is not uncommon to encounter head-injured detainees in police custody. The potential for the head injury to affect the person's ability to recall the details of the accident or assault can assume considerable importance.

Memory loss for events occurring around the time of the injury is likely to occur whenever there has been diffuse brain damage of a degree sufficient to cause concussion. In most cases loss of consciousness will accompany the head injury, but this is not invariable, and it is possible for patients to display both retrograde and posttraumatic amnesia without losing consciousness *(84)*.

Retrograde amnesia refers to the loss of memory for events that immediately precede the head injury. Individuals can often indicate with fair precision the last event that they can clearly recollect. In road traffic accidents the journey may be recalled up to a specific point, which allows an estimate of the extent of the pretraumatic gap to be made. Such amnesia is usually short in duration and can usually be counted in minutes or hours rather than days or weeks. Indeed, when the retrograde amnesia lasts for a long time the explanation is often due to hysteria.

Retrograde amnesia may render a suspect unfit for interview immediately after the head injury, but the doctor should be aware that the extent of the amnesia can change with time. At first it may be very long, but it can then shrink over the next days and weeks, eventually ending up as a matter of minutes only. Recovery from retrograde amnesia tends to occur in chronological order, with items in the distant past recovering first.

By contrast, posttraumatic amnesia refers to the period from the moment of the injury until normal continuous memory returns, the length of the amnesia providing a good index, albeit in retrospect, of the severity of the brain damage *(88)*. It should be emphasized that the amnesia only ends when the person becomes able to give a clear and consecutive account of what is happening around him or her. Sometimes "islands of memory" will be exhibited, but these should not be taken as indicating the end of the amnesia. There is a similar danger in underestimating the duration of posttraumatic amnesia in those suspects who, although aware of things going on around them, are unable to recall these events at a later date *(84)*.

A variety of behaviors may be exhibited during the period of posttraumatic amnesia, ranging from apparent normality to obvious confusion. In general, however, behavior is unremarkable, and the doctor may be easily misled into believing that there is nothing amiss. The individuals themselves are usually unaware of the abnormal memory at the time and can give superficial or made-up explanations for any defects that are discovered. On occasions these false memories can appear most convincing *(89)*.

10.6.3. Migraine

Migraine is a common and sometimes incapacitating disorder, affecting approximately 20% of women and 15% of men at some time in their lives *(90)*. Some degree of mental change is almost universal during attacks. Anxiety and irritability are common early in the attack and are often followed by drowsiness and lethargy. Cognitive impairment may occur. Cerebration is often slowed with poor concentration, and there may be marked impairment of memory *(84)*.

Detainees who claim that they suffered an attack of migraine at or around the time of the alleged offense should be questioned closely about any cognitive impairment during previous attacks. However, it should be recognized that the pattern of any such impairment can change from attack to attack in the same person.

10.6.4. Hypothyroidism

A detainee who is being adequately treated for myxedema poses no particular problem for the physician assessing fitness for interview. However, an individual with undiagnosed or undertreated hypothyroidism may exhibit mental manifestations that are as important as the physical. The typical picture is of mental lethargy, general dulling of the personality, and slowing of all cognitive functions. In particular, the hypothyroid patient shows deficits in memory, abstraction, conceptual organization, and mathematical ability *(91)*.

10.6.5. Diabetes Mellitus

Although confusion is a prominent feature in patients who are slipping into hyperglycemic coma, this condition is rarely seen in police custody. Questions relating to fitness for interview and the potential reliability of a detainee's confession are more likely to involve those with hypoglycemia.

Episodes of hypoglycemia are associated with irritability, anxiety, and panic in the early stages. As the episode develops, the individual becomes disinhibited and may exhibit childish or aggressive behavior that often mimics drunkenness. Disorientation and mental confusion are common and, in severe cases, the person may pass into a coma. Anybody suffering from hypoglycemia will prove to be a poor witness to events that occur during the episode. Most will have complete amnesia for the content of the attack and occasionally for an additional period before the attack occurred when their behavior will have appeared to be normal *(92)*. The doctor should take a clear history of any hypoglycemic episodes that may have occurred prior to arrest and should consider checking the blood sugar of any diabetic about to be interviewed by the police. The manifestations of hypoglycemia with subsequent impaired intellectual function are extremely variable, and it has been recommended that the blood sugar should be kept at 6 mmol/L or more if a diabetic person is to give a statement or be interviewed *(93)*.

10.6.6. Dementia

Dementia is a large-scale problem in the elderly. It has been estimated that 5–8% of patients aged 65 suffer from dementia to an appreciable degree, with the proportion probably exceeding 20% in 80-year-olds *(94)*. However, in many of these patients the dementia is not recognized until there is some form of crisis in their lives. Such a crisis may be precipitated by sudden illness, bereavement, or police arrest. Individuals seem able to develop strategies to cope with their daily tasks and thus appear to function normally until the crisis disrupts the status quo and exposes the degree of their dementia *(95)*.

Although there are many different causes of dementia, the clinical picture remains broadly similar, with any variation depending mainly on the age of onset of the illness, premorbid personality, and intelligence. In the custodial situation the doctor is likely to encounter only those at an early stage of the disease. This is characterized by impaired memory, loss of the sense of time, and spatial disorientation, all of which can distort a suspect's recollection of events. This distortion may be compounded by the lack of judgment that is frequently displayed by those with dementia and that can cause the suspect to misjudge the importance of providing reliable testimony *(84)*. Therefore it is important that the doctor be aware of the possibility that an elderly suspect may be suffering from dementia, even when there are reports of apparently normal social functioning prior to arrest. In such circumstances recognition of the dementia can be facilitated by using a standard test of cognitive function such as the Mini-Mental State Examination Score (*see* Appendix 5).

This test of cognitive function has been thoroughly validated *(96)*. It is called "mini" because it concentrates only on the cognitive aspects of mental functioning and excludes questions concerning mood, abnormal mental experiences, and the form of thinking. A score of 24 out of 30 was originally suggested as the lower limit of normal, but it has been repeatedly shown that performance on even this simple test is influenced very considerably by age and by educational attainment. Hence, a well-educated young adult should perform flawlessly, whereas a normal elderly subject who left school at age 14 may score as low as 22 or 23. Given this proviso, the Mini-Mental State Examination is useful in quantifying cognitive impairment and is particularly useful for grading and monitoring the severity of dementia.

References

1. See, for example, *Police and Criminal Evidence Act 1984* (s.60 (1)(a) and s.66) Codes of Practice 1995 for England and Wales. Her Majesty's Stationery Office, London.
2. British Medical Association's Medical Ethics Committee and Association of Police Surgeons (1994) *Health Care of Detainees in Police Stations*. British Medical Association, London.
3. Metropolitan Police (1997) *Medical Care of Prisoners—Person Ill or Injured*. Special Notice 37/97. Metropolitan Police, London.
4. Payne-James, J. J. (1992) Work patterns of a forensic medical examiner for the Metropolitan Police. *Police Surg.* **42,** 21–24.
5. Young, S., Wells, D., and Jackson, G. (1994) A tiered health care system for persons in police custody—the use of a forensic nursing service. *J Clin Forensic Med.* **1,** 21–25.
6. Smock, W. S. (1994) Development of a clinical forensic medicine curriculum for emergency physicians in the USA. *J Clin Forensic Med.* **1,** 27–30.
7. Hocking, G., Kalyanaraman, R., and deMello, W. F. (1998) Better drug history taking: an assessment of the DRUGS mnemonic. *J R Soc Med.* **91,** 305–306.
8. Evans,V. and Howitt, J. (1997) *The Safety and Security of the Administration of Medication in Police Custody*. Education and Research Sub-Committee of the Association of Police Surgeons, Harrogate, North Yorkshire.
9. Howitt, J. (1995) Poor conditions of detention compromise ethical standards. *J R Soc Med.* **88,** 40P,41P.
10. Brodie, M. J. (1990) Status epilepticus in adults. *Lancet.* **336,** 551,552.
11. Mathur, R. and Bell, D. (1996) Asthma management in police study. *J Clin Forensic Med.* **3,** 133–140.
12. Heller, M. B. and Vukmir, R. B. (1992) Glucagon for metabolic/endocrinologic emergencies: hypoglycaemia, in *Glucagon in Acute Medicine. Pharmacological, Clinical and Therapeutic Implications* (Picazo, J., ed.), Kluwer Academic Publishers, London.
13. Payne-James, J. J. (1993) The role of cyanoacrylate tissue adhesive (Histoacryl blue) in forensic medical practice. *Police Surg.* **43,** 30,31.
14. Marks, P. V. (1994) Acute head injury: assessment and practical management. *J Clin Forensic Med.* **1,** 43–46.
15. Jennett, B. and Teasdale, G. (1977) Aspects of coma after severe head injury. *Lancet.* **i,** 878–881.
16. Greaves, I., Dyer, P., and Porter, K. (1995). Head injury, in *Handbook of Immediate Care*, W.B. Saunders, London, p. 103.
17. Leigh, A., Johnson, G., and Ingram, A. (1998) *Deaths in Police Custody: Learning the Lessons*. Police Research Series Paper 26, Police Research Group Publications, Home Office, London.
18. Parsley, J., Fletcher, L., and Mabrook, A. F. (1997) Head injury instructions: a time to unify. *J Accid Emerg Med.* **14,** 238,239.

19. Payne-James, J. J., Keys, D. W., Wall, I., and Dean, P. J. (1994) Prevalence of HIV factors for individuals examined in clinical forensic medicine. *J Clin Forensic Med.* **1,** 93–96.
20. UK Health Departments (1998) *Guidance for Clinical Health Care Workers: Protection Against Infection with Blood-borne Viruses.* Department of Health, London, UK.
21. Regier, D. A., Farmer, M. E., Rae, D. S., Locke B. Z., Keith, S. J., Judd, L. L., et al. (1990) Comorbidity of mental disorders with alcohol and other drug abuse: results from the Epidemiologic Catchment Area (ECA) Study. *JAMA.* **264,** 2511–2518.
22. Johns, A. (1997) Substance misuse: a primary risk and a major problem of comorbidity. *Int Rev Psychiatry.* **9,** 233–241.
23. Ingram, A., Johnson, G., and Heyes, I. (1997) *Self Harm and Suicide by Detained Persons: A Study.* Police Research Group Publications, Home Office, London.
24. Norfolk, G. A. (1998) Deaths in police custody during 1994: a retrospective analysis. *J Clin Forensic Med.* **5,** 49–54.
25. Schnieden, V., Stark, M. M., and Payne-James, J. J. (1995) Violence in clinical forensic medicine. *Med Sci Law.* **35,** 333–335.
26. Schnieden, V. and Maguire J. (1993) *A Report on Violence at Work and its Impact on the Medical Profession within Hospitals and the Community.* British Medical Association, London.
27. Royal College of Psychiatrists (1997) *Using the Mental Health Act—A Training Resource for Doctors.* Gaskell, Royal College of Psychiatrists, p. 72.
28. Johns, A., Clarke, S., and Stark, M. M. (1997) Management of potentially violent detainees. *J Clin Forensic Med.* **1,** 139–144.
29. British Medical Association and Association of Police Surgeons (1999) *Guidelines for Doctors Asked to Perform Intimate Body Searches.* British Medical Association, London.
30. Stark, M. M. (1997) *Guidelines for Police Surgeons Asked to Perform Intimate Searches for Drugs.* Education and Research Sub-Committee of the Association of Police Surgeons, Harrogate, North Yorkshire.
31. Heinemann, A., Miyaishi, S., Iwersen, S., Schmoldt, A., and Puschel, K. (1998) Body-packing as cause of unexpected sudden death. *Forensic Sci Int.* **92,** 1–10.
32. Glass, J. M. and Scott H. J. (1995) "Surgical mules": the smuggling of drugs in the gastrointestinal tract. *J R Soc Med.* **88,** 450–453.
33. F v West Berkshire Health Authority (1989) 2 All ER 545.
34. Baldwin, J. and McConville, M. (1980) *Confessions in Crown Court Trials.* Royal Commission on Criminal Procedure Research Study No. 5. Her Majesty's Stationery Office, London.
35. Wald, M., Ayres, R., Hess, D. W., Schantz, M., and Whitebread, C. H. (1967) Interrogations in New Haven: the impact of Miranda. *Yale Law J.* **76,** 1519–1614.
36. R v Warickshall (1783) 1 Leach 263.
37. Inbau, F. E. and Reid, J. E. (1967) *Criminal Interrogations and Confessions,* 2nd ed. Williams & Wilkins, Baltimore.

38. Royal, R. F. and Schutt, S. R. (1976) *Gentle Art of Interviewing and Interrogation: A Professional Manual and Guide*. Prentice Hall, Englewood Cliffs, NJ.
39. Walkley, J. (1987) *Police Interrogation. A Handbook for Investigators*. Police Review Publication, London.
40. Irving, B. (1980) *Police Interrogation. A Case Study of Current Practice*. Royal Commission on Criminal Procedure, Research Study No 2. Her Majesty's Stationery Office, London.
41. Irving, B. L. and McKenzie, I. K. (1989) *Police Interrogation: The Effects of the Police and Criminal Evidence Act*. The Police Foundation, London.
42. Leiken, L. S. (1970) Police Interrogation in Colorado: the implementation of Miranda. *Denver Law J.* **47,** 1–53.
43. Kennedy, L. (1988) *10 Rillington Place*. Grafton, London.
44. Thomas, T. (1987) The Confait Confessions. *Policing.* **3,** 214–225.
45. Kee, R. (1989) *Trial and Error. The True Events Surrounding the Convictions and Trials of the Guildford Four and the Maguire Seven*. Penguin, London.
46. Brandon, R. and Davies, C. (1973) *Wrongful Imprisonment*. George Allen & Unwin, London.
47. Justice, (1994) *Unreliable Evidence? Confessions and the Safety of Convictions.* Justice, London.
48. Kassin, S. M. and Wrightsman, L. S. (1985) *The Psychology of Evidence and Trial Procedure*. Sage Publications, London.
49. Gudjonsson, G. (1992) *The Psychology of Interrogations, Confessions and Testimony*. John Wiley & Sons, Chichester.
50. See Wolchover, D. and Heaton-Armstrong, A. (1996) *On Confession Evidence*. Sweet & Maxwell, London, p. 99.
51. Gudjonsson, G. H. and Clark, N. K. (1986) Suggestibility in police interrogation: a social psychological model. *Social Behav.* **1,** 83–104.
52. Schooler, J. W. and Loftus, E. F. (1986) Individual differences and experimentation: complementary approaches to interrogative suggestibility. *Social Behav.* **1,** 105–112.
53. Gudjonsson, G. (1997) Interrogative suggestibility—can it be recognised in custody? in *Fit to be Interviewed by the Police* (Norfolk, G. A., ed.), Association of Police Surgeons, Harrogate.
54. Gudjonsson, G. H. (1989) Compliance in an interrogation situation: a new scale. *Personality Individual Differences.* **10,** 535–540.
55. Groves, T. (1991) Explaining false confessions. *BMJ.* **303,** 1087,1088.
56. Miranda v Arizona 384 US 436, 1966.
57. See for example R v Kenny (1994) Crim. L. R. 284 and R v Cox (1991) Crim. L. R. 687.
58. Norfolk, G. A. (1996) Fitness to be interviewed and the appropriate adult scheme: a survey of police surgeons' attitudes. *J Clin Forensic Med.* **3,** 9–13.
59. Norfolk, G. A. (1997) 'Fitness to be interviewed'—a proposed definition and scheme of examination. *Med Sci Law.* **37,** 228–234.
60. Norfolk, G. A. (1997) Fit to be interviewed—a police surgeon's perspective, in *Fit to be Interviewed by the Police* (Norfolk, G.A., ed.), Association of Police Surgeons, Harrogate.

61. Clarke, M. D. B. (1991) 'Fit for Interview?' *Police Surg.* **40,** 15–18.
62. Carpenter, J. A. (1980) Effects of alcohol on some psychological processes. A critical review with special reference to automobile driving skill. *Q J Stud Alcohol.* **23,** 274–314.
63. Loftus, E. F. (1980) "Did I really say that last night?" Alcohol, marijuana and memory. *Psychol Today.* **92,** 42–56.
64. Carpenter, J. A. and Ross, B. M. (1965) Effect of alcohol on short-term memory. *Q J Stud Alcohol.* **26,** 561–579.
65. Yuille, J. C. and Tollestrup, P. A. (1990) Some effects of alcohol on eyewitness memory. *J Appl Psychol.* **75,** 268–273.
66. Rogers, D. J., Stark, M. M., and Howitt, J. B. (1995) The use of an alcometer in clinical forensic practice. *J Clin Forensic Med.* **2,** 177–183.
67. Yesavage, J. A. and Leirer, V. O. (1986) Hangover effects on aircraft pilots 14 hours after alcohol ingestion: a preliminary report. *Am J Psychiatry.* **143,** 1546–1550.
68. Department of Health, Scottish Office Home and Health Department, Welsh Office (1994) *Substance Misuse Detainees in Police Custody: Guidelines for Clinical Management.* Her Majesty's Stationery Office, London.
69. Sigurdsson, J. F. and Gudjonsson, G. H. (1994) Alcohol and drug intoxication during police interrogation and the reasons why suspects confess to the police. *Addiction.* **89,** 985–997.
70. Davison, S. E. and Forshaw, D. M. (1993) Retracted confessions: through opiate withdrawal to a new conceptual framework. *Med Sci Law.* **33,** 285–290.
71. Norfolk, G. A. (1996) Fitness to be interviewed and the appropriate adult scheme: a survey of police surgeons' attitudes. *J Clin Forensic Med.* **3,** 9–13.
72. Stark, M. M. (1994) Management of drug misusers in police custody. *J R Soc Med.* **87,** 584–587.
73. Zacny, J. P. (1996) Should people taking opioids for medical reasons be allowed to work and drive? *Addiction.* **91,** 1581–1584.
74. Ross, D. F., Read, J. D., and Toglia, M. P. (Eds.) (1994) *Adult Eyewitness Testimony.* Cambridge University Press, Cambridge.
75. Gudjonsson, G. H. (1995) The vulnerabilities of mentally disordered witnesses. *Med Sci Law.* **35,** 101–106.
76. Bluglass, R. and Bowden, P. (1990) *Principles and Practice of Forensic Psychiatry.* Churchill Livingstone, Edinburgh.
77. Rix, K. J. B. (1997) Fit to be interviewed by the police? *Adv Psychiatr Treat.* **3,** 33–40.
78. Gudjonsson, G. (1995) "Fitness for interview" during police detention: a conceptual framework for forensic assessment. *J Forensic Psychiatry.* **6,** 185–197.
79. Halstead, S. (1996) Forensic psychiatry for people with learning disability. *Adv Psychiatric Treat.* **2,** 76–85.
80. Gudjonsson, G., Clare, I., Rutter, S., and Pearse, J. (1993) *The Royal Commission on Criminal Justice. Persons at Risk During Interviews in Police Custody: The Identification of Vulnerabilities.* Research Study No. 12. Her Majesty's Stationery Office, London.

81. Lyall, I., Holland, A. J., and Styles, P. (1995) Incidence of persons with a learning disability detained in police custody. A needs assessment for service development. *Med Sci Law.* **35,** 61–71.
82. Murphy, G. and Clare, I. C. H. (1998) People with learning disabilities as offenders or alleged offenders in the UK criminal justice system. *J R Soc Med.* **91,** 178–182.
83. Mayou, R. A. (1987) Emotional reactions to disorders, in *Oxford Textbook of Medicine*, 2nd ed. (Weatherall, D. J., Ledingham, J. G. G., and Warrell, D. A., eds.), Oxford University Press, Oxford.
84. Lishman, W. A. (1987) *Organic Psychiatry. The Psychological Consequences of Cerebral Disorder*, 2nd ed., Blackwell Scientific Publications, Oxford.
85. Lishman, W. A. (1996) Specific conditions giving rise to mental disorder, in *Oxford Textbook of Medicine*, 3rd ed. (Weatherall, D. J., Ledingham, J. G. G., and Warrell, D. A., eds.), Oxford University Press, Oxford.
86. Williams, D. (1963) The psychiatry of the epileptic. *Proc R Soc Med.* **56,** 707–710.
87. Laidlaw, J., Richens, A., and Chadwick, D. (Eds.) (1993) *A Textbook of Epilepsy*, 4th ed., Churchill Livingstone, Edinburgh.
88. Teasdale, G. M. (1996) Head injuries, in *Oxford Textbook of Medicine*, 3rd ed. (Weatherall, D. J., Ledingham, J. G. G., and Warrell, D. A., eds.), Oxford University Press, Oxford.
89. Whitty, C. W. M. and Zangwill, O. L., eds. (1977) *Amnesia*. Butterworths, London.
90. Pearce, J. M. S. (1996) Headache, in *Oxford Textbook of Medicine*, 3rd ed. (Weatherall, D. J., Ledingham, J. G. G., and Warrell, D. A., eds.), Oxford University Press, Oxford.
91. Droba, M. and Whybrow, P. C. (1989) Endocrine and metabolic disorders, in *Comprehensive Textbook of Psychiatry*, vol. 2, 5th ed. (Kaplan, H. I. and Sadock, B. J., eds.), Williams and Wilkins, Baltimore.
92. Deary, I. J. (1993) Effects of hypoglycaemia on cognitive function, in *Hypoglycaemia and Diabetes: Clinical and Physiological Aspects* (Frier, B. M. and Fisher, B. M., eds.), Edward Arnold, London.
93. Levy, D. (1996) Management of diabetes in clinical forensic practice. *J Clin Forensic Med.* **3,** 31–36.
94. Hodges, J. R. (1996) Dementia, Introduction, in *Oxford Textbook of Medicine*, 3rd ed. (Weatherall, D. J., Ledingham, J. G. G., and Warrell, D. A., eds.) Oxford University Press, Oxford.
95. Pearce, J. (1984) *Dementia. A Clinical Approach*. Blackwell Scientific Publications, Oxford.
96. Folstein, M. F., Folstein, S. E., and McHugh, P. R. (1975) "Mini-Mental State": a practical method for grading the cognitive state of patients for the clinician. *J Psychiatr Res.* **12,** 189–198.

Chapter 8

Substance Misuse

Margaret M. Stark and Guy Norfolk

1. Introduction

The number of individuals passing through the criminal justice system with substance misuse problems is increasing, and doctors should be aware of current drug trends in their area. In the United States there is a well-established program of research on drug testing urine samples of people arrested by the police—the Arrestee Drug Abuse Monitoring Program (ADAM), which recently replaced the Drug Use Forecasting Program (DUF) *(1)*. A smaller scale project in England, which involved testing the urine of detainees, showed high levels of recent drug consumption—61% had taken at least one drug *(2)*. The figures, similar to those found in the United States (68%), may well be higher in reality, as detainees were excluded from testing who were unfit for interview due to alcohol, drugs, or medication, or who were considered mentally disordered or potentially violent.

2. General Principles *(3)*

2.1. History and Examination

A detailed history of recent drug use including alcohol needs to be obtained to establish whether the individual is a currently dependent or recreational user (Table 1). Street names of substances will vary from country to country, within regions in the same country, with the cultural background of the user, and over time. The examination should look for signs of intoxication,

From: *Forensic Science: A Physician's Guide to Clinical Forensic Medicine*
Edited by: M. M. Stark © Humana Press, Inc., Totowa, NJ

Table 1
Substance Misuse: History

- Period of regular use
- Quantity used per day on a "typical" day
- Frequency of use
- Route of administration
- Amount used in the last 24 hours
- Time of last dose
- Prescribed drugs
- Experience of withdrawal

withdrawal, or previous drug use (Table 2). Baseline parameters are useful for reexamination if the detainee is kept in custody. Purity of illicit substances will vary between countries and from year to year; this may be reflected in the drug history obtained, with increasing amounts ingested as drug purity diminishes. Average figures from seizures available from the United States in 1993 show purity for cocaine at 72% and heroin 38% *(4)*, compared with U.K. figures in 1996 of crack 81%, cocaine 47%, heroin 44%, and amphetamine 9% *(5)*.

2.2. Harm Minimization

Information and advice should be given to the detainee by the physician on reducing the harm from continued drug misuse. Advice can be provided on a range of issues including human immunodeficiency virus (HIV) awareness, the availability of hepatitis B vaccination, and the hazards of injecting substances, especially using "shared works"; information regarding the local services involved in drug counseling and treatment can also be offered. It should be remembered that, in addition to drug-related problems, the detainee may have other medical problems that require treatment.

Brief interventions, whereby it is possible to provide advice about the risks inherent in a range of patterns of substance use and to advise reducing or stopping use as part of screening and assessment, have been found to be useful with alcohol consumption *(6)*. A person's motivation to change is important in determining the likelihood of success of any intervention *(7)*, and such motivation may alter depending on a variety of factors. For example, negative life events such as being arrested for an acquisitive crime motivated by a need to finance a drug habit can introduce conflict in the detainee's mind about substance misuse and may increase the likelihood of successful intervention.

Arrest referral schemes are partnership initiatives set up to encourage drug misusers brought into contact with the police service to voluntarily participate

Table 2
Substance Misuse: Examination

- Blood pressure
- Pulse rate
- Temperature
- Pupil size
- Pupillary reaction to light
- Conscious level—lethargy/stupor/coma
- Glasgow Coma Scale
- Orientated in time, place, and person
- Speech
- Pallor
- Flushed
- Tremor at rest
- Yawning
- Lachrimation
- Rhinorrhea
- Gooseflesh
- Sweating
- Bowel sounds
- Presence of needle tracks
- Restlessness/agitation
- Disordered perceptions
- Coordination
- Gait
- Rombergs
- Auscultation of the chest

in confidential help designed to address their drug-related problems. Early evaluation of such projects in the United Kingdom provides good evidence that such schemes can be effective in reducing drug use and drug-related crime *(8)*. In the United States it has also been recognized that point of arrest is an appropriate stage of intervention for addressing substance misuse *(1)*.

2.3. *Prescribing*

Although prompt treatment to limit or prevent the withdrawal syndrome is desirable, no central nervous system depressant medication should be given if there is evidence of intoxication with other drugs, for example, alcohol, as many substances have an additive effect. Consideration of whether the detainee is fit for detention is the priority. Most individuals are not detained in police custody for very long, and therefore medical treatment may not be required. This is particularly so if there is any question that the detainee may have recently ingested substances the full effects of which may not as yet be obvious. Reassessment after a specific period should be recommended depending on the history given by the detainee and the examination findings.

Details of medication should be verified whenever possible. Information sought should include, for example, whether the detainee is on a supervised methadone administration program as, if the methadone is taken every day on the premises, one can be reasonably sure the detainee is dependent on that dose; the detainee may of course be using other illicit substances as well. Recent urine test results should be checked with the clinic to see whether methadone or other drugs are detected on screening.

With opiate substitution treatment in particular, in the absence of withdrawal signs, confirmation of such treatment should be sought before authorizing continuation. The prescribed dose of methadone may not necessarily indicate accurately the actual amount taken each day, as part or all of the dose may be given to other individuals. If there is doubt about the daily dose then the dose can be divided and given every 12 hours. It should be remembered that giving even a small amount of methadone to a nondependent individual may be fatal. Cocaine abuse appears to accelerate the elimination of methadone; therefore higher doses of methadone need to be prescribed to individuals on maintenance regimes who continue to abuse cocaine *(9)*. Any decision to prescribe should be made on the assessment of objective signs as opposed to subjective symptoms, and a detailed record of the history and examination should be made contemporaneously.

2.4. Medical Complications of Substance Misuse

Medical complications of substance misuse may give an indication of a problem in the absence of acute symptoms or signs of intoxication. Intravenous injection may result in superficial thrombophlebitis, deep vein thrombosis and pulmonary embolus, and chronic complications of limb swelling and venous ulcers. Cellulitis and abscesses may be seen around injection sites, and deep abscesses may extend into joints, producing septic arthritis. Self-neglect, malnutrition, and dental decay may occur, as may infectious diseases such as hepatitis B, C, HIV and the acquired immunodeficiency syndrome (AIDS).

Skin manifestations of drug addiction may be seen more commonly in opiate rather than stimulant users, even though stimulant users inject more frequently *(10)*. This is partly because stimulants do not cause histamine release and are therefore seldom associated with pruritus and excoriations and also because cutaneous complications are frequently caused by the adulterants

Table 3
Drugs of Misuse: How They Work[a]

Mechanism	Transmitter[b]
Mimicking (substituting for) natural transmitters	
Opioids	Endorphin/encephalin
Alcohol	GABA-A/endorphins
Benzodiazepines	GABA-A
Cannabis	Anandamide (?)
LSD	5-HT (1,2 receptors)
Increasing endogenous transmitter release	
Cocaine	Dopamine
Amphetamine	Dopamine
Ecstasy	5-HT/dopamine
Solvents	Noradrenaline (?)
Blocking natural transmitters	
Alcohol	Glutamate
Barbiturates	Glutamate

[a]Adapted from ref. *11*.

[b]GABA-A, gamma-aminobutyric acid A type receptor; 5-HT, serotonin.

injected along with the opiates, rather than the drugs themselves. Fresh puncture sites, tattoos used to cover needle tracks, keloid formation, track marks from chronic inflammation, ulcerated areas and skin popping resulting in atrophic scars, hyperpigmentation at sites of healed abscess, puffy hands (lymphoedema with obliteration of anatomic landmarks and pitting edema absent), and histamine-related urticaria (opiates act on mast cells resulting in histamine release) may be seen.

3. Specific Drugs

The classification of drugs into their physiologic or psychological actions, e.g., stimulants and sedatives, is unsatisfactory because a single drug may have several actions; it is preferable to classify drugs according to their pharmacodynamic actions (Table 3) *(11)*.

3.1. Opiate Intoxication and Withdrawal

The characteristics of the medical syndromes in opiate intoxication, overdose, and withdrawal are given in Table 4. Opiates such as heroin may be taken orally, more usually injected, or smoked—"chasing the dragon." The start of

Table 4
Medical Syndromes in Heroin Users[a]

Syndrome (onset and duration)	Characteristics
Opiate intoxication	Conscious, sedated "nodding"; mood normal to euphoric; pinpoint pupils
Acute overdose	Unconscious; pinpoint pupils; slow, shallow respirations
Opiate withdrawal	
Anticipatory 3–4 h after the last fix (as acute effects of heroin subside)	Fear of withdrawal, anxiety, drug-craving, drug-seeking behavior
Early 8–10 h after last fix	Anxiety, restlessness, yawning, nausea, sweating, nasal stuffiness, rhinorrhea, lacrimation, dilated pupils, stomach cramps, increased bowel sounds, drug-seeking behavior
Fully developed 1–3 days after last fix	Severe anxiety, tremor, restlessness, piloerection (cold-turkey), vomiting, diarrhea, muscle spasms (kicking the habit), muscle pain, increased blood pressure, tachycardia, fever, chills, impulse-driven drug-seeking behavior
Protracted abstinence	Hypotension, bradycardia, insomnia, loss of energy and appetite, stimulus-driven opiate cravings

[a]Adapted from ref. *170*.

withdrawal will vary in time with the different opioid drugs, and it should be remembered that the severity of withdrawal symptoms is influenced greatly by psychological factors *(12)*; the environment of a police cell is likely to exacerbate these symptoms.

Chronic administration of opiate drugs results in tolerance (Table 5) to effects such as euphoria mediated by the opiate receptors and to the effects on the autonomic nervous system mediated by the noradrenergic pathways. Tolerance to heroin can develop within 2 weeks of commencing daily heroin use, occurs more slowly with methadone, and may go as quickly as it develops. With abrupt withdrawal of opiates, there is a "noradrenergic storm," which is responsible for many of the opiate withdrawal symptoms (Table 6). Cyclizine may be taken intravenously in large doses with opiates, as it is said to enhance or prolong opioid effects, also resulting in intense stimulation, hallucinations, and seizures; tolerance and dependence on cyclizine may also result *(13)*.

Table 5
Diagnostic Criteria for Opioid Dependence and Severity of Opioid Dependence[a]

1. Opioids are taken in larger amounts or over a longer period that the person intended.
2. A desire for the drug persists, or the patient has made one or more unsuccessful efforts to cut down or to control opioid use.
3. A great deal of time is spent in activities necessary to obtain opioids (such as theft), taking the drug, or recovering from its effects.
4. The patient is frequently intoxicated or has withdrawal symptoms when expected to fulfill major role obligations at work, school, or home (e.g., does not go to work, goes to school or work "high," is intoxicated while taking care of children) or when opioid use is physically hazardous (such as driving under the influence).
5. Important social, occupational, or recreational activities are given up or reduced.
6. Marked tolerance; needs greatly increased amounts of the drug—at least 50% increase—to achieve the desired effect or a notably diminished effect occurs with continued use of the same amount.
7. Has characteristic withdrawal syndrome.
8. Opioids are often taken to relieve or avoid withdrawal symptoms.

In addition some symptoms of the disturbance have persisted for at least a month or have occurred repeatedly over a longer period.

Severity of opioid dependence

Mild	Few, if any symptoms are present in excess of those required to make the diagnosis, and the symptoms result in no more than mild impairment in occupational functioning or in usual social activities or relationships with others.
Moderate	Functional impairment of symptoms is between mild and severe.
Severe	Many symptoms are present in excess of those required to make the diagnosis, and the symptoms greatly interfere with occupational functioning or usual social activities or relationship with others.
Partial remission	During the past 6 months, there has been some use of the substance and some symptoms of dependence.
Full remission	During the past 6 months, either there has been no use of opioids or opioids have been used and there were no symptoms of dependence.

[a]Adapted from ref. *170*.

Table 6
DSM-III-R Diagnostic Criteria for Opioid Withdrawal[a]

A. Cessation of prolonged (several weeks or more) moderate or heavy use of an opioid or reduction in the amount of opioid used (or administration or an opioid antagonist after a brief period of use), followed by at least three of the following:
   1. Craving for opioid
   2. Nausea or vomiting
   3. Muscle aches
   4. Lacrimation or rhinorrhea
   5. Pupillary dilation, piloerection, or sweating
   6. Diarrhea
   7. Yawning
   8. Fever
   9. Insomnia

B. Not due to any physical or other mental disorder

[a]Adapted from ref. *154*.

3.1.1. Treatment of Opiate Withdrawal

Symptomatic treatment of the opiate withdrawal syndrome can often be achieved using a combination of drugs such as benzodiazepines for anxiety and insomnia; loperamide or diphenoxylate and atropine for diarrhea; promethazine, which has antiemetic and sedative properties; and paracetamol or nonsteroidal antiinflammatories for generalized aches.

Substitution treatment may be required in more severe cases of opiate dependence using a choice of methadone, codeine, or dihydrocodeine. As street heroin varies in purity, the starting dose cannot be accurately estimated on the basis of the amount of street drug used. Therefore, substitution therapy should be titrated against the symptoms and signs of withdrawal. For example, dihydrocodeine may be commenced in a dose of 120 mg three times a day, with the dose being increased if the patient has demonstrable clinical signs of opiate withdrawal *(14)*.

Clonidine and lofexidine act as presynaptic α_2-adrenergic agonists, which inhibit the noradrenergic storm associated with opiate withdrawal. Although clonidine has been shown to be effective in reducing most symptoms of withdrawal, the drug has side effects of hypotension, sedation, and psychiatric problems, which render it unsuitable for use in police custody. By contrast, lofexidine has been used in detoxification from opiates with fewer side effects *(15)*.

Maternal opiate withdrawal syndrome may be life threatening for the fetus, and special care should be taken to ensure that a pregnant, opiate-

Table 7
Half-Lives and Observation Times Required after Acute Narcotic Overdose[a]

Opioid	Duration of action	t 1/2	Observation time (h)	iv route
Methadone (dolophine, amidone)	May be days	15–72	24–36	Single-repeated doses
Morphine	Usually 2–4 h	3	6	
Heroin	Usually 2–4 h	Short	6	Rapidly deacetylated to morphine
Codeine	2–4 h (oral)	3	6	

Note: Generally if patients remain asymptomatic 6 h after administration of naloxone, they may be discharged

[a]Adapted from ref. *171*.

dependent woman's medication is continued while she is in custody. There should be a low threshold for referral for hospital assessment, especially in the third trimester.

3.1.2. Buprenorphine (Buprenex, Temgesic)

Buprenorphine is an opioid with mixed agonist-antagonist properties that may be abused or used as an alternative to methadone in detoxification from opiates. It can be taken sublingually or by injection and is relatively safe in overdosage. An unusual property of buprenorphine is that after chronic administration the onset of the abstinence syndrome is delayed. Heroin addicts dependent on a small dose of opiate can be transferred onto buprenorphine, which can be withdrawn fairly easily because of the delayed onset of the abstinence syndrome. However, if it is given to an individual dependent on large doses of opiates, the antagonist properties precipitate withdrawal symptoms *(16)*.

3.1.3. Naloxone

Naloxone is an opioid antagonist that reverses the effects of severe intoxication (Table 7). The use of naloxone may precipitate withdrawal in addicted patients, but in initial doses of 0.4–0.8 mg it is relatively safe, with little risk of vomiting, seizures, hypotension, hypertension, or cardiac arrest *(17)*. The half-life of naloxone is shorter than that of most opiates, and therefore a period of observation in the hospital is required after administration. It is recommended to give half the dose intravenously and half intramuscularly (absorption is slower and the antidotal activity prolonged); this is useful, as often individuals discharge themselves once awakened. In the prehospital environment naloxone should only be given where there is life-threatening opiate poisoning with a respiratory rate less than 8/min, a Glasgow Coma Scale less than 8, or when the airway is at risk *(18)*. Heroin may be taken in combination with cocaine ("speedball"), and the use of naloxone in this situation may precipitate ventricular dysrhythmias *(19)*.

3.2. Benzodiazepines

Benzodiazepines produce physical and psychological dependence and are therefore only recommended for limited periods *(20)*. The drugs are commonly misused either illicitly, which usually involves high doses, or by persistent therapeutic use at a lower dose. The pharmacologic properties of the benzodiazepines are hypnotic, anxiolytic, muscle relaxant, and anticonvulsant and are produced by enhancing gamma-aminobutyric acid (GABA) transmission *(21)*.

Manifestations of intoxication and withdrawal are given in Table 8. Tolerance usually develops after continuous use, slowly for those drugs that have a long half-life but more quickly for the short-acting drugs *(22)*. Benzodiazepines are well absorbed from the gastrointestinal tract after oral administration; food can delay the rate but not the extent of absorption.

Side effects of use include daytime drowsiness, aggravation of depression, and anterograde amnesia *(23)* at therapeutic doses, the risk increasing at high dosages. Amnesic effects may be associated with inappropriate behaviors and other paradoxic behavioral responses such as increased aggression, excitement, confusion, and restlessness *(24,25)*. Rage reactions with violent behavior are most likely in people with a history of aggressive behavior or unstable emotional behavior. Anxiolytics lower tolerance to alcohol and in high doses produce mental confusion similar to alcohol intoxication. The interaction between alcohol and benzodiazepines results in a potentiation of the central nervous system (CNS) effects. In general, however, they have a very high toxic-therapeutic ratio, and doses 15–20 times therapeutic dose may not cause serious side effects *(26)*.

Sudden cessation of benzodiazepines can lead to a recognized withdrawal syndrome *(27)* with anxiety symptoms, disordered perceptions, and major complications such as seizures and psychosis *(28)*. A long-acting benzodiazepine such as diazepam or chlordiazepoxide is preferable in treating symptoms of withdrawal and preventing the major complications.

Flumazenil is a specific benzodiazepine antagonist used for the reversal of benzodiazepine-induced sedation and coma. When overdosage is suspected, it can be used in patients who would otherwise need intubation and ventilation

Table 8
Manifestations of Sedative-Hypnotic Drug Intoxication and Withdrawal

Degree	Characteristics
Mild	Sedation, disorientation, slurred speech, ataxia, nystagmus
Severe	Coma, hypoventilation, hypotension, hypothermia, depressed or absent corneal, gag, and deep tendon reflexes
Withdrawal	Anxiety, insomnia, irritability, agitation, anorexia, tremor, seizures

(29), but care should be taken when mixed overdoses are suspected *(30)*. Complications such as convulsions, dysrhythmias, heart block, and cardiac arrest suggest that its use in the prehospital environment should not be encouraged *(31)*.

3.3. Barbiturates

Barbiturates are used in the treatment of epilepsy and for the induction of anesthesia. They became less commonly misused following the introduction of benzodiazepine drugs but may be used by polydrug users. Mild intoxication may result in slurred speech, oversedation, ataxia, and nystagmus, while severe intoxication may present with coma, absent reflexes, hypothermia, hypotension, and respiratory depression. There is a narrow margin between therapeutic dose and serious toxicity. Physical and psychological dependence occurs, and the withdrawal syndrome is similar to that of benzodiazepine withdrawal, with a greater risk of seizures. Benzodiazepines may be used to prevent the withdrawal syndrome associated with barbiturates *(28)*.

3.4. Solvents

Volatile substance abuse (VSA) is the deliberate inhalation of fumes given off by volatile substances (solvents) to achieve intoxication and can occur at any age but is a particular problem among adolescents. Adhesives, aerosols, anesthetics, dry cleaning agents, fuel gases, nail varnish, and paint stripper are among the substances inhaled *(32)*, either directly from their containers, from a plastic bag placed over the nose and mouth, from impregnated rags, or sprayed directly into the mouth.

Regular users may have nasal sores, "glue-sniffer's rash" (perioral dermatitis), and have the odor of solvents on their breath. Acute effects begin within minutes *(33)* and may last 15–45 minutes; persistent abnormalities may occur in severe chronic abusers (Table 9) *(34)*.

Table 9
Manifestations of Solvent Intoxication and Abuse[a]

Degree	Characteristics
Mild	Euphoria Disinhibition Dizziness Slurred speech Lack of coordination Sneezing and coughing
Moderate	Lethargy, stupor Hallucinations Nausea, vomiting Diarrhea Nystagmus Ataxia Tremors Myalgias Paresthesia
Severe	Coma Seizures
Chronic	Cerebellar syndrome: ataxia, nystagmus, tremor (toluene) Fatigue, difficulty in concentrating Parkinsonism (toluene) Peripheral neuropathy: symmetrical, motor, mainly involving hands and feet (n-hexane and naphtha)

[a]Adapted from ref. *26*.

Most acute direct VSA-related deaths result from cardiac dysrythmias due to "sensitization" of the myocardium to adrenaline; deaths may also occur from indirect effects or may be delayed (Table 10) *(35)*. Animal experiments confirm that myocardial sensitivity may continue for hours after the initial inhalant exposure *(36)*. Tolerance may develop, and psychological dependence after long-term use and a withdrawal syndrome similar to delirium tremens has been described *(37)*.

3.5. Lysergic Acid Diethylamide

Lysergic acid diethylamide (LSD) is usually taken orally in a dose of 20–100 mg with sympathomimetic effects occuring in 5–10 minutes and psychological effects in 30–60 minutes *(38)*. There is a recovery period of 10–12 hours where there may be periods of normal perception and cognition alternating with degrees of intoxication, which may affect fitness for interview.

Table 10
Deaths from Volatile Substance Misuse[a]

		Cause
Acute		
	Direct	Immediate
		Postponed
	Indirect	Trauma
		Aspiration
		Asphyxia
		Drowning
Delayed		
	Direct	Liver failure
		Renal failure
		Liver tumors
		Bone marrow depression
		CNS involvement

[a]Adapted from ref. *35*.

Acute effects include tachycardia, hypertension, pyrexia, dilated pupils with both anisocoria (unequal size) and hippus (spasmodic rhythmical dilation and constriction), dry mouth, sweating, flushing, tremor, and hyperreflexia. Emotional lability, euphoria and anxiety, distortion of time, visual and auditory illusions (although true hallucinations can occur), and synesthesia, with a mixing of the sensory input—"seeing" sounds or "hearing" smells—may all occur *(39)*.

Both enjoyable and unpleasant effects, a "bad trip," may occur in a first-time user or with repeated use *(40)*. Five major categories of psychiatric adverse effects have been described, which include anxiety and panic attacks, self-destructive behavior, hallucinations, acute psychosis, and major depressive reactions *(41)*. Polydrug users may use benzodiazepines to alleviate anxiety and panic attacks.

Chronic toxic effects include a prolonged psychosis, major depressive illness, disruption of personality, and post-hallucinogen perceptual disorder (PHPD) *(41)* characterized by flashbacks even months or years after LSD use.

Physical dependence does not occur, and psychological dependence is uncommon and short lived. Tolerance does occur in the chronic abuser, but a few day's abstinence will restore full central nervous system sensitivity to the drug.

3.6. Phencyclidine

Phencyclidine (PCP), "angel dust," is usually smoked, although it can be taken orally, intravenously, or by nasal inhalation. It is commonly used as an additive to other drugs such as cannabis or LSD, and the symptoms and signs may vary greatly *(42)*. At low doses euphoria, relaxation, and an altered body image may occur, but at higher doses there may be agitation, bizarre behavior, and a paranoid psychosis *(43)*. Analgesia occurs, which may lead to self-injury. Physical effects include nystagmus (lateral and vertical), and with severe intoxication there is adrenergic stimulation with hypertension, tachycardia, flushing, hyperthermia, and cholinomimetic stimulation with sweating, hypersalivation, miosis, dystonia, ataxia, and myoclonus eventually resulting in coma, respiratory arrest, and circulatory collapse *(44)*. Death may also result from intoxication or from violent behavior. Chronic effects of PCP abuse include memory impairment, personality changes, and depression; however, there is probably no physical dependence.

3.7. Ecstasy (MDMA)

3,4-Methylenedioxymethamphetamine, or "ecstasy," is commonly taken in an oral dose of 75–120 mg as a recreational drug within the dance culture or "rave" scene for its central stimulant and psychedelic effects (Table 11) *(45)*. The effects last for 4–6 hours with tolerance developing to the acute effects. However, physical and psychological dependence do not occur.

Adverse effects such as a polydipsia, hyponatremia, and catatonic stupor have been reported *(46,47)*. An acute rise in antidiuretic hormone [arginine vasopressin (AVP)] accompanied by a small fall in plasma sodium has been shown following the ingestion of MDMA. Therefore, in view of the risk of hyponatremia, individuals who take such drugs should avoid drinking fluid in excess of the body's requirement. This may be difficult because MDMA reduces the perception of thirst and impairs judgment *(48)*, and people tend to overcompensate and consciously overdrink.

Regular users may habitually use chewing gum to overcome the effects on the jaw muscles. The clenching of teeth in the acidic environment caused by carbonated (fizzy) drinks will result in an increased likelihood of tooth wear on the back teeth *(49)*. Other adverse effects have been described including jaundice and hepatotoxicity *(50)*; flashbacks and psychosis *(51)*; pneumomediastinum *(52)*; urinary retention *(53)*; hyperthermia; coagulopathy *(54)*; rhabdomyolysis; and cardiovascular complications resulting in death *(55–57)*. Development of chronic paranoid psychosis has been described after heavy misuse of the drug *(58)*, and the serotonin syndrome *(59)* (altered mental state,

Table 11
Effects of MDMA (Ecstasy)

Type	Effects
Psychological	Euphoria, heightened awareness, improved sense of communication
Neuropsychiatric	Anxiety, insomnia, depression, paranoia, confusion, panic attacks, psychosis
Chronic	Depression, drowsiness, anxiety, panic disorder, aggressive outbursts, psychosis, memory disturbance
Medical	Tachycardia, hypertension, dry throat, bruxism, trismus, sweating, pyrexia, nausea, vomiting, anorexia, loss of coordination with ataxia, dilated pupils, nystagmus, hot and cold flushes, hyperreflexia

hyperthermia, and autonomic dysfunction) has also been reported following MDMA ingestion *(60)*. Evidence is emerging of possible long-term damage to the brain in the form of serotonin (5-HT) neural injury, which may result in depression, anxiety, and memory disorders *(61)*.

3,4-Methylenedioxyethamphetamine (MDEA) is an analog of MDMA with similar effects. 3,4-Methylenedioxyamphetamine (MDA) and para-methoxyamphetamine (PMA) may also be used as recreational drugs. Overdose may result in severe sympathetic stimulation and death *(62)*.

3.8. Cocaine and Crack

Cocaine occurs naturally in the leaves of the coca plant *Erythroxylum coca*, which grows predominantly in South America. Cocaine hydrochloride is a white powder that is usually snorted but can be taken orally. Crack is prepared by mixing cocaine hydrochloride with sodium bicarbonate and water and heating it. The cocaine base precipitates out and forms small "rocks" as it cools. Crack may be smoked in a pipe or heated on foil with the vapor inhaled. Both crack and cocaine may be injected.

The onset of action and plasma half-life varies depending on the route of use, very rapidly if taken intravenously or smoked compared with when snorted. The duration of effects will also vary with route of administration *(63)*. Ingestion of stimulant drugs such as cocaine or amphetamine result in activation of the sympathetic nervous system with resulting euphoria followed by irritability, depression, insomnia, and paranoia (Table 12).

Tolerance occurs to the psychological effects but not effects on the heart. Deaths may occur, most commonly from cardiac dysrhythmias, myocardial infarction, agitated delirium, and stroke. Chronic effects include perforation of

Table 12
Effects of Cocaine and Amphetamine Intoxication

Dose	Characteristics
Initial low dose	Euphoria, insomnia, dry mouth, hyperthermia, tachycardia, hypertension, increased respiration, sweating, dilated pupils
With increasing dose	Irritability, impulsivity, aggressiveness, agitated delirium, paranoia, delusions, seizures

the nasal septum and rhinorrhea, and long-term use may result in a range of psychiatric problems and vascular diseases *(64)*.

Cocaine produces a physical and psychological dependence, the severity of which will vary depending on the method of administration, being more severe if the drug is smoked or injected than if snorted. Dependence may result in a particular strong craving for the drug, followed by a withdrawal syndrome or "crash" with irritability, insomnia, depression, and anxiety on cessation. In conditions of police custody, the depression and inability to sleep may lead to acts of self-harm and suicide, and close supervision may be required, with consideration given to prescribing hypnotics and antidepressants.

3.9. Amphetamine

Amphetamine is usually found as a white powder, amphetamine sulphate, and can be taken nasally, orally, or intravenously. Clinical effects are similar to those of cocaine (Table 12), although amphetamine has a longer half-life of 10–15 hours, so the duration of euphoria is longer. "Ice" is a very pure form of methamphetamine hydrochloride (98–100% pure), which is usually smoked like crack cocaine.

Tolerance occurs with long-term use. "Speed runs" describe repeated use over a period of days with several grams of amphetamine used daily. At the end of the "run," the user may sleep for several days. Alcohol, sedative-hypnotic drugs, and heroin may be used to reduce the anxiety cause by amphetamine or, alternatively, amphetamine may be used to reduce the sedative effects of such drugs. Psychological dependence occurs, and psychosis may occur, which resolves when the drug is stopped. However, it is possible that amphetamine use may trigger latent schizophrenia.

3.10. Khat

Khat consists of the young leaves of the *Catha edulis* plant; it is usually chewed for its stimulant effect when fresh but may be drunk as an infusion of leaves. In the United Kingdom it is sold legally (it is illegal in the United States) and is used by Somali populations *(65,66)*. The main component is cathinone, with effects similar to those of amphetamine, resulting in euphoria, increased alertness, and anorexia *(67)*. There may also be mood lability, anxiety, and insomnia *(68)*.

Heavy khat consumption may result in mania-like symptoms, paranoia, and an acute schizophrenia-like psychosis, usually resolving within weeks of cessation of use *(69,70)*. Although there is no specific physical withdrawal syndrome, depression, hypersomnia, and loss of energy may occur when khat use is stopped *(68)*.

3.11. Marijuana

Marijuana is the most commonly used illicit drug in the United Kingdom and United States. It is obtained from the *Cannabis sativa* plant, and the principal active ingredient, accounting for the majority of effects, is delta-9-tetrahydrocannabinol (THC). There are a number of forms, including hashish (a resin), herbal cannabis (a green-colored preparation made from the leaves of the plant), and cannabis oil. "Skunk" is a term used to describe a potent form of the cannabis plant with high levels of THC *(71)*, which is grown indoors using hydroponic techniques, in nutrient-rich liquids rather than soil, under grow lights or greenhouse conditions. The onset of effects is reported as being more rapid, and the hallucinogenic properties are heightened. Psychotic episodes may be precipitated by relatively small quantities *(72)*.

Cannabis is usually smoked but can be ingested as, for example, "cannabis cookies." One "joint" typically contains 10–30 mg of THC and has an onset of action of 10–20 minutes with effects lasting 2–3 hours *(43)*. The acute effects of cannabis are given in Table 13 *(73)*.

Tolerance has been shown to develop to many effects of cannabis including the "high" with chronic use, and an abstinence syndrome has been described with disturbed sleep, decreased appetite, restlessness, irritability, and sweating. Withdrawal symptoms are usually mild and short-lived, although they may be more severe in heavy regular users *(74)*.

3.12. Anabolic Steroids

Anabolic steroids may be taken orally or intramuscularly by body builders or other individuals who want to enhance their physical appearance. Research has shown that injections of testosterone enathate increase muscle size and strength, especially when combined with exercise *(75)*. To achieve the desired effect, different steroids are taken in cycles, with rest periods in between, a regime known as "stacking," or, alternatively, increasing doses of

Table 13
Pharmacologic Actions of Cannabis in Humans (in Therapeutic Dosage Range)[a]

System	Characteristics
Central nervous system	
Psychological effects	Euphoria, dysphoria, anxiety, depersonalization, precipitation/aggravation of psychotic states
Effects on perception	Heightened sensory perception, distortion of space and time sense, misperceptions, hallucinations
Effects on cognition and psychomotor performance	Fragmentation of thoughts, mental clouding, memory impairment, global impairment of performance especially in complex and demanding tasks
Effects on motor function	Increased motor activity followed by inertia and incoordination, ataxia, dysarthria, tremulousness, weakness, and muscle twitching
Analgesic effects	Similar in potency to codeine (nonopioid mechanism)
Tolerance	To most behavioral and somatic effects including the euphoria with chronic use
Dependence/abstinence syndrome	Rarely observed; symptoms include disturbed sleep, decreased appetite, restlessness, irritability, and sweating
Cardiovascular system	
Heart rate	Tachycardia with acute dosage; bradycardia with chronic use
Peripheral circulation	Vasodilation, conjunctival redness, postural hypotension
Respiratory system	
Ventilation	Small doses stimulate; large doses suppress
Bronchodilatation	Coughing but tolerance develops

[a]Adapted from ref. *73*.

the same steroid are taken, a so-called drug pyramid *(76)*. Most of the steroids sold in the United Kingdom are counterfeit rather than produced by legitimate pharmaceutical companies. Consequently they may contain a different steroid from the one indicated on the bottle, and scant reliance can be placed on the reported dose as they may have little or no steroid in them at all *(77)*.

General effects of anabolic steroids *(78)* include baldness, acne (typically affecting the shoulders and upper back), raised blood pressure and heart rate, fluid retention, and a reduction in high-density lipoprotein cholesterol. Long-term effects include an increased risk of thrombosis. Gynecomastia may occur, and the prostate gland may swell, resulting in impaired micturition. Most of these effects are dose dependent and more likely with prolonged administration.

While the drug is being taken, there is a significant reduction in testosterone production by the testes so that sperm output and quality are decreased, and a return to normal can take many months after drug use is stopped. The effect on sex drive is variable, but overall it seems that the sex drive increases at the beginning of a steroid-using cycle, and then decreases to below normal after several weeks of use. Drive may remain below normal levels even after the drug is stopped until such time as the testes start producing testosterone again. There may also be a reduction in size of the testicles *(79)*.

In women menstrual irregularities are reported, with permanent enlargement of the clitoris. There may also be growth of facial and body hair, male pattern baldness, and decreased breast size. Abuse of sex steroids by recreational body builders may be an unrecognized cause of subfertility *(80)*.

Liver function tests may show abnormalities that usually return to normal once the drug is stopped. Drug-induced jaundice can be caused by temporarily impaired excretory function, and peliosis hepatitis, in which the liver tissue is replaced by blood-filled cysts, may occur, as can liver tumors *(81)* and Wilms' tumor.

Initial use may result in stimulatory effects such as increased confidence, decreased fatigue, heightened motivation, agitation, irritability, and insomnia, which may progress to argumentative and aggressive behavior and major mood disturbances including depression, mania, and hypomania *(82,83)*. "Roid rage," which may be associated with violent crimes *(84)*, seems to require a high dose of steroids over several weeks, as may occur when "stacking."

3.13. Other Body Building Drugs

Other drugs may be used by body builders including tamoxifen to reduce or prevent gynecomastia; diuretics to counteract the fluid retention caused by anabolic steroids; thyroxine to increase the rate of metabolism, which might theoretically increase the ability of anabolic steroids to boost physical strength *(85)*; and beta human chorionic gonadotrophin to alleviate testicular atrophy *(86)*. Nalbuphine (Nubain) is an opioid agonist/antagonist analgesic used for the treatment of moderate to severe pain, and dependence has been reported associated with anabolic steroid use *(87)*.

Furthermore, there has been a case report of a 21-year-old body builder who was admitted after taking excessive amounts of insulin intravenously; apparently insulin is advertised in body building magazines as having anabolic properties *(88)*. The recreational use of caffeine to toxic levels has been reported in a body builder who presented with a grand mal seizure *(89)*. Clenbuterol, which is a sympathomimetic agonist (used as a oral bronchodilator in some European countries but not licensed for human use in the United

Kingdom or United States) is said to have an "anabolic-like" effect but at high dose may cause cardiac dysrhythmias, tremor, and serious hypokalemia *(90)*.

3.14. Gamma-Hydroxy Butyrate

Gamma-hydroxy butyrate (GHB) is a naturally occurring substance in the human brain structurally related to GABA and may be a neurotransmitter *(91)*. It has been used as an anesthetic (although it has little analgesic effect), to alleviate narcolepsy, and to treat alcohol and opiate dependence *(92)*. There have been reports of abuse in the United Kingdom and United States within the dance scene and gay clubs and with body builders, as it is said to promote slow-wave sleep during which growth hormone is secreted *(93)*. It is available as a colorless, odorless liquid, powder, or capsule taken orally, rarely injected. GHB is rapidly absorbed, with peak plasma concentrations occurring after 20–45 minutes following oral administration. It has a half-life of 30 minutes *(94)*, and effects can last from 45 minutes to 8 hours *(95)*.

Initial effects include euphoria followed by profound sedation, confusion, agitation, and amnesia; nausea, vomiting, and diarrhea; ataxia, seizures, hypotonia, and tremor; vertigo and dizziness; bradycardia, hypotension, and hypothermia; coma *(96)*; respiratory collapse.

There is a narrow margin between intoxication and coma *(97)*, and the clinical effects are potentiated by use of other CNS depressant drugs such as alcohol, opiates, benzodiazepines, and neuroleptics *(98)*. Tolerance and physical dependence after high-dose use can develop with a withdrawal syndrome, which may include insomnia, muscular cramping, tremor, and anxiety *(92)*.

3.15. Ketamine

Ketamine is a commercially available anesthetic for intravenous and intramuscular use. It contains analgesic properties and is available on the street in powder, tablet, and liquid form; it can be smoked or taken intranasally ("snorted"), orally, intramuscularly or by the intravenous route *(99)*. The onset of effects depends on the route of administration; when taken orally, effects start within 20 minutes and can last up to 3 hours, whereas given intravenously, effects will be seen within 30 seconds and last about 30 minutes *(100)*. Tolerance develops after repeated use, with a decreased duration of effect *(101)*.

Physical effects may include a cocaine-like "rush," hypertension, dysrhythmias, nausea, and vomiting, slurred speech, nystagmus, lack of coordination, and seizures. On recovery, "emergence phenomema" may occur, with pyschological dissociation or out of body (flying or floating) sensations, confusion, hallucinations, synesthesia and depersonalization *(102)*. Such dissociative states may result in the individual becoming divorced from reality, and these effects, coupled with possible loss of coordination and pronounced analgesia, can result in serious accidents to users. A dose-dependent depression of respiration may occur *(103)*, and this can be a particular problem when taken with other respiratory depressant drugs such as benzodiazepines and alcohol, occasionally resulting in death *(104)*.

3.16. Alkyl Nitrites

The alkyl nitrites are volatile yellowish clear liquids that have a distinctive sweet smell. All the nitrites have vasodilatory properties and are used as a euphoric relaxant within the dance culture and to relax the anal sphincter and enhance sexual performance. The effect of inhaling the vapor, usually from the bottle or poured onto a cloth, is instantaneous and very short-lived, resulting in a "rush," but adverse effects such as dizziness, flushing, tachycardia and palpitations, headache, cold sweats, and hypotension may occur *(105,106)*. Swallowing of volatile nitrites as opposed to inhaling them may result in severe methemoglobinemia *(107)*.

4. Alcohol

Crime statistics show a clear association between heavy drinking and criminal behavior, the association being most marked in relation to violent crimes. One review found that the incidence of alcohol-related violent crime ranged from 24 to 85%, which contrasted dramatically with the 12–38% incidence of alcohol-related nonviolent crime *(108)*. While some have confirmed the association between alcohol and crime *(109,110)*, a direct causal link between the two has been disputed *(111)*. Nonetheless, alcohol assumes an importance in clinical forensic medicine because of its link with criminal activity and by virtue of the significant role it plays in a large number of assessments regarding fitness for detention *(112–114)*. Accordingly, a thorough understanding of the metabolism, effects, and problems associated with alcohol is essential for any doctor practicing in this field.

4.1. The Metabolism of Alcohol

Ethanol, hereafter referred to as alcohol, is produced by the fermentation of sugar by yeast, a process that halts at a concentration of alcohol by volume of about 15% because of the death of yeast above these levels. As a rough guide, one measure of spirits, one glass of wine, or one half-pint of beer contain 1 unit or 8 g of alcohol. However, there is a wide variation in the alcohol content of different drinks *(115)*, and any accurate assessment of intake must bear this in mind. In the EU there is now international agreement about the labeling of alcohol content, with the alcohol content of beverages being referred to by the percentage alcohol by volume (percent v/v) *(116)*. This is equivalent to the number of milliliters of pure alcohol per 100 mL of the drink. In the United States, alcoholic strengths are still measured in terms of percentage proof. U.S. proof spirit contains 50% of alcohol by volume, so to convert U.S. proof to percent v/v, one simply divides by two.

Most people who have alcohol in the body have drunk it, although it can be absorbed into the systemic circulation through the lungs (blood alcohol concentrations of up to 50 mg/100 mL have been achieved after breathing alcohol/air mixtures for several hours) *(117)*. Little or no alcohol is absorbed through the intact skin of adults.

Once ingested, alcohol is subsequently absorbed into the body by a process of passive diffusion that occurs across the mucosal surfaces of the gastrointestinal tract *(118)*. As liquids pass quickly through the mouth and esophagus, little absorption takes place until alcohol has reached the stomach. The rate of absorption is maximal in the duodenum, because its mucosa is thinner and blood supply more abundant than that of the stomach. Accordingly, any condition that delivers drink into the small intestine more quickly than normal, such as gastrectomy, will lead to more rapid absorption and an earlier, higher peak blood alcohol level *(119)*.

As soon as alcohol enters the bloodstream, mechanisms for its removal come into action. Some 5–10% of the total amount absorbed is excreted unchanged in breath, urine, and sweat *(118)*, an important factor that allows the estimation of blood alcohol concentrations from the levels in urine and breath. The remaining 90–95% of alcohol is oxidized in the liver by alcohol dehydrogenase to form acetaldehyde, and this is further metabolized to acetate (acetic acid). As alcohol dehydrogenase becomes saturated at relatively low alcohol concentrations, it soon reaches its maximum working rate, and alcohol elimination proceeds at this constant rate *(120)*.

The rate of absorption is very much faster than the rate of elimination, and this fact gives rise to the characteristic blood alcohol curve, as described by several researchers (Fig. 1) *(121–123)*. Generally speaking, the peak blood alcohol concentration is reached 30–60 minutes after drinking, although the range may be anything from 20 minutes to 3 hours. However, the peak blood alcohol concentration, the time taken to reach the peak, the area under the blood alcohol curve, and the time taken to reach a zero blood alcohol level varies from person to person and within the same person over time *(124)*. Indeed, a large number of factors can influence the kinetics of alcohol.

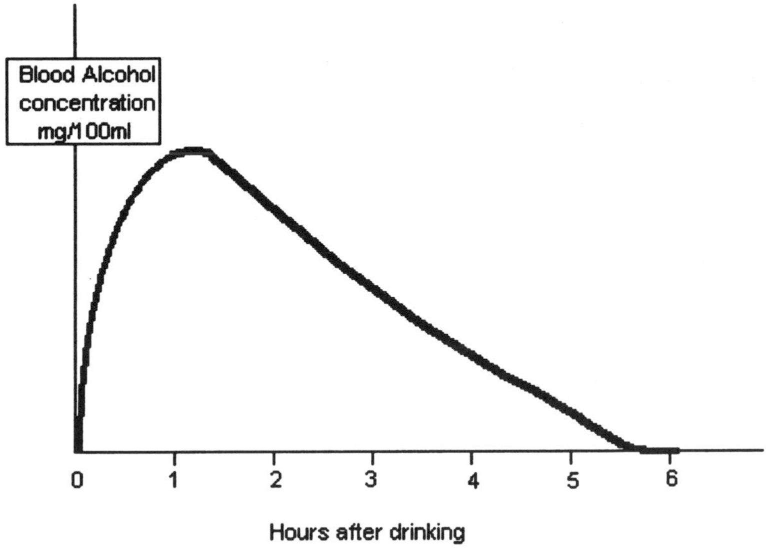

Fig. 1. The Blood-Alcohol Curve.

4.1.1. Sex and Weight

Alcohol is highly hydrophilic, so once it enters the systemic circulation it is distributed evenly throughout total body water (V_d or the volume of distribution). In general, the larger the person the larger the V_d, so that if two different sized males drink the same quantity of alcohol, a higher peak concentration will be reached in the lighter of the two because he will have a smaller V_d for the alcohol to distribute itself throughout. Similarly, because women have more body fat compared with men, and fat contains no water, higher peak alcohol levels are achieved in women than in men of the same weight. The V_d of alcohol for adult males has been shown to be about 0.70, compared with 0.60 for adult females *(118)*.

4.1.2. Duration of Drinking

If a volume of alcohol is consumed over a prolonged period, it may be eliminated almost as quickly as it is absorbed, giving rise to a much lower peak alcohol concentration.

4.1.3. Nature of the Drink Consumed

Alcohol absorption is maximal when the concentration of the ingested solution is between 10 and 20%. Because alcohol is absorbed by passive diffusion, the rate of absorption is slower with drinks of lesser strength because of a lower concentration gradient. Furthermore, the larger volumes involved may also delay gastric emptying and further slow down absorption. By contrast, the alcohol content of stronger drinks irritates the gastric mucosa and pyloric sphincter, causing increased secretion of mucus and delayed gastric emptying.

4.1.4. Food in the Stomach

Studies have shown that eating a full meal before drinking can reduce the peak alcohol level by an average of 9–23% *(118,125–127)*. The presence of food in the stomach reduces the rate of gastric emptying, dilutes the alcohol that enters the stomach, and limits the contact between the alcohol and the gastric mucosa. Alcohol absorption is slowed for all these reasons.

4.1.5. Physiologic Factors and Genetic Variation

Factors such as stomach wall permeability, blood supply to the alimentary tract, and the rate of gastric emptying will vary from person to person, and from time to time in the same person. All of these will have a bearing on the shape of the blood alcohol curve.

4.1.6. Drugs

The interaction between alcohol and drugs, either prescribed or illicit, is important because so many detained persons take other drugs in conjunction with alcohol *(2)*. Generally speaking, the most important interactions involve drugs altering the way a subject responds to a given amount of alcohol in the blood, for example, because the drug has CNS depressant effects that add to those of alcohol. However, a number of drugs may influence the rate of alcohol absorption by virtue of their affect on the rate of gastric emptying (Table 14).

4.1.7. Rate of Elimination

The rate of elimination of alcohol has been determined experimentally. Reported values range from about 10 mg/100 mL of blood per hour (mg/dL/h) to 25 mg/dL/h, with an average of 15–18.6 mg/dl/h *(120,128)* (approximately equivalent to the elimination of 1 unit of alcohol per hour in a 70-kg male). Habituation to alcohol is the single most important factor affecting the rate of elimination. One recent study reported the rate of ethanol disappearance in 22 alcoholics as ranging from 13 to 36 mg/dL/h, with an average of 22 mg/dL/h *(129)*. The increased rate of elimination is thought to be because chronic alcoholics have facilitated liver enzyme systems.

4.2. Effects of Alcohol

Alcohol acts as a CNS depressant, which in small doses interferes with cortical function, but which in larger doses may depress medullary processes.

Table 14
Drugs that Affect the Rate of Stomach Emptying and so Influence the Rate of Alcohol Absorption[a]

Drugs that slow gastric emptying
Drugs with anticholinergic actions, such as
Atropine
Chlorpromazine
Tricyclic antidepressants
Drugs with an adrenergic action, such as
Amphetamines
Drugs with an opioid action, such as
Antidiarrheal medicines
Codeine and dihydrocodeine
Diamorphine (heroin)
Methadone
Dextropropoxyphene (in co-proxamol)
Drugs that hasten stomach emptying, such as
Metoclopramide
Cisapride
Erythromycin

[a]Adapted from ref. *117*.

The apparent stimulatory effects of alcohol occur because it acts first on the so-called higher centers of the brain that govern inhibition *(130)*.

While there is general agreement on the sequence of clinical effects caused by drinking alcohol, the blood alcohol concentrations at which these effects occur vary considerably in different subjects. The difference in susceptibility is most marked between habituated and nonhabituated drinkers, but tolerance to the effects remains very variable even within these broad categories *(131,132)*. Table 15 provides a guide to the general effects. It should be noted that the effects are more pronounced when blood alcohol levels are rising than when falling. This is known as the Mellanby effect and is thought to be due to an acute tolerance to alcohol that develops during intoxication *(133)*. Some specific effects are discussed below.

4.2.1. Nystagmus

As the eye is effectively part of the CNS, it is one of the easiest parts of the body to examine in order to detect the effects of alcohol; the most extensively studied ocular effect of alcohol intoxication is nystagmus. Alcohol can cause nystagmus through at least two mechanisms. By acting on the vestibular

Table 15
Sequence of Central Nervous Depressant Effects of Alcohol

Stage of influence	Blood alcohol concentration (mg/100 mL)	Clinical effect
Sobriety	10–50	Often no obvious effect May feel "relaxed"
Euphoria	30–120	Mild euphoria with increased talkativeness Decreased inhibitions Increased self-confidence Impaired fine motor skills
Excitement	90–200	Emotional instability Poor sensory perception Impaired memory and comprehension Incoordination and loss of balance
Drunkenness	150–300	Disorientation, mental confusion Disturbances of vision (e.g., diplopia) Decreased pain sense Increased incoordination with staggering gait Slurred speech
Stupor	250–400	General inertia approaching paralysis Marked lack of response to stimuli Inability to stand or walk Vomiting, incontinence of urine and feces
Coma	350–500	Coma and anesthesia Depressed or absent reflexes Cardiovascular and respiratory depression Possible death
Death	Over 450	Death from respiratory depression

system, it can cause positional alcohol nystagmus (PAN) *(134)*, detected when the patient is lying supine with the head turned to either the left or right. Horizontal gaze nystagmus (HGN) results from the inhibition of the smooth pursuit system and the impaired ability to maintain eccentric gaze *(135)* brought about by alcohol's effect on ocular movements via neural mechanisms *(136)*.

Positional alcohol nystagmus occurs in two stages *(137)*. The first stage, PAN I, is associated with acute elevation of blood alcohol, tending to occur about 30 minutes after alcohol ingestion. In PAN I the fast phase of nystagmus is in the direction toward which the head is turned. PAN II normally occurs at about 5–6 hours after drinking and is characterized by nystagmus in the opposite direction to that seen in PAN I.

Horizontal gaze nystagmus is a jerky eye movement noted when gaze is directed to one side. The fast phase of HGN is in the direction of gaze, and it becomes intensified at a more eccentric gaze position *(136)*. Although HGN can be seen in normal individuals at extreme lateral gaze *(138)*, when detected at lesser deviations it is considered pathologic. An angle of onset of 40 degrees or less from the midline has been found to be a sensitive indicator of a blood alcohol level in excess of 100 mg/100 mL *(138)*. While some authors have maintained that blood alcohol levels of over 80 mg/100 mL are consistently associated with HGN *(139)*, others have found that it is absent in just under 40% of drivers with an average blood alcohol of 120 mg/100 mL (range 9–218 mg/100 mL) *(140)*. As HGN may be noted in a number of pathologic conditions including the ingestion of sedative and tranquilizing drugs *(141)*, its presence should not be taken as proof of alcohol intoxication. It is perhaps for these reasons that the Kansas Supreme Court, when assessing the admissibility of HGN evidence in drink driving prosecutions decided that "the reliability of HGN evidence is not currently a settled proposition in the scientific community" *(142)*.

4.2.2. Pupillary Changes

In the early stages of alcoholic intoxication the pupils are said to dilate, often becoming pinpoint as the level of intoxication advances, particularly when the state of coma is reached *(143)*. However, some commentators report the pupils as being normal-sized in alcohol intoxication *(144)*, with current advice favoring the view that pupil size may be normal or dilated *(145)*.

Alcohol may slow the pupillary response to light, such an effect being one of the more reliable eye signs of intoxication *(140,146)*.

4.2.3. Slurred Speech

Speech production is a complex motor activity. As it requires a high degree of coordination it can be a sensitive index of alcohol intoxication *(147)*. Reliable changes in speech are produced at blood alcohol levels above 100 mg/100 mL, although the effects of lower blood alcohol levels have been variable *(148)*.

4.2.4. Cardiovascular Effects

Moderate doses of alcohol cause a slight increase in blood pressure and pulse rate *(149,150)*. However, the most prominent effect with higher doses is a depression of cardiovascular functions. This depression is probably a combination of central effects and direct depression of the myocardium *(133)*.

4.2.5. Metabolic Effects

Forensic physicians need to be aware that severe hypoglycemia may accompany alcohol intoxication because of inhibition of gluconeogenesis. Alcohol-induced hypoglycemia, which develops within 6–36 hours of heavy drinking, typically occurs in an undernourished individual or one who has not eaten for the previous 24 hours. The usual features of hypoglycemia, such as flushing, sweating, and tachycardia, are often absent, and the person may present in coma.

4.3. Death from Alcohol Poisoning

Alcohol intoxication may result in death due to respiratory or circulatory failure or as a result of aspiration of stomach contents in the absence of a gag reflex. Levels of blood alcohol above 500 mg/100 mL are considered to be "probably fatal" *(151)*, although survival at much higher concentrations is now well documented. In 1982, for example, the case of a 24-year-old woman with a blood alcohol level of 1510 mg/100 mL was reported. She had gone to the hospital complaining of abdominal pain and was noted to be conscious but slightly confused. Two days later her pain had eased, her blood alcohol level fallen, and she was able to leave the hospital and return home *(152)*.

Death associated with blood alcohol levels below 350 mg/100 mL suggests that other complicating factors are present. Most commonly this will be an interaction between alcohol and some other drug that has also been ingested.

4.4 Diagnosis of Intoxication

The terms *alcohol intoxication* and *drunkenness* are often used interchangeably. However, a distinction between these terms is justified as people may exhibit behavioral changes associated with drunkenness when they believe they have consumed alcohol but actually have not *(153)*. Thus the diagnostic features of alcoholic intoxication developed by the American Psychiatric Association include a requirement that there must have been recent ingestion of alcohol (Table 16) *(154)*.

The fourth of the Diagnostic and Statistical Manual of Mental Disorders (DSM-IV) criteria requires that medical conditions likely to account for the observed condition need to be excluded before the diagnosis of alcohol intoxication is made. This is particularly important when assessing an intoxicated detainee in police custody. Indeed, the doctor's first duty in examining such individuals should be to exclude pathologic conditions that may simulate intoxication *(143)* (Table 17), as failure to do so may lead to deaths in police custody *(155)*.

Table 16
Diagnostic Criteria for Alcohol Intoxication: DSM-IV[a]

A. Recent ingestion of alcohol.
B. Clinically significant maladaptive behavioral or psychological changes (e.g., inappropriate sexual or aggressive behavior, mood lability, impaired judgment, impaired social or occupational functioning) that developed during, or shortly after, alcohol ingestion.
C. One (or more) of the following signs, developing during, or shortly after, alcohol use:
   1. Slurred speech
   2. Incoordination
   3. Unsteady gait
   4. Nystagmus
   5. Impairment in attention or memory
   6. Stupor or coma
D. The symptoms are not due to a general medical condition and are not better accounted for by another mental disorder.

[a]Adapted from ref. *154*.

Table 17
Pathologic States Simulating Alcohol Intoxication

1. Severe head injuries
2. Metabolic disorders (e.g., hypoglycemia, hyperglycemia, uremia, hyperthyroidism)
3. Neurologic conditions associated with dysarthria, ataxia, tremor, drowsiness (e.g., multiple sclerosis, intracranial tumours, Parkinson's disease, epilepsy, acute vertigo)
4. The effects of drugs, either prescribed or illicit (e.g., insulin, barbiturates, benzodiazepines, cocaine)
5. Psychiatric disorders (e.g., hypomania, general paresis)
6. High fever
7. Carbon monoxide

4.5. Alcohol Dependence

Alcohol abuse and dependence is a major risk factor for serious health, social, and economic problems *(156)*. Early identification of those who are dependent on alcohol increases the possibility of successful treatment, and brief intervention by the forensic physician seems both feasible and acceptable *(114,157)*. Although not yet validated in police custody, brief interventions have been shown to have a high acceptance among drinkers in licensed premises *(158)*.

However, obtaining accurate and reliable information about a person's drinking habits can be extremely difficult as heavy drinkers tend to underestimate or deliberately lie about their alcohol consumption *(159)*. Use of the Alcohol Use Disorders Identification Test (AUDIT) identifies persons whose alcohol consumption has become harmful or hazardous to health *(160)*; self-report questionnaires such as the MAST *(161,162)* and CAGE *(163,164)* may help identify those with alcohol dependency and should prevent the doctor falling into the trap of assuming that alcohol abuse is synonymous with alcohol dependence (Appendix 6). DSM-IV *(154)* distinguishes between these two diagnostic categories. The main features differentiating alcohol dependence from alcohol abuse are evidence of tolerance, the presence of withdrawal symptoms, and the use of alcohol to relieve or avoid withdrawal. Treatment may be required for detainees who show signs of alcohol dependence. However, there is no need to treat those who simply abuse alcohol and who do not have a history of alcohol withdrawal.

4.6. Alcohol Withdrawal

Many alcoholics develop symptoms of withdrawal when in custody. Their acquired tolerance to and physical dependence on alcohol is a manifestation of compensatory neuropsychological changes that offset the drug's CNS depressant effects. When alcohol intake is abruptly stopped on incarceration, the compensatory changes give rise to signs and symptoms of withdrawal *(165)*. The severity of the symptoms depends mainly on the amount and duration of alcohol intake, although other factors, such as concurrent withdrawal from other drugs, like benzodiazepines, may contribute to the clinical picture *(166)*.

Alcohol withdrawal may present as a mild picture of uncomplicated alcohol withdrawal or as the more severe syndrome of alcohol withdrawal delirium (DSM-IV criteria).

4.6.1. Uncomplicated Alcohol Withdrawal

This is the most frequent and benign type, usually occurring some 12–48 hours after alcohol intake is reduced, although it can develop as early as 6 hours after drinking has stopped. The essential features are a coarse tremor of the hands, tongue, and eyelids together with at least one of the following:

- Nausea and vomiting
- Malaise and weakness
- Autonomic hyperactivity (raised blood pressure and tachycardia)
- Anxiety, depressed mood, and irritability
- Transient hallucinations and illusions
- Headache and insomnia

If symptoms are mild it is quite safe to recommend simple observation, but significant tremor and agitation will usually require sedation. The drugs of choice are long-acting benzodiazepines, which will not only treat alcohol withdrawal symptoms but will also prevent later complications *(167)*. The starting dosages depend on the severity of the withdrawal, but 20 mg of chlordiazepoxide, or 10 mg of diazepam, both given four times a day, will generally be appropriate *(168)*.

Usually the benzodiazepines should not be started until such time as the blood alcohol level has reached zero *(169)*. However, detained persons with marked alcohol dependence may develop withdrawal symptoms before this point is reached. In these circumstances, it is both safe and reasonable to initiate therapy when the blood alcohol level has reached 80 mg/100 mL or thereabouts.

4.6.2. Alcohol Withdrawal Delirium

The essential diagnostic feature of this disorder is a delirium that develops after recent cessation of or reduction in alcohol consumption. Traditionally referred to as delirium tremens, this withdrawal state typically begins 72–96 hours after the last drink, so it is uncommon within the normal span of detention in police custody. The delirium is characterized by impaired attention and memory, disorganized thinking, disorientation, reduced level of consciousness, perceptual disturbances, and agitation. Vivid, and often terrifying, hallucinations may occur. Usually these are visual, but other sensory modalities (e.g., auditory or tactile) may be involved. The disorder usually coexists with other features of alcohol withdrawal, for example, autonomic hyperactivity, which is usually severe.

Alcohol withdrawal delirium is a medical emergency with a mortality rate of about 5%. Once diagnosed, the detained person with delirium requires urgent hospitalization.

4.6.3. Complications of Alcohol Withdrawal

Several complications of alcohol withdrawal have been recognized, any one of which may be encountered when alcoholics are detained in police custody *(165)*.

4.6.3.1. Withdrawal Seizures

Seizures are typically single and generalized. They tend to occur between 6 and 48 hours after the last drink and while in themselves are not life threatening, their importance lies in the fact that about one-third of those with seizures will go on to develop alcohol withdrawal delirium.

4.6.3.2. Alcoholic Hallucinosis

This is an infrequent disorder that tends to occur at about the age of 40 in those who have been drinking heavily for more than 10 years. The essential features are vivid and persistent hallucinations, which develop shortly (usually within 48 hours) after cessation of alcohol intake. The hallucinations may be auditory or visual, and their content is usually unpleasant and disturbing. The disorder may last several weeks or months and is quite different from the fleeting hallucinations observed in other forms of alcohol withdrawal.

4.6.3.3. Cardiac Arrhythmias

The frequency of tachyrhythmias in alcohol withdrawal is high, probably because of high adrenergic nervous system activity. Sudden deaths in alcohol withdrawal are most likely due to such dysrhythmias. Adequate sedation will play a part in preventing such unwanted occurrences happening in police custody, although those with severe alcohol withdrawal are best admitted to the hospital, where they can be placed on a cardiac monitor.

4.6.3.4. Metabolic Disorders

Wernicke's encephalopathy is an acute, potentially reversible neurologic disorder that is thought to be due to a deficiency of thiamine and is often secondary to chronic alcohol abuse. Features include disturbance of consciousness (ranging from mild confusion to coma), ophthalmoplegia, nystagmus, and ataxia. The disorder has a high mortality and can lead to death within 24 hours. If untreated it can progress to Korsakoff's psychosis. This is a chronic condition that usually presents as impairment of short-term memory with inability to learn new information and compensatory confabulation. Korsakoff's psychosis probably represents irreversible brain damage secondary to the combined toxicity of alcohol and metabolic derangement due to thiamine deficiency.

References

1. National Institute of Justice (1997) *1996 Drug Use Forecasting: Annual Report on Adult and Juvenile Arrestees.* U.S. Department of Justice, Washington D.C.
2. Bennett, T. (1998) *Drugs and Crime: The Results of Research on Drug Testing and Interviewing Arrestees.* Home Office Research Study 183. Home Office, London.
3. Department of Health, Scottish Office Home and Health Department, Welsh Office (1994) *Substance Misuse Detainees in Police Custody Guidelines for Clinical Management.* HMSO, London.
4. System to Retrieve Information from Drug Evidence (STRIDE). Drug Enforcement Administration 1981–96.

5. Home Office Statistical Bulletin 9th April 1998. *Statistics of Drug Seizures and Offenders Dealt With, United Kingdom 1996.* Home Office, London.
6. Wallace, P., Cutler, S., and Haines, A. (1988) Randomised controlled trial of general practitioner intervention in patients with excessive alcohol consumption. *BMJ* **297,** 663–668.
7. Prochaska, J. O. and Clemente, C. C. (1984) *The Transtheoretical Approach: Crossing Traditional Boundaries of Therapy.* Dow Jones-Irwin, Homewood, IL.
8. Edmunds, M., May, T., Hearnden, I., and Hough, M. (1998) *Arrest Referral: Emerging Lessons from Research.* Home Office Drugs Prevention Initiative Paper 23. Home Office, London.
9. Tennant, F. and Shannon, J. (1995) Cocaine abuse in methadone maintenance patients is associated with low serum methadone concentrations. *J Addic Dis.* **14,** 67–74.
10. Karch, S. B. (1996) Dermatologic sequelae of opiate abuse, in *The Pathology of Drug Abuse* (Karch, S. B., ed.), CRC Press, Boca Raton, pp. 348–353.
11. Nutt, D. J. (1996) Addiction: brain mechanisms and their treatment implications. *Lancet.* **347,** 31–36.
12. Phillips, G. T., Gossop, M., and Bradley, B. (1986) The influence of psychological factors on opiate withdrawal syndrome. *Bri J Psychiatry.* **149,** 235–238.
13. Ruben, S. M., McLean, P. C., and Melville, J. (1989) Cyclizine abuse among a group of opiate dependents receiving methadone. *Bri J Addict.* **84,** 929–934.
14. Evans, J. V. (1998) Dihydrocodeine detox regime. HMP Manchester, personal communication.
15. Washton, A. M., Resnick, R. B., and Geyer, G. (1983) Opiate withdrawal using lofexidine, a clonidine analogue with few side effects. *J Clin Psychiatry.* **44,** 335–337.
16. Ghodse, H. (1995) Drugs of abuse and dependence, in *Drugs and Addictive Behaviour—A Guide to Treatment* (Ghodse, H. ed.), Blackwell Science, Oxford, p. 82.
17. Yealy, D. M., Paris, P. M., Kaplan, R. M., Heller, M. B., and Marini, S. E. (1990) The safety of prehospital naloxone administration by paramedics. *Ann Emerg Med.* **19,** 902–905.
18. Jones, A. L. (1998) Initial management of poisoned patients in the out-of-hospital environment. *Pre-Hospital Immediate Care.* **2,** 141–149.
19. Merigian, K. S. (1993) Cocaine-induced ventricular arrhythmias and rapid atrial fibrillation temporarily related to naloxone administration. *Am J Emerg Med.* **11,** 96–97.
20. Ashton, H. (1994) Guidelines for the rational use of benzodiazepines. When and what to use. *Drugs.* **48,** 25–40.
21. Cowen, P. J. and Nutt, D. J. (1982) Abstinence symptoms after withdrawal of tranquillising drugs. Is there a common neurochemical mechanism? *Lancet.* **ii,** 360–362.
22. Bezchlibnyk-Butler, K. Z. and Jeffries, J. J. (1996) *Clinical Handbook of Psychotropic Drugs.* Hogrefe & Huber, Toronto.
23. Vgontzas, A. N., Kales, A., and Bixler, E. O. (1995) Benzodiazepine side effects: role of pharmacokinetics and pharmacodynamics. *Pharmacology.* **51,** 205–223.

24. Editorial. (1975) Tranquillisers causing aggression. *BMJ.* **1,** 113–114.
25. Gordon, E. B. (1975) Tranquillisers causing aggression. *BMJ.* **2,** 36–37.
26. Zevin, S. and Benowitz, N. L. (1998) Drug-related syndromes, in *Drug Abuse Handbook* (Karch, S. B., ed.), CRC Press, Boca Raton, pp. 559–560.
27. Ashton, H. (1984) Benzodiazepine withdrawal: an unfinished story. *BMJ.* **288,** 1135–1140.
28. Petursson, H. (1994) The benzodiazepine withdrawal syndrome. *Addiction.* **89,** 1455–1459.
29. Roald, O. K. and Dahl, V. (1989) Flunitrazepam intoxication in a child successfully treated with the benzodiazepine antagonist flumazenil. *Crit Care Med.* **17,** 1355–1356.
30. Hojer, J., Baehrendtz, S., Matell, G., and Gustafsson, L. L. (1990) Diagnostic utility of flumazenil in coma with suspected poisoning: a double blind randomised controlled study. *BMJ.* **301,** 1308–1311.
31. Katz, Y., Boulos, M., Singer, P., and Rosenberg, B. (1992) Cardiac arrest associated with Flumazenil. *BMJ.* **304,** 1415.
32. Ives, R. (1997) *Drug Notes: 6 Solvents.* ISDD, London.
33. Al-Alousi, L. M. (1989) Pathology of volatile substance abuse: a case report and a literature review. *Med Sci Law.* **29,** 189–208.
34. Ron, M. A. (1986) Volatile substance abuse: a review of possible long-term neurological, intellectual and psychiatric sequelae. *Br J Psychiatry.* **148,** 235–246.
35. Shepherd, R. T. (1989) Mechanism of sudden death associated with volatile substance abuse. *Hum Toxicol.* **8,** 287–292.
36. Taylor, G. J. and Harris, W. S. (1970) Cardiac toxicity of aerosol propellants. *JAMA.* **214,** 81–85.
37. Merry, J. and Zachariadis, N. (1962) Addiction to glue sniffing. *BMJ.* **2,** 1448.
38. Leikin, J. B., Krantz, A. J., Zell-Kanter, M., Barkin, R. L., and Hryhorczuk, D. O. (1989) Clinical features and management of intoxication due to hallucinogenic drugs. *Med Toxicol Adverse Drug Exp.* **4,** 324–350.
39. Hollister, L. E. and Hartman, A. M. (1962) Mescaline, lysergic acid diethylamide and psilocybin: comparison of clinical syndromes, effects on color perception and biochemical measures. *Compr Psychiatry.* **3,** 235–241.
40. Abraham, H. D. and Aldridge, A. M. (1993) Adverse consequences of lysergic acid diethylamide. *Addiction.* **88,** 1327–1334.
41. Schwartz, R. H. (1995) LSD. Its rise, fall and renewed popularity among high school students. *Pediatr Clin North Am.* **42,** 403–413.
42. McCarron, M. M., Schulze, B. W., Thompson, G. A., Conder, M.C., and Goetz, W. A. (1981) Acute phencyclidine intoxication: clinical patterns, complications and treatment. *Ann Emerg Med.* **10,** 290–297.
43. Brust, J. C. M. (1993) Other agents. Phencyclidine, marijuana, hallucinogens, inhalants and anticholinergics. *Neurol Clin.* **11,** 555–561.
44. Aniline, O. and Pitts Jr, F. N. (1982) Phencyclidine (PCP): a review and perspectives. *Crit Rev Toxicol.* **10,** 145–177.

45. Steele, T. D., McCann, U. D., and Ricaurte, G. A. (1994) 3,4-Methylenedioxy-methamphetamine (MDMA, "ecstasy"): pharmacology and toxicology in animals and humans. *Addiction.* **89,** 539–551.
46. Maxwell, D. L., Polkey, M. I., and Henry, J. A. (1993) Hyponatraemia and catatonic stupor after taking "ecstasy." *BMJ.* **307,** 1399.
47. Kessel, B. (1994) Hyponatraemia after ingestion of "ecstasy." *BMJ.* **308,** 414.
48. Henry, J. A., Fallon, J. K., Kicman, A. T., Hutt, A. J., Cowan, D. A., and Forsling, M. (1998) Low-dose MDMA ("ecstasy") induces vasopressin secretion. *Lancet.* **351,** 1784.
49. Redfearn, P. J., Agrawal, N., and Mair, L. H. (1998) An association between the regular use of 3,4, methylenedioxy-methamphetamine (ecstasy) and excessive wear of the teeth. *Addiction.* **93,** 745–748.
50. Shearman, J. D., Chapman, R. W. G., Satsangi, J., and Ryley, N. G. (1992) Misuse of ecstasy. *BMJ.* **305,** 309.
51. Creighton, F. J., Black, D. L., and Hyde, C. E. (1991) "Ecstasy" psychosis and flashbacks. *Bri J Psychiatry.* **159,** 713–715.
52. Levine, A. J., Drew, S., and Rees, G. M. (1993) "Ecstasy" induced pneumomediastinum. *J Rl Soc Med.* **86,** 232–233.
53. Bryden, A. A., Rothwell, P. J. N., and O'Reilly, P. H. (1995) Urinary retention with misuse of "ecstasy". *BMJ.* **310,** 504.
54. Chadwick, I. S., Curry, P. D., Linsley, A., Freemont, A. J., and Doran, B. (1991) Ecstasy, 3-4 methylenedioxymethamphetamine (MDMA), a fatality associated with coagulopathy and hyperthermia. *J Rl Soc Med.* **84,** 371.
55. Brown, C. and Osterloh, J. (1987) Multiple severe complications from recreational ingestion of MDMA ("ecstasy"). *JAMA.* **258,** 780–781.
56. Dowling, G. P., McDonough, E. T., and Bost, R. O. (1987) "Eve" and "ecstasy". A report of five deaths associated with the use of MDEA and MDMA. *JAMA.* **257,** 1615–1617.
57. Campkin, N. T. A. and Davies U. M. (1992) Another death from Ecstasy. *J Rl Soc Med.* **85,** 61.
58. McGuire, P. and Fahy, T. (1991) Chronic paranoid psychosis after misuse of MDMA (ecstasy). *BMJ.* **302,** 697.
59. Sternbach, H. (1991) The serotonin syndrome. *Am J Psychiatry.* **148,** 705–713.
60. Mueller, P. D. and Korey, W. S. Death by "ecstasy": the serotonin syndrome? *Ann Emerg Med.* **32,** 377–380.
61. McCann, U. D., Szabo, Z., Scheffel, U., Dannals, R. F., and Ricaurte, G. A. (1998) Positron emission tomographic evidence of toxic effect of MDMA ("ecstasy") on brain serotonin neurons in human beings. *Lancet.* **352,** 1433–1437.
62. James, R. A. and Dinan, A. (1998) Hyperpyrexia associated with fatal paramethoxyamphetamine (PMA) abuse. *Med Sci Law.* **38,** 83–85.
63. Resnick, R. B., Kestenbaum, R. S., Schwartz, L. K. (1977) Acute systemic effects of cocaine in man—a controlled study by intranasal and intravenous routes. *Science.* **195,** 696–698.

64. Karch, S. B. (1996) Cocaine, in *The Pathology of Drug Abuse* (Karch, S. B., ed.), CRC Press, Boca Raton, pp. 82–114.
65. Griffiths, P., Gossop, M., Wickenden, S., Dunworth, J., Harris, K., and Lloyd, C. (1997) A transcultural pattern of drug use: qat (khat) in the UK. *Br J Psychiatry.* **170,** 281–284.
66. Ahmed, A. G. and Salib, E. (1998) The Khat users: a study of khat chewing in Liverpool's Somali men. *Med Sci Law.* **38,** 165–169.
67. Joyce, H. (1994) Khat. *J Forensic Psychiatry.* **5,** 228–231.
68. Luqman, W. and Danowski, T. S. (1976) The use of khat (*Catha edulis*) in Yemen. Social and medical observations. *Ann Intern Med.* **85,** 246–249.
69. Yousef, G., Huq, Z., and Lambert, T. (1995) Khat chewing as a cause of psychosis. *Br J Hosp Med.* **54,** 322–326.
70. Pantelis, C., Hindler, C. G., and Taylor, J. C. (1989) Use and abuse of khat (*Catha edulis*): a review of the distribution, pharmacology, side effects, and a description of psychosis arributed to khat chewing. *Psychol Med.* **19,** 657–658.
71. Quinn, D. (1997) *Skunk.* Fact sheet 20 Information for Drug Workers. ISDD, London.
72. Wylie, A. S., Scott, R. T. A., and Burnett, S. J. (1995) Psychosis due to "skunk". *BMJ.* **311,** 125.
73. British Medical Association. (1997) *Therapeutic Uses of Cannabis.* Harwood Academic Publishers, Amsterdam, pp. 19–20.
74. Stephens, R. S., Roffman, R. A., and Simpson, E. E., (1993) Adult marijuana users seeking treatment. *J Consult Clin Psychol.* **61,** 1100–1104.
75. Bhasin, S., Storer, T. W., Berman, N., Callegari, C., Clevenger, B., Phillips, J., et al. (1996) The effects of superphysiologic doses of testosterone on muscle size and strength in normal men. *N Engl J Med.* **335,** 1–7.
76. Kennedy, M. (1990) Athletes, drugs and adverse reactions. *Adverse Drug Reaction Bull.* **143,** 536–539.
77. ISDD. *Drug Notes 9: Anabolic Steroids.* ISDD, London.
78. Haupt, H. A. and Rovere, G. D. (1984) Anabolic steroids: a review of the literature. *Am J Sports Med.* **12,** 469–484.
79. Stanley, A. and Ward M. (1994) Anabolic steroids—the drugs that give and take away manhood. A case with an unusual physical sign. *Med Sci Law.* **34,** 82–83.
80. Lloyd, F. H., Powell, P., and Murdoch, A. P. (1996) Anabolic steroid abuse by body builders and male subfertility. *BMJ.* **313,** 100–101.
81. Creagh, T. M., Rubin, A., and Evans, D. J. (1988) Hepatic tumours induced by anabolic steroids in an athlete. *J Clin Pathol.* **41,** 441–443.
82. Su, T., Pagliaro M., Schmidt, P. J., Pickar, D., Wolkowitz, O., and Rubinow D. R. (1993) Neuropsychiatric effects of anabolic steroids in male normal volunteers. *JAMA.* **269,** 2760–2764.
83. Pope, H. G. and Katz, D. L. (1994) Psychiatric and medical effects of anabolic-androgenic steroid use. *Arch Gen Psychiatry.* **51,** 375–382.
84. Corrigan, B. (1996) Anabolic steroids and the mind. *Med J Aust.* **165,** 222–226.
85. Perry, H. M., Wright, D., and Littlepage, B. N. C. (1992) Dying to be big: a review of anabolic steroid use. *Br J Sports Med.* **26,** 259–261.

86. Littlepage, B. N. C. and Perry, H. M. (1993) Misusing anabolic drugs: possibilities for future policies. *Addiction.* **88,** 1469–1471.
87. McBride, A. J., Williamson, K., and Petersen, T. (1996) Three cases of nalbuphine hydrochloride dependence associated with anabolic steroid use. *Br J Sports Med.* **30,** 69–70.
88. Elkin, S. L., Brady, S., and Williams, I. P. (1997) Bodybuilders find it easy to obtain insulin to help them in training. *BMJ.* **314,** 1280.
89. FitzSimmons, C. R. and Kidner, N. (1998) Caffeine toxicty in a bodybuilder. *J Accid Emerg Med.* **15,** 196–1970.
90. Perry, H. M. and Littlepage, B. N. C. (1992) Misusing anabolic drugs. *BMJ.* **305,** 1241–1242.
91. Roth, R. H. and Giarman, N. J. (1970) Natural occurrence of gamma-hydroxybutyrate in mammalian brain. *Biochem Pharmacol.* **19,** 1087–1093.
92. Galloway, G. P., Frederick, S. L., Staggers Jr, F. E., Gonzales, M., Stalcup, S. A., and Smith, D. E. (1997) Gamma-hydroxybutyrate: an emerging drug of abuse that causes physical dependence. *Addiction.* **92,** 89–96.
93. ISDD. (1995) *Drug Capsule 13—GHB.* ISDD, London.
94. Ferrara, S. D., Zotti, S., Tedeshi, L., Frison, G., Castagna, F., Gallimberti, L., et al. (1992) Pharmacokinetics of gamma-hydroxybutyric acid in alcohol dependent patients after single and repeated oral doses. *Br J Clin Pharmacol.* **34,** 231–235.
95. Luby, S., Jones, J., and Zalewski, A. (1992) GHB use in South Carolina. *Am J Public Health.* **82,** 128.
96. Thomas, G., Bonner, S., and Gascoigne, A. (1997) Coma induced by abuse of gamma-hydroxybutyrate: a case report. *BMJ.* **314,** 35–36.
97. Dyer, J. E. (1997) ER admission cases discussed, in *Getting the Scoop on GHB: The New Recreational Drug.* Presented at the 49th Annual Meeting of the American Academy of Forensic Sciences, New York.
98. Dyer, J. E., Kreutzer, R., Quatrrone, A., Kizer, K. W., Geller, R. J., Smith, J. D., et al. (1991) Multistate outbreak of poisonings associated with the illicit use of gammahydroxybutyrate. *JAMA.* **265,** 447–448.
99. ISDD (1995) *Drug Capsule 12—Ketamine.* ISDD, London.
100. Jansen, K. L. R. (1993) Non-medical use of ketamine. *BMJ.* **306,** 601–602.
101. Slogoff, S., Allen, G. W., Wessels, and J. V. (1974) Clinical experience with subanaesthetic ketamine. *Anesth Analg (Cleve).* **53,** 354–358.
102. White, P. F., Way, W. L., and Trevor, A. J. (1982) Ketamine: its pharmacology and therapeutic uses. *Anaethesiology.* **56,** 119–136.
103. ABPI Compendium of Data Sheets and Summaries of Product Characteristics (1998–99) *Ketalar.* Datapharm Publications, London.
104. Moore, K. A., Kilbane, E. M., Jones, R., Kunsman, G. W., Levine, B., and Smith, M. (1997) Tissue distribution of ketamine in a mixed drug fatality. *J Forensic Sci.* **2,** 1183–1185.
105. Sigell, L. T., Kapp, F. T., Fusaro, G. A., Nelson E. D., and Falck, R. S. (1978) Popping and snorting volatile nitrites: a current fad for getting high. *Am J Psychiatry.* **135,** 1216–1218.

106. Schwartz, R. H. and Peary, P. (1986) Abuse of isobutyl nitrite inhalation (rush) by adolescents. *Clin Pediatr.* **25,** 308–310.
107. Stambach, T., Haire, K., Soni, N., and Booth, J. (1997) Saturday night blue—a case of near fatal poisoning from the abuse of amyl nitrite. *J Accid Emerg Med.* **14,** 339–340.
108. Virkkunen, M. and Linnoila, M. (1993) Brain serotonin, type II alcoholism and impulsive violence. *J Stud Alcohol.* **Suppl. 11,** 163–169.
109. Magennis, P., Shepherd, J., Hutchison, I., and Brown, A. (1998) Trends in facial injury. *BMJ.* **316,** 325–326.
110. The All Party Group on Alcohol Abuse (1995) *Alcohol and Crime: Breaking the Link.* Alcohol Concern, London.
111. Sumner, M. and Parker, H. (1995) *Low in Alcohol. A Review of International Research into Alcohol's Role in Crime Causation.* The Portman Group, London.
112. Moore, M. R. and Moore, S. R. (1994) The potential for the use of personal computers in clinical forensic medicine. *J Clin Forensic Med.* **1,** 139–143.
113. Robertson, G. (1992) *The Role of Police Surgeons.* The Royal Commission on Criminal Justice. Research Study No 6. HMSO, London.
114. Payne-James, J. J., Keys, D. W., Wall, I., Jerreat, P. G., and Dean, P. J. (1997) Alcohol misuse in clinical forensic medicine. *J Clin Forensic Med.* **4,** 17–19.
115. Stockwell, T. and Stirling, L. (1989) Estimating alcohol content of drinks: common errors in applying the unit system. *BMJ.* **298,** 571–572.
116. EEC Directive 766/1976.
117. Ferner, R. E. (1996) *Forensic Pharmacology. Medicines, Mayhem, and Malpractice.* Oxford University Press, Oxford.
118. Baselt, R. C. (1996) Disposition of alcohol in man, in *Medicolegal Aspects of Alcohol*, 3rd ed. (Garriott, J, C., ed.), Lawyers & Judges Publishing Company, Tucson, AZ.
119. Stark, M. M. and Norfolk, G. A. (1996) Substance misuse, in *Clinical Forensic Medicine* (McLay, W. D. S. ed.), Greenwich Medical Media, London, pp. 173–179.
120. Holford, N. H. G. (1987) Clinical Pharmacokinetics of Ethanol. *Clin Pharmacokinet.* **13,** 273–292.
121. Wilkinson, P. K., Sedman, A. J., Sakmar, E., Earhart, R. H., Kay, D. R., and Wagner, J. G. (1977) Pharmacokinetics of ethanol after oral administration in the fasting state. *J Pharmacokinet Biopharm.* **5,** 207–224.
122. Jones, A. W. (1996) Biochemistry and physiology of alcohol: applications to forensic science and toxicology, in *Medicolegal Aspects of Alcohol*, 3rd ed. (Garriott, J. C., ed.), Lawyers & Judges, Tucson, AZ.
123. Drew, G. C., Colquhoun, W. P., and Long, H. A. (1959) *Effect of Small Doses of Alcohol on a Skill Resembling Driving.* Medical Research Council Memorandum No. 38. HMSO, London.
124. Jones, A. W. and Jonsson, K. A. (1994) Between-subject and within-subject variations in the pharmacokinetics of ethanol. *Br J Clin Pharmacol.* **37,** 427–431.
125. Schultz, J., Weiner, H., and Westcott, J. (1980) Retardation of ethanol absorption by food in the stomach. *J Stud Alcohol.* **41,** 861–870.

126. Jones, A. W. and Jonsson, K. A. (1994) Food-induced lowering of blood-ethanol profiles and increased rate of elimination immediately after a meal. *J Forensic Sci.* **39,** 1084–1093.
127. Sedman, A. J., Wilkinson, P. K., Sakmar, E., Weidler, D. J., and Wagner, J. G. (1976) Food effects on absorption and elimination of alcohol. *J Stud Alcohol.* **37,** 1197–1214.
128. Walls, H. and Brownlie, A. R. (1985) *Drink, Drugs & Driving*, 2nd ed. Sweet & Maxwell, London.
129. Jones, A. W. and Sternebring, B. (1992) Kinetics of ethanol and methanol in alcoholics during detoxification. *Alcohol Alcohol.* **27,** 641–647.
130. Manno, J. E. and Manno, B. R. (1996) Experimental basis of alcohol-induced psychomotor performance impairment, in *Medicolegal Aspects of Alcohol*, 3rd ed. (Garriott, J.C., ed.), Lawyers & Judges, Tucson, AZ.
131. Urso, T., Gavaler, J. S., and Van Thiel, D. H. (1981) Blood ethanol levels in sober alcohol users seen in an emergency room. *Life Sci.* **28,** 1053–1056.
132. Sullivan, J. B., Hauptman, M., and Bronstein, A. C. (1987) Lack of observable intoxication in humans with high plasma alcohol concentrations. *J Forensic Sci.* **32,** 1660–1665.
133. Garriott, J. C. (1996) Pharmacology and toxicology of ethyl alcohol, in *Medicolegal Aspects of Alcohol*, 3rd ed. (Garriott, J.C., ed.), Lawyers & Judges, Tucson, AZ.
134. Money, K. and Myles, W. (1974) Heavy water nystagmus and effects of alcohol. *Nature.* **247,** 404–405.
135. Behrens, M. M. (1978) Nystagmus. *J. Ophthalmol Clin.* **18,** 57–82.
136. Aschan, G. (1958) Different types of alcohol nystagmus. *Acta Otolaryngol (Suppl.).* **140,** 69–78.
137. Aschan, G., Bergstedt, M., Goldberg, L., and Laurell, L. (1956) Positional nystagmus in man during and after alcohol intoxication. *Q J Stud Alcohol.* **17,** 381–405.
138. Goding, G. S. and Dobie, R. A. (1986) Gaze nystagmus and blood alcohol. *Laryngoscope.* **96,** 713–717.
139. Belton, H. (1987) Lateral nystagmus: a specific diagnostic sign of ethyl alcohol intoxication. *N Z Med J.* **100,** 534,535.
140. Eakins, W. A. (1977) Clinical signs and the level of blood alcohol. *Police Surg.* **11,** 8–15.
141. Willoughby, E. W. (1987) Nystagmus and alcohol intoxication. *N Z Med J.* **100,** 640.
142. Moczula, B. (1996) Alcohol and the law: the legal framework of scientific evidence and expert testimony, in *Medicolegal Aspects of Alcohol*, 3rd ed. (Garriott, J. C., ed.), Lawyers & Judges, Tucson, AZ.
143. British Medical Association (1954) *The Recognition of Intoxication. Report of a Special Committee of the British Medical Association.* BMA, London.
144. Tennant, F. (1988) The rapid eye test to detect drug abuse. *Postgrad Med.* **84,** 108–114.

145. Fleming, P. and Stewart, D. (1998) *Drugs and Driving: Training Implications for Police Officers and Police Surgeons.* Home Office Police Policy Directorate, London.
146. Simpson-Crawford, T., and Slater, S. W. (1971) Eye signs in suspected drinking drivers: clinical examination and relation to blood alcohol. *N Z Med J.* **74,** 92–96.
147. Johnson, K., Pisoni, D. B., and Bernacki, R. H. (1990) Do voice recordings reveal whether a person is intoxicated? A case study. *Phonetica.* **47,** 215–237.
148. Martin, C. S. (1998) Measuring acute alcohol impairment, in *Drug Abuse Handbook* (Karch, S. B., ed.), CRC Press, Boca Raton, FL, pp. 309–326.
149. Potter, J. F., Watson, R. D. S., Skan, W., and Beevers, D. G. (1986) The pressor and metabolic effects of alcohol in normotensive subjects. *Hypertension.* **8,** 625–631.
150. Kelbaek, H., Gjorup, T., Brynjolf, I., Christensen, N. J., and Godtfredsen, J. (1985) Acute effects of alcohol on left ventricular function in healthy subjects at rest and during upright exercise. *Am J Cardiol.* **55,** 164–167.
151. Kaye, S. and Haag, H. B. (1957) Terminal blood alcohol concentrations in 94 fatal cases of alcoholism. *JAMA.* **165,** 451–452.
152. Johnson, R. A., Noll, E. C., and MacMillan Rodney, W. (1982) Survival after a serum ethanol level of 1.5 per cent. *Lancet.* **2,** 1394.
153. Rix, K. J. B. (1989) 'Alcohol intoxication' or 'drunkenness': is there a difference? *Med Sci Law.* **29,** 100–106.
154. American Psychiatric Association (1994) *Diagnostic and Statistical Manual of Mental Disorders.* 4th ed. American Psychiatric Association, Washington, DC.
155. Norfolk, G. A. (1998) Deaths in police custody during 1994: a retrospective analysis. *J Clin Forensic Med.* **5,** 49–54.
156. Royal College of Psychiatrists (1986) *Alcohol: Our Favourite Drug.* Royal College of Psychiatrists, London.
157. Deehan, A., Stark, M. M., Marshall, E. J., Hanrahan, B., and Strang, J. (1998) Drunken detainees in police custody: is brief intervention by the forensic medical examiner feasible? *Criminal Behav and Mental Health.* **8,** 214–221.
158. Reilly, D., Van Beurden, E., Mitchell, E., Dight, R., Scott, C., and Beard, J. (1998) Alcohol education in licensed premises using brief intervention strategies. *Addiction.* **93,** 385–398.
159. Midanik, L. (1982) The validity of self-reported alcohol consumption and alcohol problems: a literature review. *Br J Addic.* **77,** 357–382.
160. Babor, T. F., Ramon de la Fuente, J., Saunders, J., and Grant, M. (1992) *AUDIT, The Alcohol Use Disorders Identification Test: Guidelines for use in Primary Health Care.* World Health Organization, Geneva.
161. Pokorny, A. D., Miller, B. A., and Kaplan, H. B. (1972) The brief MAST: a shortened version of the Michigan alcoholism screening test. *Am J Psychiatry.* **129,** 342–345.
162. Hedlund, J. L. and Vieweg, B. W. (1984) The Michigan Alcoholism Screening Test (MAST): a comprehensive review. *J Operational Psychiatry.* **15,** 55–65.

163. Mayfield, D., McLeod, G., and Hall, P. (1974) The CAGE questionnaire: validation of a new alcoholism screening instrument. *Am J Psychiatry.* **131,** 1121–1123.
164. Ewing, J. A. (1984) Detecting alcoholism. The CAGE questionnaire. *JAMA.* **252,** 1905–1907.
165. Romach, M. K. and Sellers, E. M. (1991) Management of the alcohol withdrawal syndrome. *Annu Rev Med.* **42,** 323–340.
166. Naik, P. and Lawton, J. (1993) Pharmacological management of alcohol withdrawal. *British J Hosp Med.* **50,** 265–269.
167. Mayo-Smith, M. F. for the American Society of Addiction Medicine Working Group on Pharmacological Management of Alcohol Withdrawal (1997) Pharmacological management of alcohol withdrawal. A meta-analysis and evidence-based practice guideline. *JAMA.* **278,** 144–151.
168. Naik, P. and Lawton, J. (1996) Assessment and management of individuals under the influence of alcohol in police custody. *J Clin Forensic Med.* **3,** 37–44.
169. Linnoila, M. I. (1990) Benzodiazepines and alcohol. *J Psychiatr Res.* **24(suppl. 2),** 121–127.
170. Ling, W. and Wesson, D. R. (1990) Drugs of abuse: opiates, in addiction medicine (Special Edition). *West J Med.* **152,** 565–572.
171. Roth, B., Benowitz, N., and Olson, K. (1998) Emergency management of drug-abuse-related disorders, in *Drug Abuse Handbook* (Karch, S. B., ed.), CRC Press, Boca Raton, FL, pp. 567–639.

Chapter 9

Deaths in Custody

Richard Shepherd

1. Introduction

The forensic physician will, in all probability, have to deal with a death in police custody at some point. This chapter aims to present a broad basis for understanding the disease processes and mechanisms that may lead to death and also to present some of the current thinking behind deaths associated with restraint.

2. Definition

In considering any death associated with detention by officials of any state, caused by whatever means, each state will define, according to its own legal system, the situations categorized as being "in custody" *(1,2)*. The worldwide variations in these definitions has caused, and continues to cause, considerable confusion in any discussion of this subject. For the purposes of this chapter "in custody" relates to any individual who is either under arrest or otherwise under police control; although similar deaths may occur in prison, on psychiatric wards, or in other situations in which people are detained against their will, it is the deaths specifically associated with police detention that will form the basis for the discussion here.

Having defined the broad parameters of the subject, it is important to distinguish between the different types of custodial deaths since it is deaths that are related to direct police actions (acts of commission) that seem to cause

From: *Forensic Science: A Physician's Guide to Clinical Forensic Medicine*
Edited by: M. M. Stark © Humana Press, Inc., Totowa, NJ

the greatest concern to the family, the public, and the press. It is also important to remember that police involvement in the detention of individuals extends beyond direct physical contact and includes a "duty of care" to that individual; and "lack of care" may be termed "acts of omission." Lack of police action or "care" has also been responsible for deaths in custody. These acts are considerably harder to define and perhaps sometimes occur when members of the police are placed in, or assume, a role of caring (for instance, in states of alcoholic intoxication or acute psychiatric conditions) that are beyond their competence or that they are not equipped or trained to fulfill.

Police involvement with an individual can also include those who are being pursued by the police either on foot or by vehicle, those who have been stopped and are being questioned outside the environment of a police station, and those who have become unwell through natural causes while in contact with or in custody of the police.

The definitions of "death in custody" are therefore wide, and simple definitions are difficult to formulate. Any definition will have to cover a multitude of factors, in various circumstances and with a wide variety of individuals. The crucial point is that the police owe a duty of care to every member of the public with whom they have contact and it is essential that every police officer, whether acting or reacting to events, understands and is aware of the welfare of the individual or individuals with whom he or she is dealing.

3. Statistics

Because of the lack of a standard international definition of "death in custody," a simple comparison of the published raw data from different countries is of no value. However, the comparison of year-to-year trends from individual countries *(3,4)* may have some validity. The number of deaths recorded in England and Wales for 1990–1996 shows little evidence of a significant change in the total annual custody deaths each year during that period (Fig. 1) *(3)*. In comparison, the deaths recorded in Australia for 1986–1996 show a marked decline (Fig. 2) *(4)*. These raw data must be treated with considerable caution since the figures may not be the result of changes in policy or practice but other, undetermined factors.

4. Investigation of Deaths in Custody

4.1. Legal Framework

In the United Kingdom all deaths occurring in prison (or youth custody) *(5)* must be referred to the coroner who holds jurisdiction for that area. However, no such obligation exists concerning deaths in police custody, although

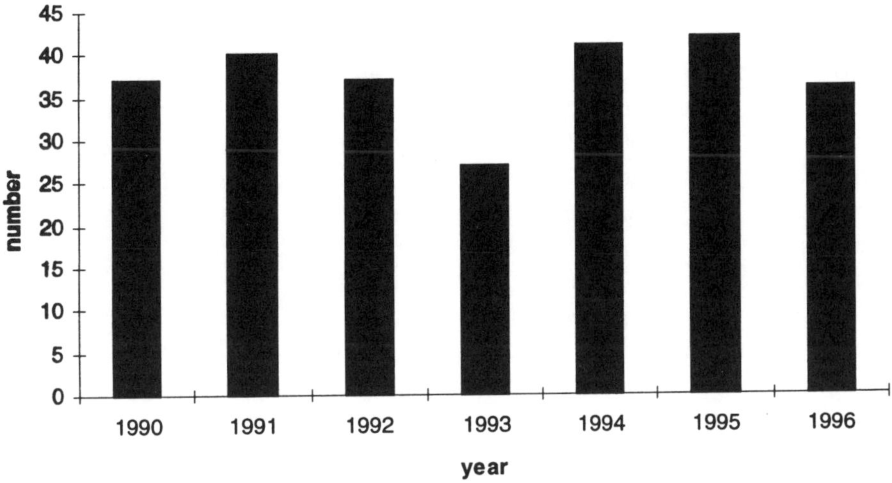

Fig. 1. Deaths in custody in England and Wales.

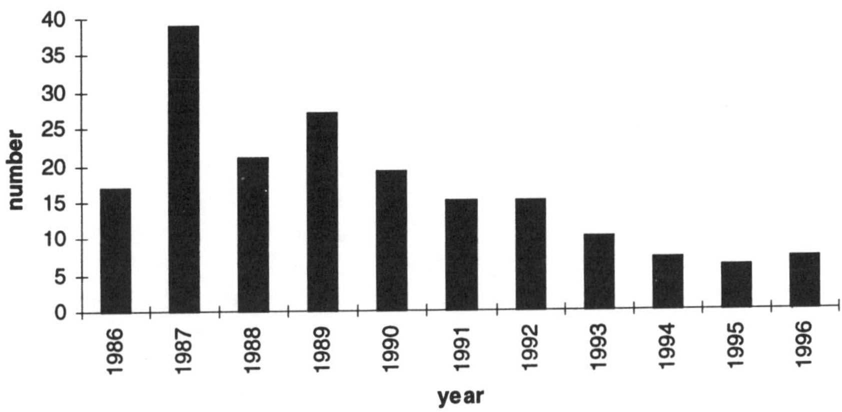

Fig. 2. Deaths in custody in Australia.

the Home Office recommends *(6)* that all deaths falling into even the widest definition of "in custody" should be subject to coronial inquest, and hence a full inquiry into the facts and a full postmortem examination should be performed. This acceptance that all deaths occurring in custody should be fully investigated and considered by the legal system represents the ideal situation; not every country will follow this procedure, and some local variations can and do occur, particularly in the United States.

4.2. Protocol

No standard or agreed protocol has been devised for the postmortem examination of these deaths; as a result, variation in the reported details of examinations is to be expected. The differences in procedures and the number and type of specialist tests results in considerable variation in the pathologic detail available as a basis for establishing the cause of death and hence available for presentation at any subsequent inquest. The absence of a defined protocol hinders considerably an analysis of the results of these examinations and makes even the most simple comparisons unreliable. There is an urgent need for a properly established academic study of such deaths (like that performed in Australia under the auspices of the Australian Institute of Criminology) *(4)* to be instituted in the United Kingdom and United States.

4.3. Terminology

In addition to the lack of reproducibility of postmortem examinations, the terminology used by pathologists to define the cause of death, particularly in the form required for the registration of the death, may often be idiosyncratic; similar disease processes may be denoted by different pathologists using many different phrases. For example, damage to the heart muscle caused by narrowing of the coronary arteries by atheroma may be termed simply ischemic heart disease, or it may be called myocardial ischemia due to coronary atheroma, or even the lay term heart attack. This marked variation in terminology may lead to considerable confusion, particularly among lay people attempting to understand the cause and the manner of death. A considerable amount of research *(1,3)* has been produced based on such lay assessments of the pathologic features of a death; this has, at times, resulted in increased confusion rather than clarification of the issues involved.

If the issues regarding the definition of "in custody," the variation in postmortem examinations and reports, and the use and analysis of subsequent specialist tests all raise problems within a single country, then the consideration of these deaths internationally produces almost insuperable conflicts of medical terminology and judicial systems.

5. Deaths Related to the Phases of the Custodial Process

In an attempt to add some clarity to the situation, it is possible to state that whatever national definition of "in custody" is used, a number of phases of the custody process can be identified and the types of deaths that occur during these phases can be analyzed. Clearly a death, either sudden or delayed, may

Table 1
Expected Types of Deaths in Different Phases of Custody

	Natural	Accidental trauma	Alcohol	Drug	Self-inflicted	Deliberately inflicted
Before arrest	++	+++	++	++	±	±
Arrest	++	+++	++	++	±	+++
Detention	+	+	+++	+++	++	++
Interview	+	+	++	++	+++	++
Charge	+	+	–	–	+++	±

occur for many reasons even in the absence of police, but since it is the involvement of police that is the *sine qua non* of "in custody" deaths, the first phase must be considered to be the presence of police officers at the scene. An arrest may be made with or without the use of restraint techniques and the prisoner will then be transported to a police station. This transport will most commonly involve a period within a police vehicle, which may be a car, a van with seating, or some other vehicle. Many factors may determine the type of transport used and the position of the individual in that vehicle. Detention in the police station will be followed by a period or periods of interview interspersed with periods of time incarcerated, usually alone, within a cell. Following an interview, the individual may be released directly, charged and then released, or detained to appear before a court. It is at this point that custody moves from the police to other authorities, usually the prison service.

When considering the types of death that can occur during each of these phases, six main groups can be identified based on the reported causes of death:

- Natural deaths
- Deaths associated with accidental trauma
- Deaths related directly to the use of alcohol
- Deaths related to the use of other drugs
- Deaths associated with self-inflicted injury
- Deaths associated with injuries deliberately inflicted by a third party

It is clear that different factors may lead directly to, or play a major part in, the death of an individual while in custody and that different factors will play their part at different phases in the period of custody (Table 1).

Acute alcohol intoxication or the deleterious effects of drugs are, in most cases, likely to have a decreasing effect as they are metabolized or excreted from the individual's body. They are therefore most likely to cause death in the post-arrest and early detention phases; it is important to note that their effects will be least visible to those with the "duty of care" while the individual is out of sight, detained within a cell—particularly if the person is alone within that cell. Similarly, the effects of trauma, whether accidentally or deliberately inflicted, are most likely to become apparent in the early phases of detention; only rarely would the effects of such trauma result in fatalities at a later stage, although this has occurred on several occasions, in particular with head injuries *(3)*. Conversely, death resulting from self-inflicted injuries are unlikely to occur in the prearrest and arrest phases of detention, but they can and do occur when the individual is placed in a cell and is not under immediate and constant supervision.

Deaths from natural causes, on the other hand, can occur at almost any time during the period of arrest and detention. It is possible that the stress (whether emotional or physical or both) associated with the initial phases of arrest and with the subsequent, more emotionally stressful, phases during detention are likely to precipitate the death of susceptible individuals through the effects of sympathetic stimulation and the release of adrenaline. Deaths from natural causes should be reduced by the medical examination and supervision of detainees from the time of initial detention and throughout the period of detention (*see* Chapter 7).

The deaths described in many reports are not "pure," that is, they are not solely attributable to any single category. Individuals with heart disease may also be under the influence of alcohol, or individuals under the influence of alcohol or drugs may also have suffered trauma, either accidental or deliberate, prior to or during their detention. In determining the cause of death it can therefore be extremely difficult to give weight to each of the factors that could be identified during the period of detention. There is clearly a great need for early assessment and accurate diagnosis of natural disease (physical or psychiatric) and of alcohol or drug intoxication, as well as for the identification, documentation, and treatment of all types of trauma.

The removal of an individual's freedom places on the police a duty of care to that individual; only by active assessment of each person entering police custody and the continuing care of that individual can the number of deaths in custody be reduced.

6. Causes of Death

6.1. Natural Causes

Apart from a few unusual cases, deaths due to natural causes while in police custody fall into the groups of disease processes that are commonly associated with sudden natural death in the community.

6.1.1. Cardiovascular Disease

The most common cause of death in the community, and of sudden death in particular, is cardiac disease; within this group those deaths recorded as being due to ischemic heart disease or coronary atheroma are the most common. The exact definitions and criteria for the pathologic diagnosis *(7)* of significant ischemic heart disease are not within the scope of this chapter. While there is a clear increase in the incidence of this cause of death with age *(8)*, it is important to remember that a small percentage of people in the younger age groups, most commonly those with hypercholesterolemia and hyperlipidemia, may also have significant coronary artery disease, and since it is the younger age groups that are more likely to be arrested by the police these few individuals may assume great significance.

The significance of coronary atheroma is that individuals with this disease are particularly prone to the development of dysrhythmias during periods of stress when their decreased ability to perfuse areas of the myocardium may result in the development of ectopic electrical foci. Death may be preceded by the development of classical cardiac chest pain, or it may present with sudden collapse and no prior warning.

Individuals suffering from significant myocardial hypertrophy due to chronic hypertension are also at greater risk during periods of stress. Once again it is the older age groups that are most commonly affected by essential hypertension, which may also render these individuals susceptible to focal lack of myocardial perfusion during periods of tachycardia. In addition to these two disease processes, there are also the much rarer diseases or syndromes that may cause sudden death; these are possibly more significant in the context of "deaths in custody" since some of them tend to affect younger age groups in particular. Congenital valvular disease (e.g., floppy mitral valve disease) and congenital myocardial disease (e.g., the cardiomyopathies) may both render an individual more susceptible to sudden cardiac death; as with ischemic or hypertensive heart disease, sudden death is more likely when the sympathetic stimulation associated with stress (emotional and/or physical) has resulted in tachycardia.

Current research is now focusing on a genetic basis for many other sudden cardiac deaths in the younger age groups. These genetically mediated disease processes (for example, prolonged QT intervals) can sometimes be diagnosed in life by electrocardiogram; however, after death their presence, and hence their possible relationship to the sudden death, can be inferred only from the detection of specific gene defects *(9)*. The examination for these specific gene markers in any sudden death in police custody must now be considered in the absence of other causes of death.

Myocarditis and rheumatic heart disease are rare causes of death in young individuals, although such deaths may occur without any prior indication of a disease process in individuals in police custody and elsewhere.

Other cardiovascular causes of sudden death are also, for the most part, age related. The rupture of atheromatous aortic aneurysms is a disease almost entirely confined to late middle and old age while the rarer forms of aortitis and collagen diseases of the aorta, which may also result in rupture, are more commonly seen in the younger age groups *(10)*.

Pulmonary emboli can cause sudden death or they may present as dyspnea and chest pain. It is most unusual for deep venous thrombosis of the leg veins to be present in a young active male; however, the association between some types of the combined oral contraceptive pill and the development of thromboses has been known for some time *(11)* and may render a small subgroup of the female population at greater risk of pulmonary emboli than the general population.

6.1.2. Central Nervous System

The stress associated with arrest and detention in custody may also have significant effects on the cerebrovascular system, which may, in susceptible individuals, precipitate intracerebral hemorrhage by the rupture of congenital or acquired aneurysms or vascular malformations. Ruptured berry aneurysms will result in the development of acute subarachnoid hemorrhages. It is less likely that these intracranial hemorrhages will result in sudden death, but they may result in sudden unconsciousness, which leads ultimately to death. Clearly the distinction between hemorrhage due to a natural disease process and that due to trauma will need to be established, and a specialist neuropathologic examination will be required should death occur.

As with the heart, the possibility that an infectious process within the central nervous system is the cause of sudden collapse and death must be considered. It is, however, unlikely that meningitis or encephalitis will present without any prodromal symptoms. Epilepsy is unlikely to develop *de novo* following arrest and detention, but epilepsy can and does lead to sudden collapse and death, and a preexisting history of epilepsy is clearly important. Any individual known to suffer from epilepsy should be monitored with the utmost care and the prescribed medication continued.

Other forms of intracranial pathology that may lead to sudden death include tumors, both benign and malignant, and such rarities as the development of colloid cysts of the ventricular system.

6.1.3. Endocrine System

Diabetes mellitus should raise concerns similar to those associated with epilepsy since poorly controlled diabetes may on occasions be the direct cause of sudden death; diabetes generally, through its association with an increased incidence of arterial disease, is a major factor in the development of coronary artery disease in the younger age groups. At postmortem examination, consideration must be given in all cases of sudden death in a young individual, but particularly when there is a history of diabetes mellitus, to the sampling of the vitreous humor in an attempt to determine the blood glucose level at the time of death. The samples need to be taken as soon after death as possible to avoid postmortem utilization of the intraocular glucose, yielding erroneous results *(12)*.

6.1.4. Other Causes

Many other natural disease processes could theoretically lead to sudden collapse and death. Among these is asthma, which is usually unlikely to lead to sudden death if individuals are adequately treated and supervised; if they are untreated, unsupervised, and in stressful circumstances they may be found dead in their cell. Other disease processes include the development of hemoptysis from tuberculosis or pulmonary malignancy or hematemesis from peptic ulceration or esophageal varices that can be life threatening and may, because of the bleeding, be considered to be the result of trauma rather than a natural disease process. These cases should present no problem to an experienced pathologist following a full postmortem examination.

6.1.5. Conclusions

The significant feature when considering possible natural causes of death of an individual in police custody is that some diseases can lead to rapid collapse and death with no prior warning in a young individual who is apparently fit and well immediately prior to the collapse. There is no method that the police can use to determine which of the individuals they encounter will be suffering from these diseases or from a genetic abnormality that may lead to electrical disturbances within the myocardium. Indeed many of these disease processes can only be diagnosed after complex medical testing following the taking of a full medical history.

The fact that many of these diseases are rare in the age group that is most likely to be detained in custody places additional burdens on the police officers required to care for these individuals and also on the doctors required to examine and treat them in the police station. The difficulty that these cases present to the pathologist lies in the need for an awareness of all possible natural causes of sudden death as well as a careful determination, and if necessary exclusion, of all these causes (cardiac, neurologic, endocrine, etc.) before forming the conclusion that some other factor has resulted in death.

6.2. Accidental Trauma

Determining whether trauma is the result of an accident or not may depend entirely on the "eye of the beholder." For example, it is impossible at postmortem examination to determine whether the injuries caused by a fall from a window during arrest were the result of an accidental fall, an intentional jump, or a deliberate push, since the points of contact during the descent and the contact with the ground will result in the same injuries whatever the initial "cause." Pathologically, the only features of relevance in determining the exact cause of initiation of the descent are the identification of specific gripping, holding, or other restraining injuries that could have occurred prior to the descent or the identification of possible marks or injuries (for instance, to the fingers) that could be ascribed to attempts to hold on to a window ledge, etc. All the injuries or marks found on the body will have to be correlated with witness statements from the police and from any other parties present at the time of the fall. Often the true interpretation of many of the injuries and marks found during the postmortem examination will only become clear when these statements are considered.

In general terms, however, accidental trauma can be caused by many events during the course of an arrest. Falls onto the ground may occur from a height or from standing. Gripping and restraining injuries are commonly present on many areas of the body. The site and significance of the injuries present will depend on the descriptions of the events before, during, and after the arrest.

It is essential that all injuries, no matter how apparently trivial, present on a detained individual be carefully documented by the forensic physician who examines the detainee whether at a police station or elsewhere. Contemporaneous photographs are always extremely helpful in these circumstances.

In terms of a cause of death, few of the minor injuries will be relevant, but they may provide an indication of the extent and degree of the force that was applied to effect an arrest; as such, they can be of immense value. Injuries present in sites that are known to be of high risk, for instance around the neck, must be examined, documented, and interpreted with particular care. All the injuries need to be interpreted in the light of witness statements and can provide very useful corroborative evidence.

7. Alcohol and Drug-Related Deaths

7.1. Alcohol

Alcohol is one of the most commonly used drugs in the world. The small ethyl alcohol molecule can pass easily through the blood–brain barrier to the central nervous system, where it has direct suppressant effects. At low concentrations the specialized cells of the cerebral cortex are affected, but as the concentration increases the depressive effects involve the higher areas of the brain, resulting in increasingly disinhibited behavior. Still higher levels of alcohol result in depressant effects involving the lower levels of brain function including the vital cardiorespiratory centers in the midbrain and the medulla, predisposing the intoxicated individual to cardiorespiratory depression or arrest. Alcohol levels in excess of 300 mg/100 mL are considered to be potentially lethal, although some individuals have survived, usually with medical attention, with far higher levels. It must be remembered that death may occur with far lower levels of alcohol in the bloodstream.

The effects of alcohol are not confined to the brain; there is also marked peripheral vasodilation resulting in increased heat loss, which may, on occasions, lead to hypothermia. The adverse effects of alcohol on the coronary circulation, particularly when associated with coronary atheroma, may lead to myocardial ischemia and the development of dysrythmias and sudden death.

Alcohol also has marked diuretic effects and when combined with the ingestion of large quantities of fluid (particularly in beer and lager drinking) may result in electrolyte disturbances, particularly hyponatremia.

The chronic effects of alcohol involve many of the internal organs; alcoholic cardiomyopathy, hepatic steatosis, and cirrhosis are the most common and can all lead to sudden death.

Alcohol may also be a major factor in causing death by predisposing the individual to accidental trauma and by obscuring the effects of that trauma. This is particularly the case in head injuries when changes in conscious level are attributed to the effects of alcohol rather than an identified or unidentified head injury.

Alcohol is also a gastric irritant and may precipitate vomiting when taken in excess. This, combined with the effects of decreased consciousness and the reduced laryngeal reflexes associated with intoxication, results in a significantly increased risk of aspiration of vomit into the airways and death. Such an event is unpredictable and, without constant supervision, unpreventable.

The anesthetic effects of alcohol may also result in deaths from asphyxiation. These deaths are the result of the intoxicated individual moving into or being placed or left in a position that impedes respiration either by occlusion of the external respiratory orifices and the internal airways (particularly the larynx) or restricting the free movement of the chest wall. These positions may result from lying face down on a bed, marked extension or flexion of the neck, or lying across an edge with the head down. Deaths resulting from impairment of respiration in this manner classically result in profound asphyxial changes involving the upper body; these deaths are ascribed to postural asphyxia.

Given the speed with which an individual under the influence of alcohol can die from either the aspiration of vomit or from postural asphyxia, it is doubtful whether a police station cell is the correct environment for recovery from intoxication.

7.2. Drugs

Drug use is now so ubiquitous in western society that any examination of a potential detainee by a forensic physician must include a very careful evaluation of recent or past drug use. The skill of the forensic physician will undoubtedly be stretched to the full in this assessment (*see* Chapter 8).

In terms of deaths in custody, all drug use, whether social, abusive, or therapeutic, is relevant, and the possibility that a detainee may have abused just one drug or a combination of drugs with or without alcohol prior to death must be positively excluded. A full drug screen on blood and, if available, urine is imperative. Some laboratories will also examine samples of bile and/or liver to detect evidence of previous drug abuse.

8. Deliberate Injuries

8.1. Baton Blows

Blows from a baton are usually easily identified in that forceful blows produce the classic "tramline" type of injuries on the skin. "Tramline" injuries are typical of a blow from a linear blunt object. The areas of the skin that are most traumatized are not those at the middle of the site of contact, where the skin is most evenly compressed, but rather at the margins of the contact site where stretching and distortion of the skin, and hence damage to the underlying tissues including the blood vessels, is most pronounced. A linear object will, almost by definition, have two such margins that run parallel, and a blow from such an object results in two linear, parallel bruises; hence the term "tramline."

Blows from a baton may also result in deeper bruising, nerve damage, and fractured bones. The deeper injuries tend to reflect the use of greater force, but it is not possible to correlate with any degree of certainty the amount of force needed to cause a particular injury in any one individual.

It is essential for both the forensic physician who examines a living victim of a blow to the head from a baton (or from any other cause) and the pathologist who performs a postmortem examination to remember that significant cerebral trauma can have been caused even in the absence of obvious external trauma or skull fractures, and it would be a matter of prudence to assess with great care anyone who has received, or complains of receiving, a head injury from a baton or any other cause and to consider carefully if referral to a hospital for a full neurologic assessment would be advisable.

8.2. Neck Holds

Pressure on and around the neck is well known to be a potentially lethal action *(12)*. Death can be caused following compression of the neck by any one of four mechanisms or by a combination of two or more.

1. Airway obstruction by direct compression of the larynx or trachea or by the pressure on the neck raising the larynx upward and causing the superior aspect of the pharynx to be occluded by the base of the tongue. This can be achieved by pressure of a forearm across the front of the neck, sometimes called the *choke hold.*
2. Occlusion of the veins in the neck. The low pressure in the venous system and the thin yielding nature of the vein walls makes venous occlusion more easily achieved than arterial occlusion; however, the large reserve capacity of the venous system makes it unlikely that rapid death would result even if complete occlusion was achieved, unless some other factor supervened.
3. Compression or occlusion of the carotid arteries. This is harder to achieve than venous occlusion due to the higher pressure in the arterial system and the thickness of the arterial walls; however, the effects of occlusion will become apparent much more quickly. Knight *(12)* records that occlusion of the carotid circulation for a period of 4 minutes or more may result in brain damage and Reay et al. *(13)* demonstrated significant changes in blood flow in the face of five individuals who were subjected to compression of the carotid arteries by the application of a "sleeper hold" in experimental conditions. A sleeper hold is applied when the upper arm compresses one side of the neck and the forearm the other and the larynx rests in the V formed by the elbow.
4. Stimulation of the vagus nerve by direct pressure in its course down the neck or as a result of stimulation of the carotid sinus. Vagal stimulation results in bradycardia, which may progress to asystole or, in some cases, immediate asystole.

Mercy et al. *(14)* reviewed 20 deaths in which neck holds had been applied and concluded that in 19 of these cases the application of the neck hold was associated with the death. Conversely Kowai *(15)* concluded that the choke hold could take between 10 and 20 seconds to cause unconsciousness and therefore it was safe. Clearly they did not experience the vagal effects of this hold in their experiments.

Neck holds are commonly used in many forms of wrestling or martial arts and in these situations they are seldom associated with fatalities, possibly because of the ability of the person held to indicate their willingness to submit to a referee and so cause the hold to be released. No such authority is present during a restraint by police, and perhaps this is why fatalities are recorded in this situation. In the United Kingdom the use of neck holds by the police during restraint is specifically prohibited, and officers are warned during their training of the potentially fatal effects of applying any pressure to the neck. In the United States, however, neck holds are an approved method of restraint.

The pathologic examination of deaths associated with compression of the neck requires a detailed and careful dissection of the neck structures *(16)*. The finding of injuries to the muscular, cartilaginous, vascular, or neural components of the neck must, however, be interpreted in the light of the events of the restraint, the actions of the restrainers, and the subsequent resuscitation (if any). Pressure on the neck to maintain an airway following cardiac or respiratory arrest may result in bruising, which could be confused with pressure prior to, or indeed causing, that arrest. Therapeutic insertion of cannulae during active resuscitation by paramedics or in the hospital commonly leads to quite marked hemorrhage into the neck, which, while it is unlikely to be confused with bruising caused by a neck hold, may mask any bruising that was present.

Pressure on the neck is not, of course, the only mechanism whereby an individual may suffer anoxia or asphyxiation. Any action that occludes, partially or completely, the mouth and/or the nose will result in difficulty in breathing and may result in asphyxiation. The features of these other causes of asphyxiation, traumatic or restraint asphyxia, will be discussed later.

8.3. Homicide

In a number of cases individuals have been murdered in the cell by another inmate; these deaths are most commonly associated with blunt trauma, but strangulation, stabbing, and other methods may be employed if suitable weapons are available. It is also evident that individuals have been deliberately assaulted and killed by police officers during arrest and detention.

The forensic physician should always be aware of the possibility that excessive force may have been applied by the police or that deliberately homicidal injuries may have been inflicted. If injuries are present on any individual in the physician's care, these injuries must be carefully documented; if they are beyond that which the physician considers reasonable in the circumstances, concerns should be expressed immediately to a senior officer, to a legal representative of the detainee, and through an official complaints procedure. The physician also has the duty to ensure that no further harm comes to that person.

9. Self-Inflicted Injuries

Suicidal deaths in custody are a cause for continuing public concern. The methods used are variable but reflect the materials available to the individual.

9.1. Hanging

To effect a hanging suicide, individuals must have two things: an object that can be made into a noose and a point to fix it to. In addition, they must be able to place their body so that the body weight can be used to apply pressure to the neck via the noose.

The materials and objects that can be made into a noose are legion and vary from the obvious (ties, belts, shoelaces, etc.) to the unusual (underwear, shirts, etc.). To attempt to reduce the possibility of hanging suicides, many cells in police stations have been redesigned, and attachment points for the noose (pipes, bars, etc.) have been removed or covered. The lack of these obvious points did not, however, deter some individuals, who placed the bed on end and used the upper end as the fixing point. Installation of fixed beds or benching should preclude the use of that method in the future. It must be remembered that hanging can still be achieved, although is clearly more difficult, from a low suspension point and that any protrusion from a wall or fitment in a cell can potentially be used as the upper attachment for the noose.

In addition to removal of the fixing points, attempts have been made to remove the items that have been used as nooses in the past, and belts, shoelaces, etc. are sometimes taken from prisoners. Paper clothing has been used, although this has not been entirely successful because it entails removing all of the individual's clothing; this is clearly impractical in many cases and may raise problems with human rights. Paper clothing made strong enough to withstand any degree of wear would also be strong enough to act as a noose.

The key to preventing hanging suicides lies in the careful evaluation of all individuals who are to be detained and in the design of the cells in which they are held to preclude any possible point for the attachment of a noose.

Given the speed with which hanging can be effected, it is most unlikely that anything other than a permanent watch over the suicidal detainee would provide a foolproof method to prevent hanging in a cell. A cycle of 15-minute checks will allow more than ample time for individuals to hang themselves and cannot be considered adequate protection against this type of suicide.

9.2. Ligature Strangulation

As the possibility of suspension is reduced by the changes in design of the cells, the possibility of other forms of self-asphyxiation is likely to increase. Self-strangulation by ligature is considered possible but difficult *(12)* since pressure has to be applied to the neck by a conscious muscular effort of the hands and arms; it follows that when consciousness is lost and the muscular tone lessens, the pressure on the ligature will decrease, the airway obstruction and/or the vascular occlusion will cease, and death will generally be averted. If, however, the ligature is knotted or if the material is "non-slip" and looped around itself, then it is possible for the individual to apply pressure to the neck and for that pressure to be maintained even after consciousness is lost; as a result, death may follow. As with hanging, the key to preventing these deaths lies in careful evaluation and, if necessary, the removal of items of clothing and observation.

9.3. Incised Injuries

All prisoners should be carefully searched before incarceration, and any sharp objects, or objects that could be sharpened, removed. The extent of the search will probably depend on the mental state of the individual; the possibility of an intimate search to exclude weapons concealed in the vagina or rectum should be considered in those individuals considered most at risk. Death from deep incised wounds to the neck or arms can occur very quickly; even if a person is found before death has occurred, the effects of profound blood loss may make death inevitable despite attempts at resuscitation.

9.4. Drugs

When considering the possibility of suicide using drugs while in police custody, the two key factors are, once again, evaluation and searching. Careful searching (possibly including intimate searches in some cases) will prevent the ingestion of drugs by individuals after they have been placed in the cell. The forensic physician must always be aware of the possibility that excessive quantities of a drug or drugs were taken prior to arrest and detention; these may exert their effects when the individual is in the cell.

10. Excited Delirium

10.1. Definition

The exact definition of this syndrome remains elusive even though many reports have apparently described similar events *(17,18)*. Indeed, the many different names given to these apparently similar conditions (Bell's mania, agitated delirium, excited delirium, acute exhaustive mania) over the years indicate that it is a syndrome that may have many different facets, not all of which may be present in any single case. All these descriptions, however, do comment on the high potential for sudden collapse and death while the individual is in the highly excited states that they all describe. It is now accepted that such a syndrome does exist, and while it is now most commonly associated with use and abuse of cocaine *(19)*, it is important to note that it was described in 1849 well before cocaine use and abuse became common *(17)*.

10.2. Features

The clinical features of excited delirium are generally accepted to be:

- A state of high mental and physiologic arousal
- Agitation
- Hyperpyrexia associated with sweating
- Violence, aggression, and hostility
- Insensitivity to physical pain or to restraint sprays

In addition to these clinically observable features, there will certainly also be significant physiologic and biochemical sequelae including dehydration, lactic acidosis, and increased catecholamine levels *(20)*. These biochemical and physiologic features may be such that they will render the individual at considerable risk from sudden cardiac arrest, and the descriptions of individuals suffering from excited delirium *(21)* indicate that sudden death is not uncommon. Shulack *(21)* also records that "*The end may come so suddenly that the attending psychiatrist is left with a chagrined surprise. . . .*" he continues "*. . . the puzzlement is intensified after the autopsy generally fails to disclose any findings which could explain the death.*" More than 50 years after the publication of that paper it still holds true—but the site of the death may have moved from the ward of a psychiatric hospital to a police station.

The findings noted in by Shulack in 1944 are also repeated today in many cases that have the features of excited delirium, the difference now being that toxicologic examination not uncommonly reveals the presence of cocaine or, in a therapeutic environment, neuroleptic drugs; as a result, it is tempting to relate the cause of death to the presence of the drug or drugs. In the context of restraint associated with death in cases of excited delirium, the presence of injuries to the neck may lead to the conclusion that death resulted from asphyxia, but this interpretation needs careful evaluation.

What is perhaps of greater importance is that in the cases described in the clinical literature *(17,18,21–23)*, there has been a prolonged period of increasingly bizarre and aggressive behavior often lasting days or weeks before admission to the hospital and subsequent death. The clinical evidence available for the deaths associated with police restraint indicates that while there may have been a period of disturbed behavior before restraint and death, the duration will have been measured in hours and not days. This change in time scale may be due to the different etiology of the cases of excited delirium now seen, and it is possible that the "natural" and the "cocaine-induced" types of excited delirium will have different time spans but a common final pathway. This feature will need to be elucidated in the future.

The conclusion that can be reached concerning individuals displaying the symptoms of excited delirium is that they clearly constitute a medical emergency. The police need to be aware of the symptoms of excited delirium and to understand that attempts at restraint are potentially dangerous and that forceful restraint should only be undertaken when individuals are a serious risk to themselves or to other members of the public.

Ideally a person displaying these symptoms should be contained and a forensic physician called to examine the individual and to give advice to the police at the scene. The possibility of treatment *in situ* by an emergency psychiatric team with resuscitation equipment and staff available will need to be discussed with the police; if such a team exists, this is probably the best and safest option. If such a team is not available, then the individual will need to be restrained with as much care as possible and taken to the hospital emergency room for a full medical and psychiatric evaluation. These individuals should not be taken directly to a psychiatric unit, where resuscitation skills and equipment may not be adequate.

11. Rapid Unexplained Deaths During Restraint

Deaths occurring while an individual is actually being restrained are extremely rare. In the U.K. Police Research Group Paper *(24)*, which covers the period 1990–1996, 16 cases are identified in which police action "may have been associated with the death," amounting to 6% of the deaths that this group studied. From consideration of the medical aspects of these deaths recorded in the report, it would appear that six of the deaths were due to natural disease and four were related to drug use or abuse. Of the remaining 6 cases, one was associated with a baton blow to the head, two with asphyxiation due to pressure to the neck, two with "restraint asphyxia" and one with a head injury. Therefore, in the deaths during the 7 years that this group considered, a total of 4 deaths, less than 1.5% of the total of 267 deaths in police custody, were apparently directly associated with asphyxia during restraint.

However, the close association of these deaths with the actions of the police in restraining the individual raises questions about the conclusions reached by the pathologists and accepted by the courts. It is very common for several pathologic opinions to be obtained in these cases; in a review of 12 in-custody deaths, an average of three opinions had been obtained (range one to seven) *(25)*. Indeed, in one of the cases cited in this report as being associated with police actions, seven pathologic opinions were sought and yet only one opinion is quoted. This points to the considerable difficulty in determining the relative significance of a number of different, and at times conflicting, areas of medical evidence that are commonly present in these cases.

The area of restraint that appears to be causing the most concern relates to asphyxiation during the act of restraint. It has been known in forensic circles for many years that individuals may asphyxiate if their ability to breathe is reduced by the position in which they are placed or into which they fall *(26)*. This type of asphyxiation is commonly associated with alcohol or drug intoxication or, rarely, with neurologic diseases that prevent individuals from extracting themselves from a position that either occludes, partially or completely, their mouth and nose or that limits the freedom of movement of the chest wall. Death resulting from these events has been described as postural asphyxia to indicate that it was the posture of the individual that resulted in the airway obstruction rather than the action of a third party.

In 1988, research by Reay et al. *(27)* was published that was initially thought to show that, in laboratory conditions, the placing of an individual in the "hog-tie" position significantly increased the time taken to return to resting blood oxygenation levels following moderate exercise. "Hog-tying" is a form of restraint by which the detainee is placed face down and the hands are tied together and then to the feet. Reay et al. concluded that this restraint had "measurable physiologic effects." In 1992, Reay et al. *(28)* concluded that six individuals had died as a result of "hog-tying" and being placed prone in police vehicles. This paper raised the possibility that asphyxiation was occurring when individuals could not move themselves to safer positions because of the type of restraint used by the police. The concept of "restraint asphyxia," albeit in a specific set of circumstances, was born.

Since the description of deaths in the prone, "hog-tied" position, the original concepts of Reay et al. have been extended to account for many deaths of individuals under restraint but not in the "hog-tied" position. The term "restraint asphyxia" has been widened to account for these sudden and unexpected deaths during restraint. Considerable pathologic and physiologic controversy exists regarding the exact effects of the prone position and "hog-tying" on respiration. Further experiments by Chan et al. *(29)* have cast considerable doubt on the thesis of Reay et al., although other experiments by Roeggla et al. *(30)* appear to support the original theory. While the physiologic controversy continues, it is clear to all those involved in the examination and investigation of these deaths that there is a small group of individuals who die suddenly and apparently without warning while being restrained.

The problem that currently faces the forensic pathologist is the determination of the cause or causes of these deaths. This is made harder since there are seldom any of the usual asphyxial signs to assist and, even if those signs are present, it is difficult to assign weight or significance to them since similar changes can be caused simply by resuscitation *(31,32)*.

The major features of asphyxiation are cyanosis, congestion, and petechial hemorrhages *(12)*. These features are seen to a greater or lesser extent in many, but not all, cases of asphyxiation. They are often completely absent in many plastic bag asphyxiations and in hanging, they have a variable presence in manual strangulation, and they are most commonly seen in ligature strangulation. Their most florid appearance is in deaths associated with postural asphyxia or crush asphyxia in which death has occurred slowly and associated with some form of pressure or force reducing the ability of the individual to maintain adequate respiratory movement, either from outside the body or from the abdominal contents splinting the diaphragm.

It is of interest then that these features if present at all in these cases are, at most, scanty and do not reflect their appearance in other cases of crush asphyxia, suggesting that different mechanisms are the causes of death in these two sets of circumstances.

The individuals who die during restraint are not infrequently under the influence of drugs (particularly cocaine) or alcohol, they may be suffering from some underlying natural disease (particularly of the cardiovascular system), or they may have suffered some trauma. These "additional" factors are sometimes seized on by pathologists and courts to "explain" the death, sometimes even in the face of expert opinion that excludes the additional factor from playing a major part in the death. It would seem that there is a subgroup of the population that is either permanently, or at times and for whatever reason, susceptible to the effects of restraint whether those effects be mediated entirely or indeed partially through decreased respiratory effort or some other factor.

There appears then to be a separate entity, the exact cause of which is not yet clear, by which otherwise fit and healthy individuals die suddenly while being restrained and yet do not show significant features of asphyxiation. It is to be hoped that further research on the physiology of restraint will elucidate the mechanisms that cause death in these cases. Until these mechanisms are established, it would seem reasonable to propose that these deaths should be classified for what they are—rapid unexplained death during restraint (RUDDR)—rather than to conclude that the cause of death cannot be determined or to ascribe a doubtful medical or toxicologic cause of death that does not bear close scrutiny. Deaths classified as RUDDR must fulfill several criteria:

1. The death must have occurred during restraint and the individual must have collapsed suddenly and without warning.
2. A full external and internal postmortem examination must have been performed by a forensic pathologist that did not reveal macroscopic evidence of significant natural disease and subsequently a full histologic examination of the tissues must have been performed that did not reveal microscopic evidence of significant natural disease.
3. Studies must not reveal genetic markers of significant disease.
4. There must be no evidence of significant trauma or of the triad of asphyxial signs.
5. A full toxicologic screen must have been performed that did not reveal evidence of drugs or alcohol, which, alone or in combination, could have caused death.

The small numbers of these deaths in any single country or indeed worldwide makes their analysis very difficult; indeed, to search for a single answer that will explain all these deaths may be futile. The bringing together of these deaths under a single classification would make identification of cases and their analysis easier.

The problem for the police is that while approaching and restraining an individual they cannot know their background or medical history nor can they have any idea of the particular (or peculiar) physiologic responses of that individual. The techniques designed for restraint and care of the individual after restraint must therefore allow for safe restraint of the most vulnerable sections of the community.

New research into the effects of restraint may possibly lead to a greater understanding of the deleterious effects of restraint and the development of safer techniques. While this experimental work is being performed the only advice that can be offered to police officers is that the prone position should be maintained for the minimum amount of time only, that no pressure should be applied to the back or the chest of a person restrained on the floor, and that that individual should be placed in a kneeling, sitting, or standing position to allow for normal respiration as soon as practical.

It should be noted that an individual who is suffering from early, or indeed late, asphyxiation may well struggle more and more in an attempt to breathe and, during a restraint, this increased level of struggling may be perceived by police officers as an renewed attempt to escape, resulting in further restriction of movement and subsequent exacerbation of the asphyxial process. Officers need to be taught that once restrained, these further episodes of struggling may signify imminent asphyxiation and not continued attempts to escape—they may represent a struggle to survive, and the police must be aware of this and respond with it in mind.

Since these matters were first brought to forensic and then public attention and improved training and advice given to police officers concerning the potential dangers of face down or prone restraints, especially if associated with any pressure to the chest or back, there appears to have been a decrease in the number of deaths during restraint. However, even one death in these circumstances is too many and it is hoped that by medical research, improved police training, and increased awareness of the dangers of restraint that these tragic deaths can be prevented.

References

1. Home Office (1996) *Consolidated Circular on Crime and Kindred Matters 35/86.* Her Majesty's Stationery Office, London.
2. Emson, H. E. (1994) Death in a restraint jacket from mechanical asphyxia. *Can Med Associ J.* **151,** 985–987.
3. Death in Custody Working Group of the Community-Police Consultative Group for Lambeth (1996) *Lessons from Tragedies. Deaths in Custody in the Metropolitan Police District 1986–95.*
4. Dalton, V. (1998) *Australian Deaths in Custody & Custody-Related Police Operations 1997–98.* http://www.aic.gov.au
5. Matthews, P., and Foreman, J., (eds.) (1993) *Jervis on Coroners*, 11th ed. Sweet & Maxwell, London.
6. Home Office (1969) Circular No 35 of 1969. Her Majesty's Stationery Office, London.
7. Davies, M. J., Robertson, W. B., Pomerance, A., and Davies, M. J. (eds.) (1975) 3. Diseases of the coronary arteries, in *The Pathology of the Heart*, Blackwell Scientific Publications, Oxford, pp. 81–126.
8. OPCS (1997) *Mortality Statistics (Cause).* London, Her Majesty's Stationery Office, London.

9. Burn, J., Camm, J., Davies, M. J., Peltonen, L., Schwartz, P., and Watkins, H. (1997) The phenotype/genotype relation and the current status of genetic screening in hypertrophic cardiomyopathy, Marfan syndrome and long QT syndrome. *Heart.* **78,** 110–116.
10. Berry, C. L., McGee, J. O., Isaacson, P. G., and Wright, N. A. (eds.) (1992) 12.6, Ateritis, in *The Oxford Textbook of Pathology.* Oxford University Press, Oxford, pp. 842–852.
11. Royal College of General Practitioners (1977) Mortality among oral contraceptive users. *Lancet.* **i,** 727–731.
12. Knight, B. (1996) *Forensic Pathology*, 2nd ed. Arnold, London.
13. Reay, D. T. and Holloway, G. A. (1982) Changes in carotid blood flow produced by neck compression. *Am J Forensic Med Pathol.* **3,** 199–202.
14. Mercy, J. A., Heath, C. W., and Rosenberg, M. L. (1990) Mortality associated with the use of upper-body control holds by police. *Violence Victims.* **5,** 215–222.
15. Koiwai, E. K. (1987) Deaths allegedly caused by the use of "choke holds" (shime-waza). *J Forensic Sci.* **32,** 419–432.
16. Vanezis, P. (1989) Techniques of examination, in *Pathology of Neck Injury*, Butterworths, London, pp. 22–27.
17. Bell, L. V. (1849) On a form of disease resembling mania and fever. *Am J Insanity.* **6,** 97.
18. Billig, O. and Freeman, W. T. (1944) Fatal catatonia. *Am J Psychiatry.* **100,** 633.
19. Karch, S. B. (1996) *The Pathology of Drug Abuse*, 2nd ed. CRC Press, Boca Raton.
20. Harries, M., Williams, C., Stanish, W. D., et al. (1996) *Oxford Textbook of Sports Medicine.* Oxford University Press, Oxford.
21. Shulack, N. R. (1944) Sudden exhaustive death in excited patients. *Psychiatr Q.* **18,** 3.
22. Kraines, S. H. (1934) Bell's mania. *Am J Psychiatry.* **91,** 29.
23. O'Halloran, R. L. and Lewman, L. V. (1993) Restraint asphyxiation in excited delirium. *Am J Forensic Med Pathol.* **14,** 289–295.
24. Leigh, A., Johnson, G., and Ingram, A. (1998) *Deaths in Police Custody—Learning the Lessons.* Home Office, London.
25. Morewood, T. C. G. (1998) In Custody Restraint Deaths, MSc Thesis, University of London.
26. Bell, M. D., Rao, V. J., and Welti, C. V. (1992) Positional asphyxiation in adults: a series of 30 cases from the Dade and Broward County, Florida Medical Examiners Offices from 1982 to 1990. *Am J Forensic Medi Pathol.* **13,** 101–107.
27. Reay, D. T., Howard, J. D., Fligner, C. L., and Ward, R. J. (1988) Effects of positional restraint on oxygen saturation and heart rate following exercise. *Am J Forensic Medi Pathol.* **9,** 16–18.
28. Reay, D. T., Fligner, C. L., Stilwell, A. D., and Arnold, J. (1992) Positional asphyxia during law enforcement transport. *Am J Forensic Medi Pathol.* **13,** 90–97.
29. Chan, T. C., Vilka, G. M., Neuman. T., and Clausen, J. L. (1997) Restraint position and positional asphyxia. *Ann Emerg Med.* **30,** 578–586.

30. Roeggla, M., Wagner, A., Muellner, M., Bur, A., Roeggla, H., Hirschl, M. M., et al. (1997) Cardiorespiratory consequences to hobble restraint. *Wien Klin Wochenschrift.* **109,** 359–361.
31. Hood, I. C., Ryan, D., and Spitz, W. U. (1988) Resuscitation and petechiae. *Am J Forensic Med Pathol.* **9,** 35–37.
32. Rao, V. J. and Welti, C. V. (1988) The forensic significance of conjunctival petechiae. *Am J Forensic Med Pathol.* **9,** 32–34.

Chapter 10

Traffic Medicine

Ian F. Wall and Steven Karch

1. Introduction

Driving a motor vehicle is a complex task requiring a reasonable level of physical fitness, accurate perception, and appropriate judgment. All these factors can be affected by drugs and alcohol, greatly increasing the risk of accidents. Many medical conditions (and their treatments) may impair fitness to drive and will first be considered.

2. Medical Aspects of Fitness to Drive

Licensing requirements depend on the type of vehicle driven, with more stringent requirements for commercial purposes and multiaxle vehicles. In many jurisdictions, including Canada, Australia, and the United Kingdom, it is the motorist's responsibility to inform the licensing authority of any relevant medical conditions. Similar requirements generally apply in the United States, except that six states (California, Delaware, Nevada, New Jersey, Oregon, and Pennsylvania) actually require physicians to report patients with seizures (and other conditions that may alter levels of consciousness), to the department of motor vehicles *(1)*. Drivers themselves have a legal responsibility to inform the licensing authority of any injury or medical condition that affects their driving ability, and physicians should take great pains to explain this obligation. Occasionally, especially when dealing with patients suffering from dementia, ethical responsibilities may require doctors to breach confidentiality and notify

From: *Forensic Science: A Physician's Guide to Clinical Forensic Medicine*
Edited by: M. M. Stark © Humana Press, Inc., Totowa, NJ

patients against their will or without their knowledge *(2)*; this situation will be considered later.

Requirements vary in different countries and in different jurisdictions within the same country. When in doubt about the appropriate course of action, physicians should consult the appropriate guidelines. In the United Kingdom, the Driver and Vehicle Licensing Agency (DVLA) has made available the *At a Glance Guide to the Current Medical Standards of Fitness to Drive (3)*. In Australia the *Austroads Guidelines for Assessing Fitness to Drive* provides similar information *(4)*. In the European Union, where EC directives have developed basic standards but allow different countries to impose more stringent requirements, there is still considerable variation from country to country. The situation is even more complicated in the United States, where each state sets its own rules, and where Federal regulations for commercial vehicles apply as well. Often, much of the required regulatory information can be acquired via the Internet, or from organizations and foundations representing patients who have the particular disease in question.

It should be assumed that all adults drive; drivers with disabilities should be given special consideration and may require modification of their vehicle or have certain personal restrictions applied.

2.1. Cardiovascular Diseases

A number of studies have demonstrated that natural deaths at the wheel are fairly uncommon and that the risk for other persons is not significant *(5,6)*. Even so, requirements for commercial drivers are generally much more rigid than for individuals, and in the United States, the Federal Highway Administration prohibits drivers with angina or recent infarction from driving. The length of prohibition varies from state to state. Restrictions for noncommercial car driving, after first acute myocardial infarction, are 4 weeks in United Kingdom, but only 2 weeks in Australia. They are entirely at the discretion of U.S. physicians. In general, ischemia itself is not considered an absolute disqualification, provided treadmill stress testing demonstrates that moderate reserves are present *(7)*. Similarly, individuals with controlled hypertension are usually considered fit to drive, although physicians, no matter what country they are in, must give serious thought to just what sort of medication is used to control hypertension; clonidine, methyldopa, reserpine, and prazosin can produce somnolence and/or impair reflex responses.

Patients with dysrhythmias, treated with medication or with the implantation of a defibrillator/pacemaker, present a special set of problems *(8)*. The tendency in the United States has been to treat such individuals as if they were epileptics, i.e., individuals with the potential to lose consciousness at the wheel.

Most states set minimum requirements for seizure-free periods. Until fairly recently, that period was 6 months in a majority of jurisdictions but is increasingly being shortened to 3 months in many locations.

2.2. Epilepsy

Epilepsy is the commonest cause of collapse at the wheel, accounting for approximately 30% of such incidents. In the United Kingdom, epilepsy is a Prescribed Disability (along with severe mental impairment, sudden attacks of disabling giddiness, and inability to meet eyesight requirements), and car driving is not allowed for at least 1 year after a seizure. Here too, restrictions vary from country to country. All 50 of the United States restrict the licenses of epileptics if their seizures are not well controlled by medication. Most states require a 6-month seizure-free period and a physician's statement confirming that the individual's seizures have, in fact, been controlled and that the individual in question poses no risk to public safety. The letter from the physician is then reviewed by a medical advisory board, which may or may not issue a licence. In the United States, even if the patient, at some later date, does have a seizure and cause an accident, the physician's act of writing to the board protects him or her from liability under American law, provided the letter was written in good faith.

Withdrawal of antiepileptic medication is associated with a risk of seizure recurrence. One study showed that 41% of patients who stopped treatment slowly developed a recurrence of seizures within 2 years compared with only 22% of patients who continued treatment *(9)*. The legal consequences of discontinuing medication, without a physician's order, can be quite devastating. Patients who stop taking antiseizure medication and then cause an accident may face future civil liability and possibly even criminal charges if they cause physical injury *(10)*. Of course, rules vary from country to country but, in general, a seizure patient who does not inform the appropriate regulatory agency may face dire consequences (including even the legitimate refusal of the insurance carrier to pay for damages).

2.3. Diabetes

Diabetes may affect the ability to drive because of loss of consciousness from hypoglycemic attacks, or from complications of the disease itself, e.g., retinopathy causing visual problems or peripheral vascular disease causing limb disabilities. In January 1998, the British government introduced new restrictions on licensing of people with insulin-dependent diabetes *(11)*. These restrictions were based on the second EU driver licensing directive (91/4389), and under most interpretations of the law, they prevent insulin-treated diabetics from driving light goods and small passenger-carrying vehicles. In response to concerns expressed by the diabetic community in Britain, the British Diabetic Association commissioned a report that found little evidence to support the new legislation; for the moment, the situation remains unsettled.

In the United States the situation varies from state to state, but in many states diabetics are subject to restrictive licensing policies that bar them from driving certain types of motor vehicles *(12,13)*. The risk of hypoglycemia, however, differs greatly among insulin-requiring diabetics, and today most insulin-dependent diabetics use self-monitoring devices to warn them when their blood glucose levels are becoming too low. Thus, a number of states have dropped blanket restrictions and allow for case-by-case evaluations to determine medical qualifications for diabetics. In some states, physicians are specifically required to notify authorities of the patient's diabetic conditions, but in all states it is the patient's responsibility to do so. As with seizure patients, failure to notify may expose the patient to both civil and criminal liability.

2.4. Vision and Eye Disorders

The two most important aspects of vision in relation to driving are visual acuity and visual fields. Visual acuity may simply be defined as the best obtainable vision with or without spectacles or contact lenses. Most countries require a binocular visual acuity greater than 6/12 for licensing purposes. In the United Kingdom the eyesight requirements are to read a car number registration plate at 20.5 m, which corresponds to between 6/9 and 6/12 on the Snellen chart. The minimum field of vision for safe driving is generally regarded as at least 120 degrees on the horizontal when measured with a Goldman IV4e target or its equivalent *(14)*.

2.5. Ethical Considerations

While it is generally a patient's responsibility to inform the licensing authority of any injury or medical condition that affects their driving, occasionally ethical responsibilities may require a doctor to inform the licensing authorities of a particular problem. If a patient has a medical condition that renders them unfit to drive, the doctor should make sure the patient understands that the condition may impair their ability to drive. If the patient is incapable of understanding this advice, e.g., due to dementia, the doctor should inform the licensing authority immediately *(15)*.

If patients continue to drive when they are not fit to do so, the doctor should make every reasonable effort to persuade them to stop, which may include informing their next of kin. If this still does not persuade the patient to stop driving, the doctor should disclose relevant medical information immediately, in confidence, to the medical adviser of the licensing authority. Before disclosing this information, the doctor should inform the patient of the decision to do so and once the licensing authority has been informed, the doctor should also write to the patient, to confirm that disclosure has been made *(15)*.

3. Alcohol and Driving

3.1. Metabolism of Alcohol

Alcohol is absorbed through the stomach and duodenum. Absorption is dependent on many factors, including sex and weight of the individual, duration of drinking, nature of the drink, and presence of food in the stomach. Alcohol dehydrogenase in the gastric mucosa may contribute substantially to alcohol metabolism (gastric first-pass metabolism), but this effect is generally only evident with low doses and after eating. Studies of alcohol dehydrogenase activity in gastric biopsies of women suggest a significant decrease in activity in women compared with men, which could explain why women have higher peak blood alcohol levels and are more susceptible to liver damage after consumption of smaller quantities of alcohol when compared with men *(16)*. Further details of alcohol metabolism are given in Chapter 8.

Once absorbed, alcohol is eliminated at a fairly constant rate, with 90% being metabolized in the liver and the remainder excreted unchanged in urine, breath, and sweat. The rate of elimination in moderate drinkers may vary between 10 to 20 mg/100 mL blood/h, with a mean of 15 mg/100 mL blood/h. Chronic alcoholics, undergoing detoxification, have elimination rates of 19 mg/100 mL blood/h or even higher *(17)*. This increased rate of alcohol burnoff is though to be a consequence of increased activity of hepatic microsomal enzymes (P450IIE).

3.2. Effects of Alcohol on Performance

Alcohol affects mood and behavior, causing euphoria (which is particularly significant in risk taking) but also depressing the central nervous system. Even at low doses, there is clear evidence that alcohol impairs performance, especially as the faculties that are most sensitive to alcohol are those most important to driving, namely complex perceptual mechanisms and states of divided attention. In a review of over 200 papers *(18)*, a variety of behavioral aspects were examined including reaction time, tracking, concentrated attention, divided attention, information processing, visual function, perception, psychomotor performance, and driver performance. Most of the studies showed impairment at 70 mg/100 mL blood, but approximately 20% showed impairment at concentrations between 10 and 40 mg/100 mL blood.

The definitive study on the relationship between risk of accident and blood alcohol concentration is that carried out in the 1960s in Grand Rapids, Michigan by Borkenstein and Dale *(19)*; data were collected on 5895 drivers involved in accidents and on 7590 drivers not involved. Comparison of the two groups disclosed that an accident was statistically more likely at blood alcohol levels greater than 80 mg/100 mL blood, with accidents occurring more frequently as follows:

Blood alcohol (mg/100 mL)	Accident occurrence
50–100	1.5 times as frequently
100–150	4 times as frequently
Over 150	18 times as frequently

Further analysis of the data by Allsop *(20)* quantified the risks for different ages and different drinking habits. On average, the risk doubles at 80 mg/100 mL, increasing sharply to a 10 times risk multiplier at 150 mg/100 mL and a 20 times risk multiplier at 200 mg/100 mL blood. For inexperienced drivers and infrequent drinkers, the sharp increase occurs at much lower levels, whereas for the more experienced drinking driver it may not occur until 100 mg/100 mL (Fig. 1).

This research has therefore encouraged some countries to have a lower blood alcohol level for legal driving and in Australia, Canada, and some states of the United States, different levels and rules are applied for younger and/or inexperienced drivers (*see* below).

3.3. Road Traffic Legislation

In the United Kingdom, this research led to the introduction of the Road Safety Act 1967, which set a legal driving limit of 80 mg/100 mL of blood (or 35 μg/100 mL of breath or 107 mg/100 mL of urine). This law also allows mandatory roadside screening tests and requires the provision of blood or urine tests at police stations. The Transport Act 1981 provided that quantitative breath tests, performed with approved devices, could be used as the sole evidence of drunk driving. Although the level for U.K. drivers is set at 80 mg/100 mL of blood, in practice drivers are not usually prosecuted at blood levels below 87 mg/100 mL of blood because, during the analysis, a series of results by gas chromatography [which must fall within 3 standard deviations (or 6%) of each other] is averaged, and then 6% (or 6 mg below 100 g/100 mL) is deducted from the result, which is then reported as not less than × mg/100 mL of blood.

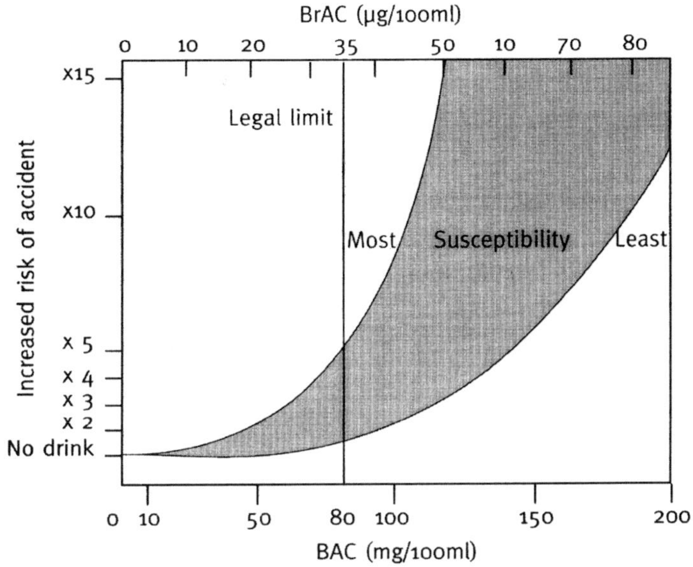

Fig. 1. Risk of road traffic accidents related to level of alcohol in the blood (BAC) and breath (BrAC). (Used with kind permission of Greenwich Medical Media.)

In the United States, permissible blood levels vary from state to state and also by age. Many states have enacted "zero tolerance" laws, and the detection of any alcohol in an individual younger than age 21 is grounds for licence revocation. Some states permit levels as high as 100 mg/100 mL, but most enforce the same limit as in the United Kingdom, and legislation to reduce the 80 mg/100 mL level further is under consideration. Repeated attempts to introduce one nationwide level have been rebuffed by the U.S. Congress.

3.4. Equivalent Limits in Other Body Fluids

Statutes have been used to establish blood alcohol concentration equivalents in other tissues and breath. Not infrequently, alcohol concentrations will be measured in accident victims taken for treatment at trauma centers. However, there are two very important differences between alcohol measurements made in hospitals and those made in forensic laboratories; first, in hospitals, standard international units (SI) are the norm, the mole is the unit of mass, the liter is the unit of volume, and alcohol concentrations are reported in mmol/L. In forensic laboratories, results are expressed as gram/deciliter or liter, or even milligrams per milliliter, and measurements are made in whole blood, not serum or plasma. Because 1 mL of whole blood weighs, on average, 1.055 g, a blood alcohol concentration of 100 mg/dL is actually the same as 95 mg/100 g or 21.7 mmol/L *(17)*.

There is another, even more important, difference between serum/plasma and whole blood. The former contains 91.8% water, while the latter contains only 80.1% water. Because alcohol has a very large volume of distribution, this difference in water content means that alcohol concentrations measured in serum/plasma will be higher than concentrations measured in whole blood by approximately 14%. In practice, if plasma alcohol concentrations are to be introduced as evidence, they should be related back to whole blood concentrations using an even higher ratio (1.22 : 1), which corresponds to the mean value, ± 2 standard deviations. As mentioned earlier, if whole blood is tested, drivers are not usually prosecuted at blood levels below 87 mg/100 mL of blood *(17)*.

Breath testing is equally problematic. The instruments used are calibrated to estimate the concentrations of alcohol in whole blood, not plasma or serum. To estimate the serum or plasma alcohol concentration from breath measurements, a plasma/breath ratio of 2,600 : 1 must be used (because, as explained above, whole blood contains 14% less alcohol!). In Europe, but not necessarily in the United States, two specimens of breath are taken for analysis, and the specimen with the lower proportion of alcohol should be used as evidence.

Bladder urine, because it contains alcohol (or other drugs) that may have accumulated over a long period, is generally not considered a suitable specimen for forensic testing, especially since the presence of alcohol in the urine only proves that alcohol is present in the body. Alcohol concentrations in bladder urine cannot be used to infer the blood levels reliably. Even so, U.K. legislation and most U.S. states still allow drivers the option of providing breath, blood, or urine specimens, but as of 1999, the State of California has dropped the option of providing urine samples, and other states are considering similar actions. Under the new California provisions, police can still request a urine test if a suspect's breath test is negative *(21)*.

Other options are available in the case of alcohol-related fatalities. Comparison of alcohol concentrations in vitreous and blood can provide a good indication of whether concentrations were rising or falling at the time of death (alcohol is distributed mainly in water and the water content of vitreous is lower than that of blood). Urine obtained from the kidney pelvis can also be used, since its alcohol content can be precisely related to blood concentration *(22)*.

Table 1
Prescribed Blood Alcohol Levels in Various Jurisdictions

Australia	50	Austria	80	Belgium	80
Bulgaria	0	Canada	80	Czechoslovakia	80
Denmark	80	Eire	80	Finland	50
France	50	Germany	80	Greece	50
Hungary	0	Italy	80	Luxembourg	80
Netherlands	50	Norway	50	Poland	20
Romania	0	Russia	0	Sweden	20
Spain	80	Turkey	0	USA	100*
Yugoslavia	50				

*Some states in the US have reduced the legal level to 80 mg/100 mL blood.

3.5. Legal Limits in Other Jurisdictions

Table 1 shows permissible alcohol limits for various countries. All figures are the maximum permissible amount in milligrams per 100 mL of blood (in the United States, referred to as deciliters and abbreviated dL). Although legislation has been introduced to enforce uniform standards, these standards have not been enacted, and in the United States permissible alcohol levels vary from state to state.

3.6. Countermeasures

A number of measures have already been taken to discourage drivers from drinking, and they have had a considerable degree of success.

3.6.1. Lowering the Legal Limit

When the legal limit was reduced in Sweden from 50 to 20 mg, there was a fall in casualties *(23)*. It has been estimated that a similar reduction in the United Kingdom would save 50 lives, prevent 250 serious injuries, and eliminate another 1200 slight injuries each year. A cost/benefit analysis suggests that this would save £75 million a year *(24)*.

3.6.2. Widening Police Breath Testing Powers

At present, in the United Kingdom, a police officer may stop any person driving a motor vehicle on the road, but that does not necessarily mean that the officer can administer a breath test. As is the case in the United States, police officers can require a breath test only if there is reasonable cause to suspect that the person detained has alcohol in their body, has committed a moving traffic offense, or has been involved in an accident.

In Finland, random breath testing along with a legal limit of 50 mg/100 mL of blood was introduced in 1977; highly visible check points are established and typically, 8–12 policemen with breath alcohol screening devices are placed along the center of the road, the sites being chosen so that it is impossible for a driver to avoid being tested. All drivers are tested except those of emergency vehicles. The procedure takes only seconds to perform, the system receives general public support *(25)*, and it has resulted in a marked reduction in the number of accidents and injuries.

In the state of Victoria, Australia, "booze buses" are set up along with a roadblock—any driver who fails a roadside breath test is taken into the bus and given an evidentiary breath test (Drager 7100 machine). Every driver in Victoria is said to be tested on average at least once a year *(26)*.

3.6.3. Ignition Interlocks for Repeat Drink-Drive Offenders

These devices prevent the car ignition from being started unless the concentration of breath alcohol blown into the device is below a predetermined level, often well below the legal limit. Thereafter, during the journey, the driver is required to undertake random rolling retests. A failure of these tests activates the vehicle's lights and horn. These devices have been used in several states of the United States and also in Alberta, Canada. They are generally applied to repeat offenders, either as an alternative to disqualification or in succession to a period of disqualification. Results in the United States have shown that repeat offenses occur rapidly once the restriction is removed *(27)*. However, in Alberta, where there is closer supervision of the program, supplemented by counseling, more long-term improvements have been experienced.

3.6.4. High Risk Offender Scheme

A special program in England, Wales, and Scotland was introduced in 1983, and the criteria widened in 1990, to cover drivers who were convicted of having a blood alcohol concentration (BAC) in excess of 200 mg/100 mL blood, or refusing to provide an evidential specimen, or two offenses involving BACs in excess of 80 mg/100 mL blood within a 10-year period. This group accounts for about 30–40% of drunk driving offenders in Britain. To regain their licences at the end of a period of disqualification, the drivers must undergo a medical examination (including blood tests to discover biochemical evidence of excessive alcohol consumption) to demonstrate with reasonable certainty that they are not alcohol abusers *(3)*. Similar statues apply in the United States. In California, drivers found to have a blood alcohol concentration greater than 200 mg/100 mL, in addition to whatever other sanctions are imposed, are required to attend a 6-month educational program *(21)*. In the United States, penalties for drunk driving may be "enhanced" under special circumstances, such as a second conviction for drunk driving, or speeding at the time of arrest, or the presence of a child in the car, or the causation of property damage or injury.

3.7. Procedural Issues

While the procedures involved may seem very simple, numerous technical defenses have been raised in most countries around the world. Not surprisingly, many of these challenges are very similar, no matter the country in which they are offered. Challenges to the U.K. Road Traffic Act are illustrative of the problem.

3.7.1. Definitions

Section 5(1) of the Road Traffic Act 1988 (subsequently referred to as RTA) states that: if a person drives or attempts to drive a motor vehicle on a road or other public place, or is in charge of a motor vehicle on a road or other public place, after consuming so much alcohol that the proportion of it in his or her breath, blood, or urine exceeds the prescribed limit, he or she is guilty of an offense. Unfortunately, the word "drive" is not actually defined, but in fact, three points need to be proved: first, that the person is in the driving seat or has control of the steering, second, that the person charged must have something to do with the propulsion of the vehicle, and finally, that what the individual was doing must fall within the normal meaning of driving.

Attempting to drive has produced an abundance of case law, but it has been held that acts of mere preparation, e.g., checking the engine, finding keys, or opening the car door do not amount to attempting to drive. However, steps on the way to what would have been driving, if not interrupted, may amount to an attempt, e.g., putting the key in the ignition.

In Section 185(1) of the RTA, a motor vehicle is defined as a "mechanically propelled vehicle intended or adapted for use on a road"—the words "mechanically propelled" are intended to have a very wide meaning and will cover any transmission of power from the engine to the wheels by mechanical means. Similar regulations are to be found throughout the EU, and if further evidence is needed as to just how vague the definition of "mechanically propelled" may be, one needs only to consider the arrest, in 1997, of a paraplegic Scandinavian who was arrested (and tried) for unsafe driving of his wheelchair.

In Section 192(1) of the RTA, the word "road" is defined as any highway and any other road to which the public has access and includes bridges over which a road passes. Public place is a question of fact for the court to determine. In English law, a car park attached to a public house was held, during opening hours, to be a public place as it was attached to a tavern that offered its services to all members of the public, whereas the same car park would not be regarded as a public place if it were attached to a private club *(28)*.

"In charge" is a question of fact, not law. As a general rule, the person remains in charge until he or she takes the vehicle off the road unless some intervening act occurs, e.g., handing keys to another person prevents him or her from retaining control. There is a statutory defense in that a person shall be deemed not to be in charge if he or she can prove that at the time, the circumstances were such that there was no likelihood of his or her driving the vehicle while the proportion of alcohol in the blood was over the prescribed limit. The fact that the driver was injured or that the vehicle was damaged may be disregarded by the court if it is put forward as a defense. The court is therefore entitled to consider what the position would have been had the defendant not been prevented from driving by damage or injury. Of course, the state must always prove that the defendant was actually driving the car. That may prove difficult if, as is the case in many accidents, there are no witnesses.

3.7.2. Breath Testing

Section 6(1) of the RTA conferred the power to require a breath test only to officers in uniform. The courts have already ruled against a challenge where the officer was not wearing his helmet *(29)*. In the United Kingdom the breath test may be taken either at or near the place where the officer makes a request for one. Normally, that would be at the roadside but not necessarily at the scene of the offense. If an accident occurs owing to the presence of a motor vehicle on a road or other public place, a police officer may require any person who he or she has reasonable cause to believe was driving or attempting to drive, or in charge of the vehicle at the time of the accident, to provide a specimen of breath for a breath test. The test may be taken at or near the place where the requirement was made or, if the police officer thinks fit, at a police station specified by the officer. In the United States, roadside breath testing, with nonevidentiary screening devices, is permitted only in "zero tolerance" states, with drivers under age 21 years.

In the United Kingdom, a person failing to provide a specimen of breath without reasonable excuse is guilty of an offense. A reasonable excuse would include someone who is physically or mentally unable to provide a sample, or if the act of providing the sample would, in some way entail risk to health. In most U.S. states, refusal to submit to a breath (or blood or urine) test is admissible as evidence in criminal proceedings, and, as a rule, leads to licence suspension, even if guilt is not proved in court. In some states, refusal is actually considered a separate crime. This somewhat strange situation comes about because most U.S. states, and most other countries, have *per se* laws for alcohol: an alcohol level above some preset limit is, by law, proof of intoxication *(30,31)*.

Section 6 of the RTA allows police officers to arrest a driver without a warrant if the breath test is positive, or if the driver fails or refuses to provide a specimen of breath, and the officer has reasonable cause to suspect alcohol in his or her body. Additionally, if an accident occurs owing to the presence of a motor vehicle on a road or public place, and a police officer reasonably suspects that the accident involved injury to another person, then for the purpose of requiring a breath test or arresting a person, the officer may enter (by force if need be) any place where that person is or where the officer reasonably suspects the person to be.

3.7.3. Hospital Procedure

In the United Kingdom, patients at a hospital do not have to produce a breath test or provide a specimen for a laboratory testing unless the practitioner in immediate charge of their case has been notified and does not object on the grounds that the requirement would be prejudicial to the proper care and treatment of the person. In the United Kingdom, but not in America, forensic blood samples cannot be taken from unconscious patients who are not able to give informed consent. After death, a coroner can order that the blood alcohol level be measured (remembering always that the value measured will be 14% lower than had serum or plasma been measured at a clinical laboratory). In the United States, when bodily harm has resulted, or when there is evidence of criminal activity (such as leaving the scene of an accident), then it is within the power of the officer to order that blood be drawn, even if the suspect is unwilling or unconscious.

3.7.4. Police Station Procedure

Police may require a suspect to provide either two breath samples, for analysis by means of an approved device, or a sample of blood or urine for laboratory testing. This is usually done at a police station, since it is almost unheard of for a hospital in the United Kingdom or the United States to be equipped with an evidentiary breath testing device. Blood or urine samples can only be collected at a police station or hospital. In the United Kingdom such a request cannot be made at a police station unless the constable making the requirement has reasonable cause to believe that, for medical reasons, a specimen of breath cannot be provided, or at the time the requirement is made, an approved breath analysis device is not available, or not practical to use, or that the suspected offense is one under Section 3A or 4 of the RTA, and the constable making the requirement has been advised by a doctor that the condition of the person might be due to some drug. This situation does not occur in the United States where, if appropriate staff are available, both blood and urine may be obtained at the police station.

In the United Kingdom, if a specimen other than breath is required police may demand either a urine or blood test. If blood cannot be obtained as, for example, might well be the case in a chronic intravenous drug abuser, then a urine sample must be provided within 1 hour of the request for its provision being made and after the provision of a previous specimen of urine. In the United States, urine specimens are generally not considered admissible proof of intoxication. A very large number of studies have shown that the ratio between blood alcohol and pooled urine is highly unreliable and unpredictable *(32,33)*. Ureteral urine, on the other hand, has an alcohol concentration 1.3 times greater than blood *(22)*. Collection of ureteral urine is often attempted at autopsy but, for obvious reasons, is not an option with living patients.

Breath samples can only be analyzed with approved devices. Those currently in use include the Camic Breath Analyser, Lion Intoximeter 3000, Lion Intoxilyzer 6000, and Drager Alcotest 7100 (Australia). Only officers trained to use the machine are allowed to carry out the intoximeter procedure, and the lower of two readings is taken. The subject must not have smoked for 10 minutes or have consumed alcohol or used a mouth spray or mouthwash, taken any medication, or consumed any food for 20 minutes before the breath test.

If the reading is below the prescribed limit of 35 μg of alcohol per 100 mL of breath, no action is taken unless impairment through drugs is suspected. If that is the case, a police surgeon should be called. If the level is between 36 and 39, no prosecution can occur unless there is impairment. If the level is between 40 and 50, the person is given the option of having the breath sample reading replaced by a specimen of blood or urine, but it is for the police officer to decide which, in accordance with Section 7 above. At levels over 51, the person is charged with an offense. Different rules and regulations, but with much the same intent, apply in other countries.

3.7.5. Blood Samples

It is wise to have a standardized routine for this procedure, if only to help prevent some of the technical defenses that are frequently raised in court. RTA blood alcohol kits are available with all the necessary equipment, and similar kits are sold in the United States, although their use is not mandatory. Whether or not a kit is used, appropriate chain of custody forms must be completed, and the record must reflect that alcohol-containing swabs were *not* used to cleanse the skin (actually, studies have shown that alcohol swabs contribute negligibly to the final result, but the issue is routinely raised in court) *(34)*.

The police officer should identify the doctor to the person, and the doctor should obtain witnessed informed consent. The physician must then determine whether there are any medical reasons why a sample of blood cannot be taken. It is for the doctor to decide where the sample of blood is taken from. The sample should be divided equally between the two bottles and shaken to disperse the preservative (an additional needle through the rubber membrane helps to equalize the pressure). The bottles should be labeled and placed in the secure containers and caps applied. The driver is allowed to retain one sample, which is placed in an envelope and sealed. The driver is then given a list of analysts.

Under U.S. law, blood may be taken even if the driver objects, providing the driver has been involved in an accident leading to injury, or a crime has been committed. Most U.S. states have statutes that excuse hemophiliacs and patients taking anticoagulants from blood testing *(21)*. Under British law, a police surgeon may make up to three unsuccessful attempts at taking blood before the driver can reasonably refuse to give blood on grounds that the defendant has lost confidence in the doctor. No such protection exists in U.S. law.

3.7.6. Section 4, RTA

The medical examination and procedure to be adopted when it is suspected that a person is unfit through drink or drugs will be considered later in this chapter under Section 4., Drugs and Driving.

3.8. Complex Defenses

Numerous technical defenses have been advocated over the years, and doctors should be aware of the most common. Failure to provide a sample of breath or blood will be considered separately.

3.8.1. Failure to Provide a Sample of Breath

Unless there is a reasonable excuse, failure to provide a specimen of breath, blood or urine is an offense under Section 7 of the RTA. In the United States, refusal leads to automatic licence suspension and, in some states, may actually constitute a separate crime; police are under an obligation to make sure that drivers are made aware of that fact. The motorist must understand the mandatory warning of prosecution if a specimen is not produced. Failure to understand, at least in the United Kingdom, is a reasonable excuse for the nonprovision of a sample *(35)*. The decision as to whether there is a medical reason not to supply a sample of breath is left to the police officer and is summarized in case law. There is no provision or requirement at that stage for a doctor to be summoned or to give an opinion.

Examples of medically acceptable reasons include mouth, lip, or facial injury, tracheotomy, rib injury, and neurologic problems; case law has stated that fear of AIDS not amounting to phobia *(36)*, shock *(37)*, and even intoxication *(38)* can, in certain circumstances, be regarded as reasonable excuses.

Many cases have been challenged on the basis that the person was unable to blow into the intoximeter due to respiratory problems. Research has now clarified some of these situations. Spirometry has shown that if a person has a forced expiratory volume in 1 second (FEV_1) of less than 2.0 L and a forced vital capacity (FVC) of less than 2.6 L, then that person would generally be unable to use a breath alcohol testing device *(39)*. A further study of healthy people of small stature (less than 166 cm tall) showed that if their FEV_1, FVC, and peak expiratory flow rate (PEFR) were greater than 2.31, 2.61, and 330 L/min, respectively, then they should be capable of supplying a suitable breath sample *(40)*. This paper was particularly useful as most police surgeons do not have access to spirometry but do have access to a simple peak flow reading in the custody situation.

A more recent study in Victoria, Australia showed that persons with an FEV_1 greater than 1.51 could provide an adequate screening sample on the Lion Alcolmeter SD2 roadside screening device *(41)* and that with an FEV_1 greater than 1.0 and FVC greater than 1.75 individuals were able to provide adequate samples on the Drager Alcotest 7110 (as used in Victoria) evidentiary breath testing machine.

In the future, it is likely that versions of software in the new Lion Intoxilyzer 6000 will have the capability of reporting both volume and flow rate of expired air during any unsuccessful attempt a subject may make in trying to provide a specimen of breath.

A recent fashionable defense is that the presence of a metal stud through a hole pierced in the tongue invalidates the breath alcohol test because of the prohibition against foreign substances in the mouth and because of the potential for the jewelery to retain alcohol and interfere with the breath test. However, experimental work has shown that the rates of elimination of mouth alcohol were no different in subjects with a tongue stud as opposed to controls and that for the purposes of breath alcohol testing, oral jewelery should be treated the same as metallic dental work and left in place without affecting the outcome of the breath test *(42)*.

3.8.2. Failure to Provide a Sample of Blood

First, there must be a definite request to provide a sample of blood. In Kuldip Singh Gill v. DPP *(43)*, it was held that a driver could not be convicted of failing to supply a specimen of blood or urine if he or she was not requested to do so. Where the sample of blood is taken from is solely the choice of the police surgeon (or, in the United States, the emergency room physician). In Solesbury v. Pugh *(44)*, the defendant was found guilty of failing to supply a specimen as he would only allow a sample to be taken from his big toe, which the doctor was not prepared to do.

It is reasonable for the person to request that his or her own doctor take the sample of blood, providing this does not delay the sample being taken *(45)*. In the United Kingdom, if the patient's own doctor and police surgeon are both present, the person can choose which doctor took the sample. Similar rules apply in the United States, where statutes generally spell out that financial responsibility for such services rests with the driver and not the state. In the United Kingdom, and probably in the United States as well, if a sample of blood is provided but the doctor spills the sample, then the law has been complied with on the basis that removal of the syringe from the vein by the doctor completes the provision of the specimen by the defendant *(46)*. In the United Kingdom a minimum of 2 mL of blood is required (the laboratory requires a minimum of 1 mL for analysis) for an adequate sample *(47)*. If less than this is obtained, the sample should be discarded and another one attempted or the police officer advised that there is a medical reason why a sample of blood should not be provided and the urine option can then selected. In the United States, minimum quantities are generally not written into statute. As indicated previously, alcohol swabs should not be used. In the early 1980s, one police force purchased and used swabs containing alcohol with the result that numerous convictions were later quashed *(48)*.

Probably the most common defense for failure to provide a sample of blood is that of needle phobia. If this is alleged, a full medical history should be obtained and enquiry made of whether the person has had blood tests before, whether ears or other parts of the body have been pierced, or whether there have been foreign travel immunizations or any other medical or dental procedure undertaken in which an injection may have been administered. Specific enquiry about the phobia should be made. British appellate judges *(49)* have stated that "no fear short of phobia recognized by medical science to be as strong and as inhibiting as, for instance, claustrophobia can be allowed to excuse failure to provide a specimen for a laboratory test, and in most if not all cases where the fear of providing it is claimed to be invincible the claim will have to be supported by medical evidence." Rix gives some very practical advice to police surgeons: be able to distinguish between repugnance and phobia, be able to distinguish between unwillingness and inability, document the history and examination with emphasis on the presence or absence of signs of anxiety, and be sure the decision is based on firm medical evidence *(50)*. Finally, record all this information, specifically note in the police record whether or not a medical condition has been identified, and then communicate this opinion to the police officers verbally *(50)*.

Another common defense is that of consuming alcohol after the offense—the hip flask defense *(51)*. It is used almost universally and is based on the fact that while it is unlawful to have an excessive blood alcohol concentration at the time of driving, it is *not* unlawful to have an elevated blood alcohol at the time of being tested. In the United Kingdom, Section 15(3) of the RTA allows for a driver to prove that he or she had imbibed alcohol after ceasing to drive and that the amount of such consumption was the sole reason for being over the legal limit or unfit to drive, at the time he or she gave a sample for analysis. It will be necessary for a scientist to prove that it was only the postdriving consumption that caused the analysis to reveal an alcohol level above the prescribed limit. The quantity of alcohol in the after-drink, the time of intake, and the age, sex, height, and body weight of the driver can all be used to calculate the theoretical expected blood alcohol concentration *(52)*. Backcalculations can only ever be approximate as they are based on average values and while they are reasonable estimates for most people, they may, on occasions, fail to reflect accurately the situation of a particular individual, regardless of whether the calculation is for pre- or postincident drinking.

3.8.3. Failure to Provide a Sample of Urine

If a woman is requested to provide a sample of urine, it is important to have a female officer present as it has been held that because of the embarrass-

Table 2
Top 10 Defense Challenges for Driving Under the Influence of Alcohol

1	Drinking after the offence - the hip flask defence
2	Laced drinks
3	Inhalation of ethanol vapours from the work environment
4	Pathological condition or trauma
5	Use of skin antiseptics containing ethanol
6	Alleged mix-up of blood specimens
7	Post-sampling formation of alcohols
8	Drug-alcohol interactions
9	Consumption of elixirs or health tonics containing alcohol
10	Infusion of blood or other liquids during surgical emergency treatment.

ment that it could involve, the refusal to supply a sample of urine could be regarded as a reasonable excuse *(53)*. However, any embarrassment at having to urinate in front of an officer of the same sex is not regarded as a reasonable excuse for not having supplied a specimen. Similar statutes apply in the United States. Methadone and other opiates are known to have an effect on the bladder sphincter and can thus cause delayed bladder emptying; this effect could be considered a reasonable excuse for failing to provide a urine sample *(54)*. In Sweden, Jones *(51)* reported the top ten defense challenges for driving under the influence of alcohol (Table 2). This situation may be subject to some change, since medications such as tolterodine (Detrusitol), and other muscarinic receptor antagonists are being increasingly prescribed for treatment of patients with symptoms of an unstable bladder. This may explain why California has already dropped urine from its list of testing options.

3.9. Postmortem Alcohol Measurements

This topic has recently been reviewed in depth by Pounder and Jones *(22)*. High postmortem alcohol concentrations do not imply that impairment was evident during life. Of 32 alcoholics presented at an emergency room for medical treatment, only 23 had apparent behavioral abnormalities, 6 were confused, and 3 were drowsy, even though the mean alcohol concentration was 313 mg/100 mL (range 180–450 mg/100 mL) *(55)*. Alcohol can be measured in a number of tissues, but the most accurate picture is usually obtained when multiple sites are sampled, e.g., vitreous, gastric contents, blood, and urine (particularly if ureteral urine is available) and the alcohol concentrations compared.

Since the eye is anatomically isolated, putrefaction is delayed, and there is little problem with postmortem redistribution, vitreous measurements can be used to confirm values obtained from whole blood and urine, to distinguish postmortem alcohol production from antemortem ingestion, and to determine whether blood alcohol concentrations were rising or falling at the time of death. Vitreous contains more water than blood so that the blood/vitreous alcohol ratio is less than 1. Ratios greater than 1 suggest that death occurred before equilibrium had been reached, i.e., blood alcohol was still rising *(56)*. Vitreous alcohol concentrations can be related to blood concentrations; however, there is so much intraindividual variation that extrapolation in an individual case is probably unwise and unsound scientifically.

As previously mentioned, serum and plasma contain more water than whole blood, and it follows that the alcohol content of the former will be 10–15% higher than the latter. Since postmortem measurements are made with whole blood, and since the water content of the cadaver begins to decrease almost immediately after death, estimating antemortem values with any precision is difficult, especially if only blood has been sampled. However, if samples from multiple sites are obtained, and vitreous, blood, and urine (urine as it is being formed contains 1.3 times as much alcohol as whole blood) are all analyzed, it may be possible to make a reasonable estimate of what the alcohol concentration was at the time of death *(22)*.

4. Drugs and Driving

4.1. The Problem

Increasing alcohol levels are associated with increased risk of accidents, but fatigue, drug abuse, and even the use of prescription medication can also increase risk *(57)*. The danger associated with sedatives and hypnotics is readily appreciated, but other drugs, such as anticholinergics, antidepressants, antihistamines, and antihypertensive medications may occasionally cause drowsiness. Patients should be warned about this and, after starting therapy, or after a significant change in dose, should avoid driving until it is known that unwanted effects do not occur *(58,59)*.

4.2. The Scale of the Problem

The size of the problem is not really known. In the United Kingdom in 1997, over 860,000 breath tests for alcohol were carried out with a refusal (presumed positive) rate of 12% (103,000) *(60)*. During that same period, the Forensic Science Service dealt with only 1850 drugs/driving submissions. In a 2-week period in August 1996, the Forensic Science Service received 270 blood specimens for testing for driving with excess alcohol. Further examination revealed that 18% contained one or more drugs and of those that fell below the legal alcohol limit, a further 18% were positive for drugs. If this 18% figure were applied to those 103,000 cases in 1997, over 18,000 cases would have been identified in which drivers had drugs in their body *(61)*.

In January 1998, the U.K. Department of Environment, Transport and the Regions published the findings of the first 15 months of a 3-year study into the incidence of drugs in road accident fatalities *(62)*. There were a total of 619 road user fatalities including drivers, riders of two-wheeled vehicles (21 of them cyclists), passengers in vehicles, and pedestrians; over 6% tested positive for medicinal drugs, 18% for illicit drugs (mainly cannabis), and 34% for alcohol.

In this study urine was tested by immunoassay for the following drugs: alcohol, amphetamines, methyl amphetamines (including ecstasy), cannabis, cocaine, opiates, methadone, LSD, benzodiazepines, and tricyclic antidepressants. The incidence of medicinal drugs likely to affect driving had not significantly changed from the 1985–87 study. However, illicit drug taking in drivers had increased sixfold in percentage terms, and there was a comparable increase among passengers. In addition, an increasing number had taken more than one illicit drug. In 1997 drugs were detected in approximately 90% of samples submitted to the U.K. Forensic Science Service for analysis (Table 3).

4.3. Effects of Different Drugs

The peak effect, half-life, duration of action, and times of detection of commonly taken drugs can be found in Appendix 7. The effects on driving of different drugs will now be considered.

4.3.1. Cannabis

Numerous studies have been undertaken to examine the effects of cannabis on driving. One large meta-analysis of over 150 studies showed that cannabis impairs the skills important for driving, including tracking, psychomotor skills, reaction time, and performance, with the effects most marked in the first 2 hours after smoking and with attention, tracking, and psychomotor skills being affected the most *(63)*. The study also showed that impairment is most marked in the absorption phase as opposed to the elimination phase, and that frequent cannabis users become less impaired than infrequent users. These are, for the most part, older studies, done during the 1970s. Impairment is dosage

Table 3
Type of Drug Detected in Samples Submitted to the FSS in 1997

Amphetamine	13%	Methyl Amphetamine	3%
Cannabis	28%	Cocaine	6%
Opiates	16%	Methadone	7%
Benzodiazepines	24%	Others	3%

dependent, and externally observable symptoms, e.g., impairment of psychomotor skills or the impression of absent-mindedness, disappear quickly during the early elimination phase. More recent studies *(64)* carried out with volunteer marijuana smokers who were actually driving found that the main effect of marijuana was to increase lateral movement of the vehicle moderately within the driving lane on a highway *(65,66)*.

4.3.2. Opiates

Single doses of narcotics can have marked effects on performance, such as reaction time. However, most studies of opiates among regular users suggest that they do not present a hazard or exist as a significant factor in driving. One study compared the effects of alcohol, diazepam, and methadone on clients commencing or stabilized on a methadone program. The battery of tests showed no evidence for an effect of the acute dose of methadone; thus clients on a methadone program should not be considered impaired in their ability to perform complex tasks such as driving a motor vehicle. Thus, in the United Kingdom, persons on a stable methadone program who have not abused other drugs for 1 year and who have clear urine drug screening tests on a regular basis are allowed a driving license subject to annual review. However, it should be remembered that users of heroin are also prone to heavy use of other psychoactive drugs, such as cocaine, alcohol, and tranquilizers, all dangerous when it comes to driving.

This problem is illustrated by a more recent study from Germany. Thirty-four methadone substitution patients, all of them volunteers, were subjected to a battery of psychological tests and the results compared with those of a control group. The methadone group ($n = 34$) consisted of 25 men and 9 women (age range 18–38 years). Urine samples of approximately two-thirds of the methadone patients tested positive for multiple drug use, the most frequent drug ($n = 14$) being cannabis. On psychological testing the methadone substitution patients achieved lower scores on almost all tests. Performance deficits were particularly conspicuous in sustained attention, sensori-motor coordination, and reaction capability. Deficits were minimal in the 12 methadone patients who were, in fact, taking only methadone. The authors conclude that under certain conditions, long-term methadone maintenance patients under strict medical supervision do not suffer significant driving impairment, providing that no other drugs have been taken.

4.3.3. Cocaine and Methamphetamine

Although the argument often goes unchallenged in court, all drugs do not, by definition, produce impairment. Even though some U.S. states define "being under the influence" as synonymous with the presence of any drug, some drugs do improve performance. In fact, low to moderate acute doses of cocaine and amphetamine can be expected to increase positive mood, energy, and alertness, especially in nontolerant individuals *(67)*. It has been known since World War II that use of d-amphetamine can increase the ability to sustain attention over prolonged periods when performing monotonous tasks. For that very reason, radar operators and pilots of both Allied and Japanese armies were issued supplies of amphetamine. Many of the performance tasks related to driving can be improved, at least in the laboratory, by treatment with stimulants *(68)*. Although the results of one retrospective autopsy study suggest that methamphetamine users seem more likely to be involved in traffic accidents *(69)*, the effects of stimulant drugs have never been tested on actual drivers, even in simulated conditions! It seems likely that abrupt discontinuation of either drug in a chronic user could result in driving impairment, but that situation has never been tested either *(65)*. Very large doses can result in toxic psychosis with symptoms indistinguishable from paranoid schizophrenia, a condition that is extremely unlikely to improve driving performance.

4.3.4. Sedative-Hypnotics

Benzodiazepines impair psychomotor performance in nontolerant individuals, generally in a dose dependent-manner. Most of the widely prescribed benzodiazepines increase lateral lane movement and slow response time to a lead car's change in speed. Several of the benzodiazepines (oxazepam 50 mg, flurazepam 30 mg, and lormetazepam 2 mg) predictably impair driving the morning after. Diazepam (15 mg) impaired performance on a clinical test for drunkenness, which comprised 13 tests assessing motor, vestibular, mental, and behavioral functioning *(70,71)*.

Acute doses of many benzodiazepines slow response time in simple or choice visual reaction time tests and impair attentional performance and cause deficits that are not due to sedation. In fact, the impairment of sustained attention and vigilance in benzodiazepine users seems to be the direct result of some, as yet uncharacterized, direct action on perceptual sensitivity *(65)*.

4.3.5. Multiple Drug Use

Polydrug use is common and can result in complex interactions, with the drugs having additive, antagonistic, or overlapping effects. Alcohol is commonly consumed in addition to abused drugs. In a study on alcohol and cannabis *(72)*, it has been shown that when they are administered together the result was one of additive impairment. In the laboratory, however, setting, simultaneous administration of alcohol and cocaine seems to minimize alcohol-related deficits *(68)*.

4.3.6. Antidepressants

There are many side effects associated with the use of the tricyclic antidepressants (TCAs), e.g., amitriptyline, that are relevant to the ability to drive, such as blurred vision, slow visual accommodation, disorientation, and eye-hand coordination; the most important are the induction of drowsiness, lethargy, and sedation. An analysis of 500 road traffic accidents showed that victims who had taken TCAs had a relative accident risk 2.2 times greater than non-TCA users and that patients using TCAs with a daily dose greater than or equivalent to amitriptyline 125 mg had a sixfold increase in road traffic crash risk *(73)*. The newer antidepressants drugs of the 5-HT re-uptake inhibitor class, e.g., fluoxetine, paroxetine or the selective serotonin and noradrenaline re-uptake inhibitors (venlafaxine, for example), have been shown to not generally affect driving performance and are safe for use by patients who drive *(74)*.

4.3.7. Over-the-Counter Preparations

An increasing number of drugs can now be bought over the counter from pharmacies. Many of these preparations, e.g., cough mixtures and decongestants, contain drugs that can cause sedation, particularly the older antihistamines, e.g., chlorpheniramine. The newer nonsedating antihistamines such as terfenadine and astemizole generally do not appear to impair driving. However, one study that measured driving performance across differing doses of terfenadine found that performance was impaired at very high doses (240 mg), stressing the need to establish the behavioral effects of drugs over a range of doses *(75)*. The second-generation group of antihistamines is less lipophilic than the previous generation and thus cross the blood–brain barrier less readily, which accounts for the lower levels of sedation observed with the newer drugs. Thus, while the second-generation antihistamines generally produce less sedation than first-generation compounds, if therapeutic doses are exceeded, the so-called non-sedating antihistamines become sedating and can impair driving.

4.4. Assessment in the Field by Police

In the United Kingdom, if a police officer stops a driver, for whatever reason, and feels the driver is unfit to drive, it is highly likely that a roadside breath test will be carried out. That is not the case in the United States, where field breath testing is only permitted in some states, and then only for drivers under the age of 21 *(21)*. The laws of the United States also prevent random breath testing. Under the Fourth Amendment, searches and seizures must be reasonable. Stopping a vehicle is a seizure, but it may be construed as reasonable if the police officer has a justifiable suspicion that an offense is being committed. The procedures American officers follow in Driving Under the Influence (DUI) cases are surprisingly similar to the procedures under the United Kingdom Section 4 RTA. To gain powers to carry out further tests, officers in most U.S. states first have to be satisfied that the driver is impaired. This then gives them the probable cause to carry out subsequent tests similar to the Section 4 procedure to prove impairment.

If breath testing is negative, impairment due to drugs or medical illness must be considered. In the United Kingdom, police traffic officers receive little or no training in the recognition of signs and symptoms of drug effects. However, a pilot study was carried out in England and Wales in 1999, whereby police officers were trained to perform roadside impairment tests; this study is currently being evaluated. This contrasts dramatically with the United States, where in 1979, the Drug Recognition Expert Program was introduced. Police officers were trained to observe and document known indicators of drug use and impairment.

Instead of breath testing, a series of Standardized Field Sobriety Tests, which include psychomotor and divided attention tests, is conducted. If alcohol is suspected, the following tests are carried out: Walk and Turn Test, One Leg Stand, and the Horizontal Gaze Nystagmus Test. In addition, if drugs are suspected, a Romberg Balance Test is also carried out. Unlike chemical tests (with refusal to submit possibly resulting in immediate licence suspension), drivers in the United States are not legally required to take any Field Sobriety Tests; if the driver submits, however, the results can be introduced as additional evidence of impairment.

These tests are all divided attention tests, which assesses the individual's balance and coordination as well as the ability to follow simple instructions, i.e., to divide attention between multiple tasks. They are as follows:

- Horizontal Gaze Nystagmus: nystagmus may be caused by any number of conditions, but its presence could indicate drugs or alcohol.
- Walk and Turn: nine steps heel to toe are taken in one direction, and then the individual turns and repeats the process in the other direction. Eight impairment

indicators are measured; if two of the eight are present, impairment would be indicated.
- One Leg Stand: the subject has to stand on alternate feet for 30 seconds while counting aloud. Failing two of the four recognized indicators would indicate impairment.
- Romberg Balance Test: the subject stands with eyes closed and estimates a period of 30 seconds during which body sway is estimated. Some drugs alter the body's internal clock and make the person act faster or slower than normal. The test allows for a tolerance of ±10 seconds.

If impairment is identified, and alcohol is suspected, the driver is breathalyzed and a similar procedure to the United Kingdom Section 5 RTA procedure is carried out. However if drugs are suspected, the police officer would call on a drug recognition expert (DRE) to carry out a more detailed examination.

The DRE will use a 12-step procedure as follows:

1. Breath alcohol test: this is carried out by the arresting officer; if the reading is not consistent with the degree of impairment, the DRE is called in.
2. Interview with the arresting officer: the purpose is to ascertain baseline information including the circumstances of the arrest, whether an accident occurred, whether drugs were found, and if so, what they looked like.
3. Preliminary examination: the purpose of the preliminary examination is to determine whether if there is sufficient reason to suspect a drug offense and to try to exclude any underlying medical problems. General observations and details of any current medical problems are ascertained, and the first measurement of the pulse is taken. If no signs of drug influence are found, the procedure is terminated; if any medical problems are found, a medical assessment is obtained and if drugs are still suspected, a full assessment is carried out. If at any time during the assessment a serious medical condition is suspected, a medical opinion will be obtained.
4. Eye examination: the driver is assessed for horizontal gaze nystagmus, vertical gaze nystagmus, and convergence.
5. Divided attention tests: once at a police station, the Romberg Balance Test, Walk and Turn Test, One Leg Stand Test, and Finger to Nose Test are carried out. These are all examples of divided attention tests whereby balance and movement tests are performed in addition to remembering instructions.
6. Vital signs examination: blood pressure, temperature, and a second recording of the pulse are carried out.
7. Darkroom examination: pupil size is measured in room light and then in near total darkness, using both indirect artificial light and direct light. The mouth and nose are also examined for evidence of drug use.
8. Muscle tone: limb tone is assessed as some drugs cause rigidity whereas others, e.g., alcohol, cause flaccidity.

9. Injection sites examination: the purpose is to seek evidence of intravenous or injection drug abuse. A third pulse reading is taken.
10. Interrogation: a structured interview about the use of drugs is carried out.
11. Opinion: based on all the previous assessments, the DRE forms an opinion as to drug impairment and also the type of drug causing the problem, the legal standard being a reasonable degree of certainty.
12. Toxicology testing: at the same time, samples are obtained for toxicologic examination, either a blood or urine sample being taken for analysis of common drugs.

Initial studies, suggesting very high sensitivity and specificity for DRE examination *(76)*, have not been confirmed in controlled laboratory studies. The results of the few studies that have been performed suggest that the accuracy of DRE assessment in general may not be sufficiently good to provide evidence in court fairly *(65,66)*. Several field studies have indicated that a DRE's opinions were confirmed by toxicologic analysis in 74–92% of cases when DREs concluded that suspects were impaired. However, published controlled trials, in which blood levels were measured before and during DRE examination, have shown that except in the case of alcohol, DRE assessment agreed with toxicology findings only 32–44% of the time.

There are other options for roadside screening tests. Both sweat and saliva have been used *(77)*. Devices are already available, and some have been approved by the U.S. Department of Transportation for the testing of commercial drivers. The mere detection of a drug does not prove impairment unless, of course, the jurisdiction has *per se* laws whereby the detection of drugs at some predetermined level is ruled, by law, to be proof of impairment.

4.5. Medical Examination Under Section 4, RTA

In the United Kingdom it is not necessary to prove impairment, as Section 7(3)(c) of the RTA states that "the suspected offence is one under Section 3A or 4 of this Act and the constable has been advised by a medical practitioner that the condition of the person required to provide the specimen *might* [author's emphasis] be due to some drug." It is for the court to decide whether the driver is unfit to drive on the evidence before it.

Whether the examination is carried out by a police surgeon in London, or an emergency room physician in San Francisco, the aim of the examination is to exclude any medical condition other than alcohol or drugs as the cause of the driver's behavior. The differential diagnosis is very wide and includes head injury, neurologic problems (e.g., epilepsy, stroke, cerebral tumour, multiple sclerosis), metabolic problems (e.g., hypoglycemia), hepatic or renal failure, and mental illness. The procedure should include introductory details, full medical history, and clinical examination. In Scotland, police surgeons use form F97. Appendix 8 contains a form that has been found useful. Similar forms are not available in the United States, but there is nothing to prevent any emergency department in the United States from drafting and providing a similar document. Even if no special form is provided, most of the relevant material will have been (or at least should be) recorded in the emergency department record.

4.5.1. Introductory Details

These should include the name, address, and date of birth of the driver and the name and number of the police officer as well as the place and date the examination took place and various times including time doctor contacted, time of arrival at police station/hospital, and time the examination commenced and ended.

The doctor will need to know brief details of the circumstances leading to arrest and the results of any field impairment tests that may have been carried out by the police officer. Informed consent should be obtained.

4.5.2. Full Medical History

Details of any current medical problems and details of recent events, particularly whether there was a road traffic accident that led to the event, should be recorded. Past medical history (with specific reference to diabetes, epilepsy, asthma, visual and hearing problems), past psychiatric history, and alcohol and drug consumption (prescribed, over the counter, and illicit) should be noted.

4.5.3. Clinical Examination

This should include general observations on demeanor and behavior, a note of any injuries, speech, condition of the mouth, hiccoughs, and any smell on the breath. The cardiovascular system should be examined and pulse, blood pressure, and temperature recorded. Signs of drug abuse should be looked for, e.g., needle marks. Examination of the eyes should include state of the sclera, state of the pupils including size, reaction to light, convergence, and the presence of both horizontal or vertical nystagmus.

A series of divided attention tests should be performed including the Romberg Test, Finger Nose Test, One Leg Stand Test, and Walk and Turn Test. The mental state should be assessed and a sample of handwriting obtained. Fitness for detention is of paramount importance, and any person who is not fit to be detained because of illness or injury should be transferred to hospital and not subjected to a Section 4 assessment. If the person refuses to consent to an examination it is prudent to make observations on his or her manner, possible unsteadiness, etc. and make written note of these.

At the end of the examination the doctor should decide whether there is a condition present that might be due to some drug. In the case of very short-acting drugs, the observations of the police officer or other witnesses can be of crucial importance. In a recent case a person was found guilty of driving while unfit through drugs on the basis of the officer's observations and the results and opinion of the toxicologist—the police surgeon was not called to give evidence *(78)*. Similarly, if the police officer reports that the person was swerving all over the road but the doctor later finds only minimal physical signs, this may be sufficient to indicate that a condition may be present due to some drug, e.g., cannabis, and that it is appropriate to proceed to the next part of the procedure.

The doctor should inform the police officer whether there is a condition present that might be due to a drug and if so, the police officer will then continue with the blood/urine option as in Section 5, previously described. Consent will need to be obtained for a blood specimen. On this occasion, 10 mL of blood should be taken and divided equally into two septum-capped vials as the laboratory requires a greater volume of blood for analysis because of the large number of drugs potentially affecting driving performance and their limited concentration in body fluids; indeed, if the driver declines the offer of a specimen, both samples should be sent.

References

1. Finucane, A. K. (1999) Legal aspects of epilepsy. *Neurol Clin.* **17,** 235–243.
2. Fitten, L. J. (1997) The demented driver: the doctor's dilemma. *Alzheimer Dis Assoc Disord.* **11 (suppl 1.),** 57–61.
3. Driver and Vehicle Licensing Agency (1998) *For Medical Practitioners: At a Glance Guide to the Current Medical Standards of Fitness to Drive.* Drivers Medical Unit. DVLA, Swansea.
4. Austroads (1998) *Assessing Fitness to Drive: Austroads Guidelines for Health Professionals and Their Legal Obligations. Austroads*, Sydney.
5. Osawa, M., Nagasawa, T., Yukawa, N., Nakajima, Y., Seto, Y., Ohki, T., et al. (1998) Sudden natural death in driving: case studies in the western area of Kanagawa. *Nippon Hoigaku Zasshi.* **52,** 315–318.
6. Cheng, L. H. and Whittington, R. M. (1998) Natural deaths while driving: would screening for risk be ethically justified? *J Med Ethics.* **24,** 248–251.
7. Belkic, K., Emdad, R., and Theorell, T. (1998) Occupational profile and cardiac risk: possible mechanisms and implications for professional drivers. *Int J Occup Med Environ Health.* **11,** 37–57.
8. Conti, J. B., Woodard, D. A., Tucker, K. J., Bryant, B., King, L. C., and Curtis, A. B. (1997) Modification of patient driving behavior after implantation of a cardioverter defibrillator. *Pacing Clin Electrophysiol.* **20 (9 Pt. 1),** 2200–2204.

9. Medical Research Council Antiepileptic Drug Withdrawal Study Group (1993) Prognostic index for recurrence of seizures after remission of epilepsy. *BMJ.* **306,** 1374–1378.
10. Krumholz, A. (1994) Driving and epilepsy: a historical perspective and review of current regulations. *Epilepsia.* **35,** 668–674.
11. MacLeod, K. M. (1999) Diabetes and driving: towards equitable, evidence-based decision-making. *Diabetes Med.* **16,** 282–290.
12. Ehrlich, E. N. (1991) Diabetes and the license to drive. *Wis Med J.* **90,** 115–118.
13. Distiller, L. A. and Kramer, B. D. (1996) Driving and diabetics on insulin therapy. *S Afr Med J.* **86 (8 suppl.),** 1018–1020.
14. Charman, W. N. (1997) Vision and driving—a literature review and commentary. *Ophthalmic Physiol Opt.* **17,** 371–391.
15. General Medical Council (1995) *Duties of a Doctor—Confidentiality. Guidance from the General Medical Council.* GMC, London.
16. Ellenhorn, M. J., et al. (1997) *Ellenhorn's Medical Toxicology: Diagnosis and Treatment of Human Poisoning.* Williams & Wilkins, Baltimore.
17. Jones, A. and Pounder, D. (1998) Measuring blood-alcohol concentration for clinical and forensic purposes. *Drug Abuse Handbook* (Karch, S., ed.), CRC Press, Boca Raton, pp. 327–356.
18. Noordzij, P. C. and Roszbach, R. (1987) Alcohol, drugs, and traffic safety, in T86: Proceedings of the 10th International Conference on Alcohol, Drugs, and Traffic Safety, Amsterdam, September 9–12, 1986. Excerpta Medica, New York.
19. Borkenstein, R. F. and Dale, A. (1964) The role of the drinking driver in traffic accidents. *Department of Police Administration, Indiana University,* Bloomington.
20. Allsop, R. (1996) Alcohol and road accidents: a discussion of the Grand Rapids study: *RRL 6 Crowthorne: Transport and Road Research Laboratory.*
21. California Code of Regulations (1999) Title 13, Motor Vehicles. State of California.
22. Pounder, D. and Jones, G. (1998) Measuring alcohol post-mortem, in *Drug Abuse Handbook* (Karch, S., ed.), CRC Press, Boca Raton, pp. 356–374.
23. Aberg, L. (1993) Behaviours and opinions of Swedish drivers before and after the 0.02% legal BAC limit of 1990, in T9: proceedings of the 12th International Conference on Alcohol, Drugs, and Traffic Safety; Cologne, 1992 (Utzelmann, H. D. and Berghaus, G., eds.).
24. Department of Environment, Transport and the Regions (1998) *Combating Drunk-Driving—Next Steps.* A Consultation Document. DETR, U.K.
25. Dunbar, J. A., Penttila, A., and Pikkarainen, J. (1987) Drinking and driving: success of random breath testing in Finland. *BMJ.* **295,** 101–103.
26. Marsden, A. (1996) Accidental injury and traffic medicine, in *Clinical Forensic Medicine* (McLay, W. D. S., ed.), Greenwich Medical Media, London, p. 231.
27. Coben, J. H. and Larkin, G. L. (199) Effectiveness of ignition interlock devices in reducing drunk driving recidivism. *Am J Prev Med.* **16(1 suppl.),** 81–87.
28. Pugh v Knipe. R.T.R. 286. 1972.
29. Wallwork v. Giles. 114 S.J. 36. 1969.

30. Krause, K. R., Howells, G. A., Bair, H. A., Bendick, P. J., and Glover, J. L. (1998) Prosecution and conviction of the injured intoxicated driver. *J Trauma.* **45,** 1069–1073.
31. McArthur, D. L. and Kraus, J. F. (1999) The specific deterrence of administrative per se laws in reducing drunk driving recidivism. *Am J Prev Med.* **16(1 suppl.),** 68–75.
32. Kaye, S. and Cardona, E. (1969) Errors of converting a urine alcohol value into a blood alcohol level. *Am J Clin Pathol.* **52,** 577–584.
33. Winek, C. L. and Esposito, F. M. (1981) Comparative study of ethanol levels in blood versus bone marrow, vitreous humor, bile and urine. *Forensic Sci Int.* **17,** 27–36.
34. Carter, P. G. and McConnell, A. A. (1990) Alcohol in drink driving swabs: does it make any difference? [letter]. *Med Sci Law.* **30,** 90.
35. Chief Constable of Avon and Somerset v. Singh. R.T.R. 107. 1988.
36. D.P.P. v Kinnersley. The Times, December 29 D.C. 1992.
37. D.P.P. v Pearman. R.T.R. 407. 1992.
38. Young v D.P.P. R.T.R. 328. 1992.
39. Gomm, P. J., Osselton, M. D., Broster, C. G., Johnson, N. M., and Upton, K. (1991) Study into the ability of patients with impaired lung function to use breath alcohol testing devices. *Med Sci Law.* **31,** 221–225.
40. Gomm, P. J., Broster, C. G., Johnson, N. M., and Hammond, K. (1993) Study into the ability of healthy people of small stature to satisfy the sampling requirements of breath alcohol testing instruments. *Med Sci Law.* **33,** 311–314.
41. Odell, M., McDonald, C., Farrar, J., Natsis, J. S., and Pretto, J. F. (1998) Breath testing in patients with respiratory disability. *J Clin Forensic Med.* **5,** 45–48.
42. Logan, B. K. and Gullberg, R. G. (1998) Lack of effect of tongue piercing on an evidential breath alcohol test. *J Forensic Sci.* **43,** 239–240.
43. Kuldip Singh Gill v D.P.P. January 16, 1995.
44. Solesbury v Pugh. 1 W.L.R. 1114. 1969.
45. Bayliss v. Thames Valley Police Chief Constable. (1978) Criminal Law Review. p. 363.
46. Beck v Watson. R.T.R. 91. 1980.
47. Robinson, S. P. (1996) Road traffic offences, in *Principles of Forensic Medicine* (Robinson, S. P., ed.), Greenwich Medical Media, London. Distributed worldwide by Oxford University Press, pp. 139–147.
48. R v Bolton JJ. Ex p Scally 1 Q.B. 537. 1991.
49. R v Harding. R.T.R. 325. 1974.
50. Rix, K. (1996) Blood or needle phobia as a defence under the Road Traffic Act of 1988. *J Clin Forensic Med.* **3,** 173–177.
51. Jones, A. W. (1991) Top ten defence challenges among drinking drivers in Sweden. *Med Sci Law.* **31,** 229–238.
52. Jones, A. and Logan, B. (1998) DUI defenses, in *Drug Abuse Handbook* (Karch, S., ed.), CRC Press, Boca Raton, pp. 1006–1046.
53. Rowland v. Thorpe. 3 All E.R. 195. 1970.

54. Acevedo, C. G., Tamayo, L., and Contreras, E. (1986) Effects of morphine in the isolated mouse urinary bladder. *Gen Pharmacol.* **17,** 449–452.
55. Davis, A. R. and Lipson, A. H. (1986) Central nervous system tolerance to high blood alcohol levels. *Med J Aust.* **144,** 9–12.
56. Felby, S. and Olsen, J. (1969) Comparative studies of postmortem ethyl alcohol in vitreous humor, blood, and muscle. *J Forensic Sci.* **14,** 93–101.
57. Seppala, T., Linnoila, M., and Mattila, M. J. (1979) Drugs, alcohol and driving. *Drugs.* **17,** 389–408.
58. Mattila, M. J., Vanakoski, J., Kalska, H., and Seppala, T. (1998) Effects of alcohol, zolpidem and some other sedatives and hypnotics on human performance and memory. *Pharmacol Biochem Behav.* **59,** 917–923.
59. Ramaekers, J. G. (1998) Behavioural toxicity of medicinal drugs. Practical consequences, incidence, management and avoidance. *Drug Saf.* **18,** 189–208.
60. Rowe, D. (1999) Personal communication. DETR.
61. Osselton, M. D., Owen, P., and Fysh, R. (1996) *Drugs and Driving*, Forensic Science Service Report No. TN816. Forensic Science Service. London, p. 3.
62. Department of the Environment, Transport, and the Regions (1998) *Press Notice 94/Transport.* DETR, February 11.
63. Berghaus, G., Scheer, N., and Schmidt, P. (1995) Effects of cannabis on psychomotor skills and driving performance—a meta-analysis of experimental studies, in T95 Proceedings of the 13th International Conference on Alcohol, Drugs, and Traffic Safety, Adelaide, 1994.
64. Chait, L. and Pierri, J. (1992) Effects of smoked marijuana on human performance: a critical review, in *Marijuana/Cannabinoids: Neurobiology and Neurophysiology* (Murphy, L. and Bartke, A., eds.), CRC Press, Boca Raton.
65. Heishman, S. and Karch, S. (2000) Drugs and driving, in *Encyclopaedia of Forensic Sciences* (Siegel, J., Saukko, P., and Knupfer, G., eds.), Academic Press, London.
66. Heishman, S. J., Singleton, E. G., and Crouch, D. J. (1998) Laboratory validation study of drug evaluation and classification program: alprazolam, d-amphetamine, codeine, and marijuana. *J Anal Toxicol.* **22,** 503–514.
67. Koelega, H. S. (1993) Stimulant drugs and vigilance performance: a review. *Psychopharmacology.* **111,** 1–16.
68. Farre, M., Llorente, M., Ugena, B., Lamas, X., and Cami, J. (1991) Interaction of cocaine with ethanol. *NIDA Res Monogr.* **105,** 570–571.
69. Logan, B. K. (1996) Methamphetamine and driving impairment. *J Forensic Sci.* **41,** 457–464.
70. O'Hanlon, J. F., Vermeeren, A., Uiterwijk, M. M., van Veggel, L. M., and Swijgman, H. F. (1995) Anxiolytics' effects on the actual driving performance of patients and healthy volunteers in a standardized test. An integration of three studies. *Neuropsychobiology.* **31,** 81–88.
71. Barbone, F., McMahon, A. D., Davey, P. G., Morris, A. D., Reid, I. C., McDevitt, D. G., et al. (1998) Association of road-traffic accidents with benzodiazepine use [see comments]. *Lancet.* **352,** 1331–1336.

72. Chesher, G. B., Dauncey, H., Crawford, J., and Horn, K. (1996) *The Interaction Between Alcohol and Marijuana.* Report to the Australian Federal Office of Road Safety. Department of Pharmacology, University of Sydney, Sydney.
73. Hindmarch, I. (1993) *Psychiatry in Practice* (Winter). pp. 23–25.
74. O'Hanlon, J. F., Robbe, H. W., Vermeeren, A., van Leeuwen, C., and Danjou, P. E. (1998) Venlafaxine's effects on healthy volunteers' driving, psychomotor, and vigilance performance during 15-day fixed and incremental dosing regimens. *J Clin Psychopharmacol.* **18,** 212–221.
75. Bhatti, J. Z. and Hindmarch, I. (1989) The effects of terfenadine with and without alcohol on an aspect of car driving performance. *Clin Exp Allergy.* **19,** 609–611.
76. Burns, M. and Adler, E. (1995) Study of a Drug Recognition Expert (DRE) program, in T95: Proceedings of the 13th International Conference on Alcohol, Drugs, Traffic Safety, Adelaide, 1994.
77. Kidwell, D. A., Holland, J. C., and Athanaselis, S. (1998) Testing for drugs of abuse in saliva and sweat. *J Chromatogr B Biomed Sci Appl.* **713,** 111–135.
78. Leetham v. D.P.P. Q.B. 488. 1998.

APPENDICES

From: *Forensic Science: A Physician's Guide to Clinical Forensic Medicine*
Edited by: M. M. Stark © Humana Press, Inc., Totowa, NJ

PREFACE

The attached appendices include international ethical documents and samples of forms used in clinical forensic practice as well as guidance notes on key topics.

The appendices contain useful information for a worldwide audience of physicians working in the field of clinical forensic medicine. They provide comparative data and are not meant to be exhaustive.

APPENDIX 1
ETHICAL DOCUMENTS

DOCUMENT 1

Code of Conduct for Law Enforcement Officials
(Adopted by the United Nations General Assembly, 17 December 1979)
G.A. res. 34/169, annex, 34 U.N. GAOR Supp. (No. 46) at 186, U.N. Doc. A/34/46 (1979)

Article 1

Law enforcement officials shall at all times fulfil the duty imposed upon them by law, by serving the community and by protecting all persons against illegal acts, consistent with the high degree of responsibility required by their profession.

Commentary:
(a) The term "law enforcement officials," includes all officers of the law, whether appointed or elected, who exercise police powers, especially the powers of arrest or detention.
(b) In countries where police powers are exercised by military authorities, whether uniformed or not, or by State security forces, the definition of law enforcement officials shall be regarded as including officers of such services.
(c) Service to the community is intended to include particularly the rendition of services of assistance to those members of the community who by reason of personal, economic, social or other emergencies are in need of immediate aid.
(d) This provision is intended to cover not only all violent, predatory and harmful acts, but extends to the full range of prohibitions under penal statutes. It extends to conduct by persons not capable of incurring criminal liability.

Article 2

In the performance of their duty, law enforcement officials shall respect and protect human dignity and maintain and uphold the human rights of all persons.

Commentary:
(a) The human rights in question are identified and protected by national and international law.
Among the relevant international instruments are the Universal Declaration of Human Rights, the International Covenant on Civil and Political Rights, the

Declaration on the Protection of All Persons from Being Subjected to Torture and Other Cruel, Inhuman or Degrading Treatment or Punishment, the United Nations Declaration on the Elimination of All Forms of Racial Discrimination, the International Convention on the Elimination of All Forms of Racial Discrimination, the International Convention on the Suppression and Punishment of the Crime of Apartheid, the Convention on the Prevention and Punishment of the Crime of Genocide, the Standard Minimum Rules for the Treatment of Prisoners and the Vienna Convention on Consular Relations.
(b) National commentaries to this provision should indicate regional or national provisions identifying and protecting these rights.

Article 3

Law enforcement officials may use force only when strictly necessary and to the extent required for the performance of their duty.

Commentary:
(a) This provision emphasizes that the use of force by law enforcement officials should be exceptional; while it implies that law enforcement officials may be authorized to use force as is reasonably necessary under the circumstances for the prevention of crime or in effecting or assisting in the lawful arrest of offenders or suspected offenders, no force going beyond that may be used.
(b) National law ordinarily restricts the use of force by law enforcement officials in accordance with a principle of proportionality. It is to be understood that such national principles of proportionality are to be respected in the interpretation of this provision. In no case should this provision be interpreted to authorize the use of force which is disproportionate to the legitimate objective to be achieved.
(c) The use of firearms is considered an extreme measure. Every effort should be made to exclude the use of firearms, especially against children. In general, firearms should not be used except when a suspected offender offers armed resistance or otherwise jeopardizes the lives of others and less extreme measures are not sufficient to restrain or apprehend the suspected offender. In every instance in which a firearm is discharged, a report should be made promptly to the competent authorities.

Article 4

Matters of a confidential nature in the possession of law enforcement officials shall be kept confidential, unless the performance of duty or the needs of justice strictly require otherwise.

Commentary:
By the nature of their duties, law enforcement officials obtain information which may relate to private lives or be potentially harmful to the interests, and especially the reputation, of others. Great care should be exercised in safeguarding and using such information, which should be disclosed only in the performance of duty or to serve the needs of justice. Any disclosure of such information for other purposes is wholly improper.

Article 5

No law enforcement official may inflict, instigate or tolerate any act of torture or other cruel, inhuman or degrading treatment or punishment, nor may any law enforcement official invoke superior orders or exceptional circumstances such as a state of war or a threat of war, a threat to national security, internal political instability or any other public emergency as a justification of torture or other cruel, inhuman or degrading treatment or punishment.

Commentary:
(a) This prohibition derives from the Declaration on the Protection of All Persons from Being Subjected to Torture and Other Cruel, Inhuman or Degrading Treatment or Punishment, adopted by the General Assembly, according to which: "[Such an act is] an offense to human dignity and shall be condemned as a denial of the purposes of the Charter of the United Nations and as a violation of the human rights and fundamental freedoms proclaimed in the Universal Declaration of Human Rights [and other international human rights instruments]."
(b) The Declaration defines torture as follows:
". . . torture means any act by which severe pain or suffering, whether physical or mental, is intentionally inflicted by or at the instigation of a public official on a person for such purposes as obtaining from him or a third person information or confession, punishing him for an act he has committed or is suspected of having committed, or intimidating him or other persons. It does not include pain or suffering arising only from, inherent in or incidental to, lawful sanctions to the extent consistent with the Standard Minimum Rules for the Treatment of Prisoners."
(c) The term "cruel, inhuman or degrading treatment or punishment" has not been defined by the General Assembly but should be interpreted so as to extend the widest possible protection against abuses, whether physical or mental.

Article 6

Law enforcement officials shall ensure the full protection of the health of persons in their custody and, in particular, shall take immediate action to secure medical attention whenever required.

Commentary:
(a) "Medical attention," which refers to services rendered by any medical personnel, including certified medical practitioners and paramedics, shall be secured when needed or requested.
(b) While the medical personnel are likely to be attached to the law enforcement operation, law enforcement officials must take into account the judgement of such personnel when they recommend providing the person in custody with appropriate treatment through, or in consultation with, medical personnel from outside the law enforcement operation.
(c) It is understood that law enforcement officials shall also secure medical attention for victims of violations of law or of accidents occurring in the course of violations of law.

Article 7

Law enforcement officials shall not commit any act of corruption. They shall also rigorously oppose and combat all such acts.

Commentary:
(a) Any act of corruption, in the same way as any other abuse of authority, is incompatible with the profession of law enforcement officials. The law must be enforced fully with respect to any law enforcement official who commits an act of corruption, as Governments cannot expect to enforce the law among their citizens if they cannot, or will not, enforce the law against their own agents and within their agencies.
(b) While the definition of corruption must be subject to national law, it should be understood to encompass the commission or omission of an act in the performance of or in connection with one's duties, in response to gifts, promises or incentives demanded or accepted, or the wrongful receipt of these once the act has been committed or omitted.
(c) The expression "act of corruption" referred to above should be understood to encompass attempted corruption.

Article 8

Law enforcement officials shall respect the law and the present Code. They shall also, to the best of their capability, prevent and rigorously oppose any violations of them. Law enforcement officials who have reason to believe that a violation of the present Code has occurred or is about to occur shall report the matter to their superior authorities and, where necessary, to other appropriate authorities or organs vested with reviewing or remedial power.

Commentary:

(a) This Code shall be observed whenever it has been incorporated into national legislation or practice. If legislation or practice contains stricter provisions than those of the present Code, those stricter provisions shall be observed.

(b) The article seeks to preserve the balance between the need for internal discipline of the agency on which public safety is largely dependent, on the one hand, and the need for dealing with violations of basic human rights, on the other. Law enforcement officials shall report violations within the chain of command and take other lawful action outside the chain of command only when no other remedies are available or effective. It is understood that law enforcement officials shall not suffer administrative or other penalties because they have reported that a violation of this Code has occurred or is about to occur.

(c) The term "appropriate authorities or organs vested with reviewing or remedial power" refers to any authority or organ existing under national law, whether internal to the law enforcement agency or independent thereof, with statutory, customary or other power to review grievances and complaints arising out of violations within the purview of this Code.

(d) In some countries, the mass media may be regarded as performing complaint review functions similar to those described in subparagraph (c) above. Law enforcement officials may, therefore, be justified if, as a last resort and in accordance with the laws and customs of their own countries and with the provisions of article 4 of the present Code, they bring violations to the attention of public opinion through the mass media.

(e) Law enforcement officials who comply with the provisions of this Code deserve the respect, the full support and the cooperation of the community and of the law enforcement agency in which they serve, as well as the law enforcement profession.

Document 2

Declaration on the Police
(extract from Resolution 690 of the Parliamentary Assembly of the Council of Europe, 1979)

The Assembly

1. Considering that the full exercise of human rights and fundamental freedoms, guaranteed by the European Convention on Human Rights and other national and international instruments, has as a necessary basis the existence of a peaceful society which enjoys the advantages of order and public safety;
2. Considering that, in this respect, police play a vital role in all the member states, that they are frequently called upon to intervene in conditions which are dangerous for their members, and that their duties are made yet more difficult if the rules of conduct of their members are not sufficiently precisely defined;
3. Being of the opinion that it is inappropriate for those who have committed violations of human rights whilst members of police forces, or those who have belonged to any police force that has been disbanded on account of inhumane practices, to be employed as policemen;
4. Being of the opinion that the European system for the protection of human rights would be improved if there were generally accepted rules concerning the professional ethics of the police which take account of the principles of human rights and fundamental freedoms;
5. Considering that it is desirable that police officers have the active moral and physical support of the community they are serving;
6. Considering that police officers should enjoy status and rights comparable to those of members of the civil service;
7. Believing that it may be desirable to lay down guidelines for the behavior of police officers in case of war and other emergency situations, and in the event of occupation by a foreign power;
8. Adopts the following Declaration on the Police, which forms an integral part of this resolution;
9. Instructs its Committee on Parliamentary and Public Relations and its Legal Affairs Committee as well as the Secretary General of the Council of Europe to give maximum publicity to the declaration.

Appendix
Declaration on the Police

Ethics

1. A police officer shall fulfil the duties the law imposes upon him by protecting his fellow citizens and the community against violent, predatory and other harmful acts, as defined by law.

2. A police officer shall act with integrity, impartiality and dignity. In particular he shall refrain from and vigorously oppose all acts of corruption.
3. Summary executions, torture and other forms of inhuman or degrading treatment or punishment remain prohibited in all circumstances. A police officer is under an obligation to disobey or disregard any order or instruction involving such measures.
4. A police officer shall carry out orders properly issued by his hierarchical superior, but he shall refrain from carrying out any order he knows, or ought to know, is unlawful.
5. A police officer must oppose violations of the law. If immediate or irreparable and serious harm should result from permitting the violation to take place he shall take immediate action, to the best of his ability.
6. If no immediate or irreparable and serious harm is threatened, he must endeavour to avert the consequences of this violation, or its repetition, by reporting the matter to his superiors. If no results are obtained in that way he may report to higher authority.
7. No criminal or disciplinary action shall be taken against a police officer who has refused to carry out an unlawful order.
8. A police officer shall not cooperate in the tracing, arresting, guarding or conveying of persons who, while not being suspected of having committed an illegal act, are searched for, detained or prosecuted because of their race, religion or political belief.
9. A police officer shall be personally liable for his own acts and for acts of commission or omission he has ordered and which are unlawful.
10. There shall be a clear chain of command. It should always be possible to determine which superior may be ultimately responsible for acts or omissions of a police officer.
11. Legislation must provide for a system of legal guarantees and remedies against any damage resulting from police activities.
12. In performing his duties, a police officer shall use all necessary determination to achieve an aim which is legally required or allowed, but he may never use more force than is reasonable.
13. Police officers shall receive clear and precise instructions as to the manner and circumstances in which they should make use of arms.
14. A police officer having the custody of a person needing medical attention shall secure such attention by medical personnel and, if necessary, take measures for the preservation of the life and health of this person. He shall follow the instructions of doctors and other competent medical workers when they place a detainee under medical care.
15. A police officer shall keep secret all matters of a confidential nature coming to his attention, unless the performance of duty or legal provisions require otherwise.
16. A police officer who complies with the provisions of this declaration is entitled to the active moral and physical support of the community he is serving.

Document 3

Declaration of Tokyo
Guidelines for Medical Doctors concerning Torture and Other Cruel, Inhuman or Degrading Treatment or Punishment in relation to Detention and Imprisonment
(Adopted by the 29th World Medical Assembly, Tokyo, Japan, October 1975)

Preamble

It is the privilege of the medical doctor to practise medicine in the service of humanity, to preserve and restore bodily and mental health without distinction as to persons, to comfort and to ease the suffering of his or her patients. The utmost respect for human life is to be maintained even under threat, and no use made of any medical knowledge contrary to the laws of humanity.
For the purpose of this Declaration, torture is defined as the deliberate, systematic or wanton infliction of physical or mental suffering by one or more persons acting alone or on the orders of any authority, to force another person to yield information, to make a confession, or for any other reason.

Declaration

The doctor shall not countenance, condone or participate in the practice of torture or other forms of cruel, inhuman or degrading procedures, whatever the offence of which the victim of such procedure is suspected, accused or guilty, and whatever the victim's belief or motives, and in all situations, including armed conflict and civil strife.

The doctor shall not provide any premises, instruments, substances or knowledge to facilitate the practice of torture or other forms of cruel, inhuman or degrading treatment or to diminish the ability of the victim to resist such treatment.

The doctor shall not be present during any procedure during which torture or other forms of cruel, inhuman or degrading treatment are used or threatened.

A doctor must have complete clinical independence in deciding upon the care of a person for whom he or she is medically responsible. The doctor's fundamental role is to alleviate the distress of his or her fellow men, and no motive whether personal, collective or political shall prevail against this higher purpose.

Where a prisoner refuses nourishment and is considered by the doctor as capable of forming an unimpaired and rational judgement concerning the consequences of such voluntary refusal of nourishment, he or she shall not be fed artificially. The decision as to the capacity of the prisoner to form such a judgement should be confirmed by at least one other independent doctor. The consequences of the refusal of nourishment shall be explained by the doctor to the prisoner.

The World Medical Association will support, and should encourage the international community, the national medical associations and fellow doctors to support the doctor and his or her family in the face of threats or reprisals resulting from a refusal to condone the use of torture or other forms of cruel, inhuman or degrading treatment.

Document 4

Principles of Medical Ethics Relevant to the Role of Health Personnel, Particularly Physicians, in the Protection of Prisoners and Detainees against Torture and Other Cruel, Inhuman or Degrading Treatment or Punishment
G.A. res. 37/194, annex, 37 U.N. GAOR Supp. (No. 51) at 211, U.N. Doc. A/37/51 (1982)

Principle 1

Health personnel, particularly physicians, charged with the medical care of prisoners and detainees have a duty to provide them with protection of their physical and mental health and treatment of disease of the same quality and standard as is afforded to those who are not imprisoned or detained.

Principle 2

It is a gross contravention of medical ethics, as well as an offence under applicable international instruments, for health personnel, particularly physicians, to engage, actively or passively, in acts which constitute participation in, complicity in, incitement to or attempts to commit torture or other cruel, inhuman or degrading treatment or punishment.

Principle 3

It is a contravention of medical ethics for health personnel, particularly physicians, to be involved in any professional relationship with prisoners or detainees the purpose of which is not solely to evaluate, protect or improve their physical and mental health.

Principle 4

It is a contravention of medical ethics for health personnel, particularly physicians:

(a) To apply their knowledge and skills in order to assist in the interrogation of prisoners and detainees in a manner that may adversely affect the physical or mental health or condition of such prisoners or detainees and which is not in accordance with the relevant international instruments;

(b) To certify, or to participate in the certification of, the fitness of prisoners or detainees for any form of treatment or punishment that may adversely affect their physical or mental health and which is not in accordance with the relevant international instruments, or to participate in any way in the infliction of any such treatment or punishment which is not in accordance with the relevant international instruments.

Principle 5

It is a contravention of medical ethics for health personnel, particularly physicians, to participate in any procedure for restraining a prisoner or detainee unless such a procedure is determined in accordance with purely medical criteria as being necessary for the protection of the physical or mental health or the safety of the prisoner or detainee himself, of his fellow prisoners or detainees, or of his guardians, and presents no hazard to his physical or mental health.

Principle 6

There may be no derogation from the foregoing principles on any ground whatsoever, including public emergency.

Document 5

The Nurse's Role in the Care of Detainees and Prisoners
(International Council of Nurses, 1975)

At the meeting of the Council of National Representatives of the International Council of Nurses in Singapore in August 1975, a statement on the role of the nurse in the care of detainees and prisoners was adopted. The text, last reviewed in 1991, is as follows:

The International Council of Nurses (ICN) Code for Nurses[1] states that:

1. The fundamental responsibility of the nurse is fourfold: to promote health, to prevent illness, to restore health and to alleviate suffering.
2. The nurse's primary responsibility is to those people who require nursing care.
3. The nurse when acting in a professional capacity should at all times maintain standards of personal conduct which reflect credit upon the profession.
4. The nurse takes appropriate action to safeguard the individual when his care is endangered by a co-worker or any other person.

ICN has reaffirmed its support of the Geneva Conventions of 1949[2], and the additional protocols, which state that, in case of armed conflict of international as well as national character (i.e. internal disorders, civil wars, armed rebellions):

1. Members of the armed forces, prisoners and persons taking no active part in the hostilities
   a) shall be entitled to protection and care if wounded or sick,
   b) shall be treated humanely, that is:
      - they may not be subjected to physical mutilation or to medical or scientific experiments of any kind which are not justified by the medical, dental or hospital treatment of the prisoner concerned and carried out in his interest;
      - they shall not be wilfully left without medical assistance and care, nor shall conditions exposing them to contagion or infection be created;
      - they shall be treated humanely and cared for by the party in conflict in whose power they may be, without adverse distinction founded on sex, race, nationality, religion, political opinion or any other similar criteria.

---

[1]International Council of Nurses, Code for Nurses, Geneva, ICN, Adopted 1973, Reaffirmed in 1989.

[2]International Committee of the Red Cross, Rights and Duties of Nurses under the Geneva Convention of August 12, 1949, Geneva, ICRC, 1970.

2. The following acts are and shall remain prohibited at any time and in any place whatsoever with respect to the above mentioned persons:
   a) violence to life and person, in particular murder of all kinds, mutilation, cruel treatment and torture;
   b) outrages upon personal dignity, in particular humiliating and degrading treatment.

ICN has endorsed the United Nations Universal Declaration of Human Rights[3] and, hence, accepted that:

i) Everyone is entitled to all the rights and freedoms, set forth in this Declaration, without distinction of any kind, such as race, colour, sex, language, religion, political or other opinion, national or social origin, property, birth or other status (Art. 2),

ii) No one shall be subjected to torture or to cruel, inhuman or degrading treatment or punishment (Art. 5).

In relation to detainees and prisoners of conscience, interrogation procedures are increasingly being employed resulting in ill effects, often permanent, on the person's mental and physical health. ICN condemns the use of all such procedures harmful to the mental and physical health of prisoners and detainees.

Nurses having knowledge of physical or mental ill-treatment of detainees and prisoners must take appropriate action including reporting the matter to appropriate national and/or international bodies.

Nurses employed in prison health services do not assume functions of prison security personnel, such as body search for prison security reasons.

Nurses participate in clinical research carried out on prisoners only if the freely given consent of the patient has been secured after a complete explanation and understanding by the patient of the nature and risk of the research.

The nurse's first responsibility is towards the patients, notwithstanding considerations of national security and interest.

[3]United Nations Universal Declaration of Human Rights, United Nations, Adopted 10 December 1948.

Document 6

Relevant Articles of the European Convention on Human Rights

Article 2

1. Everyone's right to life shall be protected by law. No one shall be deprived of his life intentionally save in the execution of a sentence of a court following his conviction of a crime for which this penalty is provided by law.
2. Deprivation of life shall not be regarded as inflicted in contravention of this article when it results from the use of force which is no more than absolutely necessary:
   (a) in defence of any person from unlawful violence;
   (b) in order to effect a lawful arrest or to prevent the escape of a person lawfully detained;
   (c) in action lawfully taken for the purpose of quelling a riot or insurrection.

Article 3

No one shall be subjected to torture or to inhuman or degrading treatment or punishment.

Article 5

1. Everyone has the right to liberty and security of person. No one shall be deprived of his liberty save in the following cases and in accordance with a procedure prescribed by law:
   (a) the lawful detention of a person after conviction by a competent court;
   (b) the lawful arrest or detention of a person for non-compliance with the lawful order of a court or in order to secure the fulfilment of any obligation prescribed by law;
   (c) the lawful arrest or detention of a person effected for the purpose of bringing him before the competent legal authority on reasonable suspicion of having committed an offence or when it is reasonably considered necessary to prevent his committing an offence or fleeing after having done so;
   (d) the detention of a minor by lawful order for the purpose of educational supervision or his lawful detention for the purpose of bringing him before the competent legal authority;
   (e) the lawful detention of persons for the prevention of the spreading of infectious diseases, of persons of unsound mind, alcoholics or drug addicts or vagrants;
   (f) the lawful arrest or detention of a person to prevent his effecting an unauthorised entry into the country or of a person against whom action is being taken with a view to deportation or extradition.
2. Everyone who is arrested shall be informed promptly, in a language which he understands, of the reasons for his arrest and of any charge against him.

3. Everyone arrested or detained in accordance with the provisions of paragraph 1(c) of this article shall be brought promptly before a judge or other officer authorised by law to exercise judicial power and shall be entitled to trial within a reasonable time or to release pending trial. Release may be conditioned by guarantees to appear for trial.
4. Everyone who is deprived of his liberty by arrest or detention shall be entitled to take proceedings by which the lawfulness of his detention shall be decided speedily by a court and his release ordered if the detention is not lawful.
5. Everyone who has been the victim of arrest or detention in contravention of the provisions of this article shall have an enforceable right to compensation.

Article 6

1. In the determination of his civil rights and obligations or of any criminal charge against him, everyone is entitled to a fair and public hearing within a reasonable time by an independent and impartial tribunal established by law. Judgment shall be pronounced publicly but the press and public may be excluded from all or part of the trial in the interests of morals, public order or national security in a democratic society, where the interests of juveniles or the protection of the private life of the parties so require, or to the extent strictly necessary in the opinion of the court in special circumstances where publicity would prejudice the interests of justice.
2. Everyone charged with a criminal offence shall be presumed innocent until proved guilty according to law.
3. Everyone charged with a criminal offence has the following minimum rights:
   (a) to be informed promptly, in a language which he understands and in detail, of the nature and cause of the accusation against him;
   (b) to have adequate time and facilities for the preparation of his defence;
   (c) to defend himself in person or through legal assistance of his own choosing or, if he has not sufficient means to pay for legal assistance, to be given it free when the interests of justice so require;
   (d) to examine or have examined witnesses against him and to obtain the attendance and examination of witnesses on his behalf under the same conditions as witnesses against him;
   (e) to have the free assistance of an interpreter if he cannot understand or speak the language used in court.

Article 7

1. No one shall be held guilty of any criminal offence on account of any act or omission which did not constitute a criminal offence under national or international law at the time when it was committed. Nor shall a heavier penalty be imposed than the one that was applicable at the time the criminal offence was committed.

2. This article shall not prejudice the trial and punishment of any person for any act or omission which, at the time when it was committed, was criminal according to the general principles of law recognised by civilized nations.

Article 8

1. Everyone has the right to respect for his private and family life, his home and his correspondence.
2. There shall be no interference by a public authority with the exercise of this right except such as in accordance with the law and is necessary in a democratic society in the interests of national security, public safety or the economic wellbeing of the country, for the prevention of health or morals, or for the protection of the right and freedoms of others.

APPENDIX 2
GUIDANCE NOTES ON STATUTORY PROVISIONS GOVERNING ACCESS TO HEALTH RECORDS

Data Protection Act 1998

The 1998 Act replaces the 1984 Act, making some important changes including extending the provisions of the Act to "relevant filing systems," whether manual (paper-based) or computerized. The 1998 Act, when fully in force, will regulate the processing, use, and storage of information relating to individuals including the obtaining, holding, use, or disclosure of such information, which is "being processed by means of equipment operating automatically in response to instructions given for that purpose" (that is, data held on computers). It will give them rights of access to personal data and to know how they are stored and processed. All those who control data (that is, determine the purposes for which data are stored and the manner in which data are processed) must comply with the provisions of the Act. Comparable provisions extend throughout the European Union, giving effect to the Data Protection Principles.[1]

The individual whose data is stored has rights of access to check what is held and to require correction of inaccurate information. Those who suffer financial loss as a consequence of inaccurate information can seek compensation. Those who operate the data systems (and this may include doctors who use computers to record information about patients) must ensure that they comply with the provisions of the legislation, including the rights of data subjects to have access to personal data.

There are exceptions for the processing of sensitive personal data (as defined in section 2 of the Act) for medical purposes by a health professional (as defined in section 69). Medical purposes include the provision of preventative medicine, medical diagnosis, medical research, the provision of care and treatment, and the management of health care services. Readers are referred to texts on the provisions of the Act for a more detailed exposition of its provisions and ramifications.

---

[1]Schedule 1, Part 1 of the Data Protection Act 1998

Access to Medical Reports Act 1988

This Act, not to be confused with the Access to Health Records Act (see below), gave individuals a new right of access to any medical report prepared for insurance or employment purposes by a doctor "who is or has been responsible for the patient's care" provided that allowing the individual to see the report will not endanger his or her health or disclose information about another person who is not a health professional. If access is denied on this ground the individual has a right of challenge in the county court (England and Wales) or Sheriff's court (Scotland).

Individuals who exercise their right of access but dispute the content of the report may request amendments. If these are not agreed to by the doctor, the individual may either refuse to allow the report to be despatched or may request that it be accompanied by a statement prepared by the individual.

The statute applies only to reports prepared by a doctor who is or has been responsible for the care of the patient and not to an independent occupational physician who has not provided care. Where the doctor occupies a dual role (e.g., as both general practitioner and as part-time occupational physician or insurance medical examiner), the provisions of the Act do apply.

Access to Health Records Act 1990

The 1984 Data Protection Act gave patients a new right of access to data (including health data) held about them on computers but no right of access to manual records. The 1990 Act made prospective provision for a right of access to health records made on or after November 1, 1991. Health record is given a very wide definition and covers entries made by any health professional (as defined now in section 69 of the Data Protection Act 1998). A health record is any record consisting of information relating to the physical or mental health of an individual who can be identified from that information, or from that and other information in possession of the holder of the record and has been made by or on behalf of the health professional in connection with the care of that individual. Health professionals are widely defined and cover just about everyone from registered medical practitioners to "music therapists employed by a health service body."

Applications to see health records may be made by a patient or by anyone authorized by the patient, a parent, or guardian in the case of a child and by certain other defined persons or officials and are made to the record holder in writing. There is a 21-day time limit for disclosure of records made within the previous 40 days and a 40-day time limit for records made more than 40 days previously. A fee may be charged for access and a charge made for photocopies requested by the applicant.

Applications for access may be denied if disclosure of the record is likely to cause serious harm to the physical or mental health of the patient or if access would reveal information about another identifiable individual other than a health professional (e.g., a documented family history). Access to records of a deceased patient may be denied if the record holder believes that the information was provided or obtained from the patient in the expectation that it would not be disclosed to the applicant.

If, following disclosure, the applicant disputes the content of the record, he or she may ask the record holder to amend the record. If the record holder is content to make the amendment, it may be effected immediately; if not, the applicant may request that his objection be noted in the same part of the health record.

In the case of any dispute about access or amendments to the record that cannot be resolved between the applicant and the record holder, the matter may be resolved by application to the courts.

Human Rights Act 1998

This Act, which received royal assent in November 1998, will have a most profound impact on the rights of the individual in European Community member states and on the interpretation of U.K. statute law (*see* Appendix 1 for relevant Articles). It will come into effect at some future date (unknown at the time of writing), and the Act will give effect to rights and freedoms guaranteed under the European Convention on Human Rights. U.K. primary and subordinate legislation "so far as it is possible to do so . . . must be read and given effect in a way which is compatible with the Convention rights." When the Act is in force, by section 19, "A Minister of the Crown in charge of a Bill in either House of Parliament must, before second reading of the Bill—(a) make a statement to the effect that in his view the provisions of the Bill are compatible with the Convention Rights" or must make clear that he or she cannot make such a statement but wishes in any event to proceed with the Bill. It will assuredly have a far-reaching and wide-ranging impact on U.K. law and practice.

APPENDIX 3
MANAGEMENT OF HEAD-INJURED DETAINEES

Glasgow Coma Scale

Symptom	Score
Eye opening	
Spontaneous	4
To speech	3
To painful stimulus	2
None	1
Best motor response	
Obeys commands	6
Localizes painful stimulus	5
Withdraws (normal flexion)	4
Flexes abnormally (spastic flexion)	3
Extension	2
No response	1
Best verbal response	
Orientated	5
Confused	4
Says inappropriate words	3
Makes incomprehensible sounds	2
No verbal response	1
Maximum	15

Reproduced from Jennett, B., and Teasdale, G. (1997) Aspects of coma after severe head injury. *Lancet.* i, 878–881.

Head Injury Warning Card for Adults

Ensure that a responsible person is available to keep an eye on you for the next 24 hours.
DO take painkillers such as paracetamol to relieve pain and headache.
DO NOT drink alcohol for the next 24 hours.
DO take your normal medication but DO NOT take sleeping tablets or tranquilizers without consulting your doctor first.

If any of the following symptoms occur then you should return or be brought back to hospital or the hospital telephoned immediately:

Headache not relieved by painkillers such as paracetamol
Vomiting
Disturbance of vision
Problems with balance
Fits
Patient becomes unwakeable

Adapted from Parsley, J., Fletcher, L., and Mabrook, A. F. (1997) Head injury instructions: a time to unify. J Accid Emerg Med. 14, 238–239.

Health Care of Prisoners—4Rs Observation Checklist

If any prisoner fails to meet any of the following criteria, a doctor or paramedic MUST be called; when assessing the level of rousability consider the following:

Rousability—can they be woken?

- Go into the cell
- Call their name
- Shake gently

Response to questions—can they give appropriate answers to questions such as:

- What's your name?
- Where do you live?
- Where do you think your are?

Response to commands—can they respond appropriately to commands such as:

- Open your eyes!
- Lift one arm, now the other arm!

Remember—take into account the possibility or presence of other illnesses, injury, or mental condition.
A person who is drowsy and smells of alcohol may also have the following:

- Diabetes
- Epilepsy
- Head injury
- Drug intoxication or overdose
- Stroke

Reproduced from Metropolitan Police (1997) Medical care of prisoners—person ill or injured. Special Notice 37/97. Metropolitan Police, London.

APPENDIX 4
APPROPRIATE ADULTS

Code C1.7 of the Police and Criminal Evidence Act 1984 (s.60(1)(a) and s.66) Codes of Practice 1995 states:
In this code "the appropriate adult" means:

(a) In the case of a juvenile:
  (i) his parent or guardian (or, if he is in care, the care authority or voluntary organization. The term "in care" is used in this code to cover all cases in which a juvenile is "looked after" by a local authority under the terms of the Children Act 1989)
  (ii) a social worker
  (iii) failing either of the above, another responsible adult aged 18 or over who is not a police officer or employed by the police

(b) In the case of a person who is mentally disordered or mentally handicapped:
  (i) a relative, guardian or other person responsible for his care or custody;
  (ii) someone who has experience of dealing with mentally disordered or mentally handicapped people but who is not a police officer or employed by the police (such as an approved social worker as defined by the Mental Health Act 1983 or a specialist social worker); or
  (iii) failing either of the above, some other responsible adult aged 18 or over who is not a police officer or employed by the police.

Notes:

1. The custody officer is responsible for calling the appropriate adult (C1.4).
2. Appropriate adults should advise the person being interviewed, observe whether the interview is being conducted properly, and fairly and facilitate communication with the person being interviewed (C.11.16).

APPENDIX 5
THE MINI-MENTAL STATE EXAMINATION

	Score
Orientation	
What is the (year) (season) (date) (day) (month)	..../5
Where are we: (country) (state) (county) (town) (police station)	..../5
Registration	
Examiner names three objects (e.g. orange, key, ball) Patient asked to repeat the three names Score one for each correct answer	..../3
Then ask the patient to repeat all three names three times	
Attention	
Serial 7's. Stop after 5 correct answers. Alternatively, if patient makes errors on serial subtraction: spell 'world' backwards: D L R O W Score best performance on either task	..../5
Recall	
Ask for the names of the objects learnt earlier	..../3
Language	
Show and ask the patient to name a pencil and a watch	..../2
Repeat the phrase 'No ifs, and, or buts'	..../1
Give a three-stage command. Score one for each stage (e.g. 'Take this piece of paper in your right hand, fold it in half, and place it on the chair next to you')	..../3
Ask patient to read and obey a written command on a piece of paper stating: 'Close your eyes'	..../1
Ask the patient to write a sentence. Score correct if it has a subject and a verb.	..../1
Copying	
Ask patient to copy intersecting pentagons. Score as correct if they overlap and if each has five sides	..../1

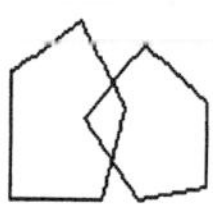

Total Score	..../30

From: Folstein, M. F., Folstein, S. E., McHugh, P. R. (1975) "Mini-Mental State" A practical method for grading the cognitive state of patients for the clinician. *J Psychiat Res.* **12,** 189–98.

APPENDIX 6
ALCOHOL ASSESSMENT QUESTIONNAIRES

The Brief MAST

Questions	Yes (Score)	No
1. Do you feel you are a normal drinker?	0	2
2. Do friends or relatives think you're a normal drinker?	0	2
3 Have you ever attended a meeting of Alcoholics Anonymous?	5	0
4. Have you ever lost boyfriends/girlfriends because of drinking?	2	0
5. Have you ever got into trouble at work because of drinking?	2	0
6. Have you ever neglected your obligations, your family or your work	2	0
for more than 2 days in a row because you were drinking?	2	0
7. Have you ever had DTs, severe shaking, heard voices or seen things that weren't there after heavy drinking?	2	0
8. Have you ever gone to anyone for help about your drinking?	5	0
9. Have you ever been in hospital because of drinking?	5	0
10. Have you ever been arrested for drunk driving or driving after drinking?	2	0

The brief MAST is useful as a quick screening instrument to distinguish between alcohol dependent (a score of 6 or above) and non-alcohol dependent individuals.

Pokorny, A. D., Miller, B. A., Kaplan, H. B. (1972) The Brief MAST: A shortened version of the Michigan Alcoholism Screening Test. *Amer. J. Psychiat.* 129, 342-345

The CAGE Questionnaire

1. Have you ever felt you should **C**ut down on your drinking?
2. Have people **A**nnoyed you by criticising your drinking?
3. Have you ever felt bad or **G**uilty about your drinking?
4. Have you ever had a drink first thing in the morning to steady your nerves, or to get rid of a hangover (**E**ye-opener)?

Two or more positive responses sensitive indicator of alcohol dependence.

Mayfield, D., McLeod, G., and Hall, P. (1974) The CAGE Questionnaire: Validation of a new Alcoholism Screening Instrument. *Am J Psychiatry.* **131,** 1121–1123.

THE AUDIT QUESTIONNAIRE
Circle the number that comes closest to the patient's answer.

1. How often do you have a drink containing alcohol?
(0) NEVER (1) MONTHLY OR LESS (2) TWO TO FOUR TIMES A MONTH (3) TWO TO THREE TIMES A WEEK 4) FOUR OR MORE TIMES A WEEK

2. How many drinks containing alcohol do you have on a typical day when you are drinking? (CODE NUMBER OF STANDARD DRINKS)
(0) 1 OR 2 (1) 3 OR 4 (2) 5 OR 6 (3) 7 OR 8 (4) 10 OR MORE

3. How often do you have six or more drinks on one occasion?
(0) NEVER (1) LESS THAN MONTHLY (2) MONTHLY (3) WEEKLY (4) DAILY OR ALMOST DAILY

4. How often during the last year have you found that you were not able to stop drinking once you had started?
(0) NEVER (1) LESS THAN MONTHLY (2) MONTHLY (3) WEEKLY (4) DAILY OR ALMOST DAILY

5. How often during the last year have you failed to do what was normally expected from you because of drinking?
(0) NEVER (1) LESS THAN MONTHLY (2) MONTHLY (3) WEEKLY (4) DAILY OR ALMOST DAILY

6. How often during the last year have you needed a first drink in the morning to get yourself going after a heavy drinking session?
(0) NEVER (1) LESS THAN MONTHLY (2) MONTHLY (3) WEEKLY (4) DAILY OR ALMOST DAILY

7. How often during the last year have you had a feeling of guilt or remorse after drinking?
(0) NEVER (1) LESS THAN MONTHLY (2) MONTHLY (3) WEEKLY (4) DAILY OR ALMOST DAILY

8. How often during the last year have you been unable to remember what happened the night before because you had been drinking?
(0) NEVER (1) LESS THAN MONTHLY (2) MONTHLY (3) WEEKLY (4) DAILY OR ALMOST DAILY

9. Have you or someone else been injured as a result of your drinking?
(0) NO (2) YES, BUT NOT IN THE LAST YEAR (4) YES, DURING THE LAST YEAR

10. Has a relative or friend or a doctor or other health worker, been concerned about your drinking or suggested you cut down?
(0) NO (2) YES, BUT NOT IN THE LAST YEAR (4) YES, DURING THE LAST YEAR

* In determining the response categories it has been assumed that one "drink" contains 10g alcohol. In countries where the alcohol content of a standard drink differs by more than 25% from 10g, the response category should be modified accordingly.

Record sum of individual item scores here ______

A score of 8 produces the highest sensitivity; a score of ten or more results in higher specificity. In general high scores on the first three items in the absence of elevated scores on the remaining items suggest hazardous alcohol use. Elevated scores on items 4 through 6 imply the emergence of alcohol dependence. High scores on the remaining items suggest harmful alcohol use.

For details see: Babor, T. F., Ramon de la Fuente, J., Saunders, J., Grant, M. (1992) *AUDIT The Alcohol Use Disorders Identification Test: Guidelines for use in Primary Health Care*. World Health Organisation.

APPENDIX 7
PEAK EFFECT, HALF-LIFE, DURATION OF ACTION, AND TIMES FOR DETECTION OF COMMON DRUGS[a]

Drug	Peak effect	Half-life	Duration	Detection
Cannabis	10–30 min	4 h	2–3 h	Up to 12 days in blood Up to 46 days in urine
Dihydrocodeine	1.5–2 h	3–4.5 h	3–6 h	12 h in blood
Methadone	1–5 h	12–18 h after single dose. 15–60 h after multiple doses	36–48 h	48 h in blood and urine
Morphine	1 h	3 h	3–6 h	18 h in blood 2 days in urine
Diamorphine	30 min after oral dose	3 min	3–6 h	40 h in urine
Diazepam	30 min–2 h	20–50 h	4–8 h	48 h in blood 1–2 days in urine
Temazepam	45 min–5 h	13 h	4–8 h	48 h in blood 1–2 days in urine
Ecstasy	2 h	7 h	4–6 h	48 h in blood 2–4 days in urine
Amphetamine	Variable	12 h	2–4 h	48 h in blood 2–4 days in urine
LSD	30 min–8 h	2–5 h	3–12 h	2–3 days in urine
Cocaine				
Snort	30–40 min	1 h	60–90 min	12 h in blood
iv	10–20 min			12 h–3 days in urine

[a]Figures are approximate and may vary from individual to individual.

APPENDIX 8 - DRINK/DRUGS DRIVING IMPAIRMENT ASSESSMENT FORM

Sec 4 Road Traffic Act 1991

Date:	**Custody Record No:**
Time called:	Name
Time arrived:	Address
Examination started:	
Examination completed:	Date of Birth:
Case completed:	OIC:
Where examined:	Examined in presence of:

Reason for detention:		
Reason for examination:		
Time of arrest :	Roadside breath test:	Intoximeter readings:
INFORMATION FROM ARRESTING OFFICER		
FIELD IMPAIRMENT TEST RESULT		
INFORMATION FROM CUSTODY OFFICER		
Consent: written/verbal in presence of:		

Medication	Dose	Duration	Route	Last taken	Allergies
Prescribed					
OTC medicines					Date of last tetanus
Non-prescribed					

Current problems			
Memory of recent events			
Past Medical History			
Visual problems		**Hearing problems**	
Diabetes	Epilepsy	**Asthma**	**Hepatitis**
Past Psychiatric History			
Self harm:			

Alcohol:	**Social:**	**Education:**
Weekly		
Last 24 hours		

EXAMINATION FINDINGS

General demeanour/behaviour:	**Examined in presence of:**
	All body surfaces examined: Yes/No
State of clothing:	**Area excluded:**

Speech	Tongue	Hiccoughs
Mouth	Breath	

ADDICTION	
Needle Marks	
Sweating	
Shivering	
Yawning	
Rocking	
Rhinorhoea	
Gooseflesh	

CVS	**RS**	**GIT**
Pulse:	PN:	Soft:
BP:	BS:	Tender:
Heart Sounds:	Added Sounds:	LKKS:
Temp:	PEFR:	BS:

Co-ordination Tests

Eye signs	Conjunctiva	Pupil Size	Direct	Indirect	Fundi	Nystagmus	Convergence	Yes	No
Right							Spectacles	Yes	No
Left							Contact Lens	Yes	No

Pupil Size (mm): 1.0 1.5 2.0 2.5 3.0 3.5 4.0 4.5 5.0 5.5 6.0 6.5 7.0 7.5 8.0 8.5 9.0

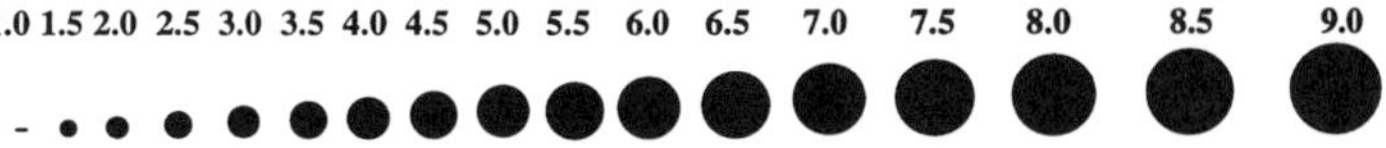

Romberg Test
Estimate body sway:
Front to Back **Side to Side**

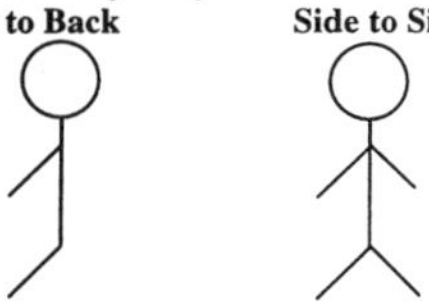

Internal clock 30 secs at………………..

Finger to Nose Test

2 1
4 3
5 6

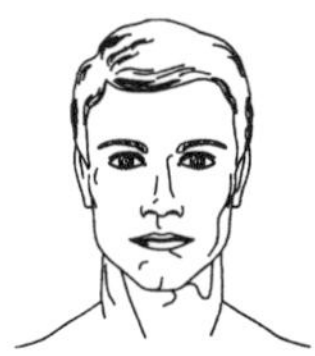

Indicate each result above

One Leg Stand

	Left	**Right**
Sways		
Raises Arms		
Hops		
Puts foot down		
Fails Instructions		

Walk and Turn Test

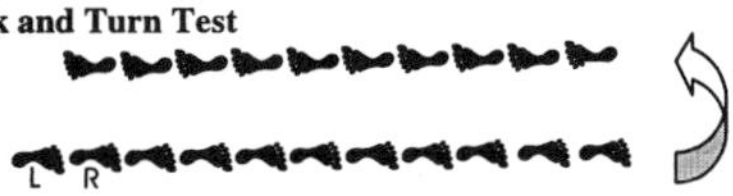

Start too soon	**Y/N**	Starting Balance	**Normal/Impaired**
Stops walking	**Y/N**	Turn	**Normal/Impaired**
Misses heel/toe	**Y/N**	Steps off line	**Y/N**
Raises arms	**Y/N**	Correct step count	**Y/N**

Psych

Memory of recent events : Mental State:

Orientation: Time: Place

Handwriting

Opinion:

Is person fit to be detained? YES/NO. If no, action taken:

If fit to be detained, is there a condition present that might be due to a drug? YES/NO

Conditions present:

Consent for blood in presence of:

Further action/Comments:

Blood sample taken: Time Site Given to: Time: Ref

Index

B

C

T